THE OBESITY REALITY

ALSO FROM NAHEED ALI

Diabetes and You: A Comprehensive, Holistic Approach

THE OBESITY REALITY

A Comprehensive Approach to a Growing Problem

Naheed Ali, M.D.

ROWMAN & LITTLEFIELD PUBLISHERS, INC.
Lanham • Boulder • New York • Toronto • Plymouth, UK

Published by Rowman & Littlefield Publishers, Inc.
A wholly owned subsidary of The Rowman & Littlefield Publishing Group,
Inc.
4501 Forbes Boulevard, Suite 200, Lanham, Maryland 20706
www.rowman.com

10 Thornbury Road, Plymouth PL6 7PP, United Kingdom

British Library Cataloguing in Publication Information Available

Library of Congress Cataloging-in-Publication Data
Ali, Naheed, 1981–
  The obesity reality : a comprehensive approach to a growing problem /
Naheed Ali.
    p. ; cm.
  Includes bibliographical references and index.
  ISBN 978-1-4422-1446-0 (cloth : alk. paper)—ISBN 978-1-4422-1448-4
(electronic)
  I. Title.
  [DNLM: 1. Obesity. WD 210]
  616.3'98—dc23   2012002512

∞™ The paper used in this publication meets the minimum requirements of
American National Standard for Information Sciences—Permanence of Paper
for Printed Library Materials, ANSI/NISO Z39.48-1992.
Printed in the United States of America

The Obesity Reality is dedicated to my students,
to obesity victims, and to all who provided
encouragement and support
throughout this project.

CONTENTS

DISCLAIMER

This book represents reference material only. It is not intended as a medical manual, and the data presented here is meant to assist you in making informed choices regarding your wellness. This book is not a replacement for treatment(s) that may have been suggested by your personal physician. If you believe you are experiencing a medical issue, it is recommended that you seek professional medical help. Mention of particular products, companies, or authorities in this book does not entail endorsement by the publisher or author.

PROLOGUE

In *Diabetes and You*, I explained what irregular sugar levels in the body are really all about. My quest to uncover diabetes in such a manner has led me to examine one of its major spinoffs: obesity. For centuries, people have been searching for ways to stay in shape and get thin, but why does obesity still pose a problem? Let's face it: The world is getting fatter in spite of all our palpable efforts to bring obesity to a standstill. The World Health Organization (WHO), in a 2000 report titled "Obesity: Preventing and Managing the Global Epidemic," classified obesity as a growing epidemic.[1] More than a decade later, we find obesity to be truly a global phenomenon. It's no longer a plague of the "well-fed" developed world. It is increasingly seen everywhere, adding to national burdens across the globe to the point where a new word, "globesity," has been coined.

Figures from a 2005 WHO report show that 1.5 billion adults from around the planet were overweight and 400 million were obese.[2] WHO believes that by 2015, there will be slightly higher than 2 billion adults around the world who are overweight. Over 700 million of them will be considered medically obese.

There's no doubt that obesity negatively affects the health of a person, and both old and recent research findings confirm this fact. New studies only add more detail to the saddening picture. What's not so clear however, is how an obese population can affect the health of a city, a region, or a nation, and we need to figure out how the social fabric of a nation adds to the burden of obesity.

It is not publicly well documented how obesity can place a heavier burden on medical and health systems and on economic welfare of city and national governments. Throughout this book, I refer to obesity as a disease but not a condition, since in 2004 Medicare agreed to reimburse the healthcare community for its treatment using the former term.[3] Looking at obesity on a scale much grander than government funding is a new experience for everyone. Calculating its impacts mean treading unknown territory and perceiving the unknown. The way in which this disease contributes to loss of productivity is no walk in the park, but some have attempted to unearth as much as possible, even out of simple curiosity.

The hidden costs of obesity that companies have to bear in serving increasingly obese populations became even clearer with a 2009 news article appearing in the *Sydney Daily Telegraph* titled "Too Fat to Fly: $60m Cost of Obesity to NSW Ambulance Service."[4] The report goes on to suggest that many Australians are now extremely overweight, and the new NSW Ambulance Service may have to increase spending by over $60 million on larger planes, simply for transporting overweight people to medical centers in and around the country. Stretchers on the planes are now required to be able to hold people that weigh up to around 570 pounds. Interestingly, this new weight limit is nearly double that of the existing weight limit that was standardized as a baby elephant or small aircraft. The overweight and obese Australians include over 7.5 million adults that cost the health care system more than 8 billion Australian dollars each year.[5]

I have thought about it over and over again: How long of a shadow does obesity really cast? While the health care industry and its institutions address the growing problem of obesity in their own ways, the real answer to whether obesity can undermine the positives of our world is yet to be determined. We are all inclined to address the issue of obesity in the world and explore how this could affect our well-being in the long run.

Let's look at all the key aspects of the obesity problem in such a way that it enables key decision makers to gain a broader understanding of the disease and its impacts. While the exact definition of obesity is discussed further along in the book, I prefer to break the ice with the idea that obesity means "fatness above average." The WHO defines both overweightness and obesity as having enough fat to pose a risk to your health.[6] Make that *serious* risk. If you're overweight or obese, you face an ominously higher risk of suffering from chronic diseases such as diabetes, cardiovascular diseases, and cancer, to mention just a few.

Keep in mind that body mass index (BMI) is a popular but rough measure for determining overweightness and obesity. You can get your BMI, which estimates the body fat mass, by simply dividing your kilograms of weight by the square of your height in meters. In general, a person with a BMI of 25 or more is considered overweight, but a person with a BMI of 30 or more is considered obese by some standards. BMI makes a lot more sense if branded together with your waist to hip ratio and all the cardiovascular risk factors you face as an obesity victim.

It is also necessary to consider the body type or condition of each individual before concluding obesity or overweightness. A person whose body contains a lot more muscle protein than excessive fat, such as a body builder, could be classified overweight if only his or her BMI measurement is taken into account.

Professional research conducted at Vrije University in Amsterdam in The Netherlands suggests that it is helpful to combine your BMI together with age and gender if you want to accurately estimate your body fat percentage.[7] In children, obesity is expressed in weight percentages, categorized by age and gender category. A child whose BMI is 95 percent above normal for his or her age and gender is overweight. A child whose BMI falls between 85 to 95 percent for his or her age category is considered, by the director of a major weight-loss clinic, to be at risk.[8]

Throughout the course of my study, I was able to identify the many causes and contributing factors for obesity. While there are genetic and hormonal factors that cause an increase in fat for some people, obesity occurs at the physiological level when you take in more calories than metabolized through activity. Your body stores the excess calories in fat tissue and leads to weight gain and obesity.

Obesity often surfaces from inactivity and lack of regular exercise. An unhealthy fast food diet that's rich in calories is a key contributing factor to obesity. Unhealthy eating habits, such as skipping a morning meal or eating high-calorie meals at night, also cause weight gain that contributes to obesity.

When reading this book, keep in mind that certain drugs and medical conditions can also contribute to weight gain, especially in the absence of dietary controls or physical activity. Some antidepressants, antipsychotic medications, antiseizure medications, diabetes drugs, and steroid treatments have been found to cause weight gain in people. Obesity also arises in some cases due to medical causes. Medical problems such as Prader-Willi syndrome, Cushing's syndrome, polycystic ovary syndrome, and other diseases and conditions could lead to weight gain.[9] Issues such as arthritis, which lead to decreased activity, also contribute to weight gain. Pregnancy causes a natural and necessary weight gain. Many women find it difficult to lose this weight after the birth of their baby. Lack of sleep is also known to cause changes in hormones that increase appetite, which in turn leads to weight gain.[10]

The Mayo Clinic reports that obesity-related symptoms can include the following: sleep difficulties, snoring, sleep apnea, pain in the back or joints, excessive sweating, and always feeling hot. Obesity can also cause rashes or infection in skin folds, shortness of breath with even minor exertion, daytime sleepiness or fatigue, and depression.[11] Whoever thought that obesity could do all of this? It's a very scary—but not impossible—reality to confront.

I have always leaned on the saying, "Prevention is better than cure." Obesity is no exception to this maxim since the disease is mostly lifestyle based in most people, regardless of a person's age. Obesity victims, who are who they are due to genetics or medical or health related conditions, need to be treated specifically based on their clinical history. I believe that treatment or prevention of obesity needs to focus on multiple lifestyle factors. Better success can be achieved through multipronged approaches in weight-related treatment regimes. These include changes in diet and nutrition, a focus on fitness and exercise, and making positive lifestyle changes.

Those who are already overweight and obese face significant emotional and psychological issues. They need support and therapy that guides them toward a cure. For example, they could suffer from body image issues and as a result, have difficulty from a social context. It really doesn't help those suffering from obesity to know that our society places great value on physical attributes that may seem unattainable to the individual. Treatment for obesity needs to address these societal issues as well. As you'll read in chapter 12, motivational support will also contribute in a positive way toward obesity treatment.

According to the WHO, obesity has reached unprecedented levels. WHO stated that in 1995, there were over 200 million obese adults across seven continents. By 2005, that number ballooned to over 400 million with no end in sight.[12] Obesity also increases the risk of breast cancer in both women and men, and many other medical conditions can be traced back to obesity. Being overweight and physically inactive greatly increases the chance of heart attack. Other diseases where risk factors involve obesity include esophagus cancer, gallstones, and arthritis. The US Health and Human Services reports that obesity results in 300,000 additional deaths a year. The cost to treat obesity-related health conditions exceeded $100 billion.[13] This book will reflect on the dangers of obesity and some methods on how to fight back.

Those who are overweight or obese should consider the health-risk factors. Some diseases are extremely dangerous. From my research on obesity, I gained insight on one of the largest projects ever to look at obesity prevalence across the globe, published in the American Heart Association (AHA) journal *Circulation*.[14] Scientists found that more than 60 percent of men and 50 percent of women were either overweight or obese. The experiment included around 70,000 men and approximately 98,000 women from more than sixty countries representing five different continents. Yes, that's *five* different continents. The subjects were evaluated for body weight, height, diabetes, cardiovascular disease (heart disease or stroke), and waist circumference. They concluded that obesity is a very obvious and evident problem around the world. A researcher from the French health organization Institut National de la Santé et de la Recherche Médicale (National Institute of Health and Medical Research, or INSERM) suggests that excess body weight is a huge pandemic, with at least half the individuals in the study being overweight or obese.[15] The United States was not part of the study.

Nestlé, a major candy producer in the United States, claims that the lifestyle changes that have taken place around the world since the last half of the twentieth century are a key reason for the obesity epidemic.[16] Consider factors such as the decrease in physical activity, an increased sedentary lifestyle, and the increased use of motorized transport due to increased urbanization. Education policies have also changed, making physical education less important at the same time that the food industry has been offering more energy-packed, cheaper items. All these factors taken together may have brought the world to its current unhealthy state.

Obesity is galloping in the United States. A study shows that obesity rates rose in twenty-three of the fifty states during 2008.[17] The rates *fell* in none. Colorado was the only state where the adult obesity rate was below 20 percent. In 1980, the US national average for adult obesity was 15 percent. No state had an adult obesity rate above 20 percent in 1991. The percentage of obese and overweight children has surpassed 30 percent in thirty US states. Childhood obesity rates have more than tripled since 1980.[18]

A major news agency interviewed the director of one of the organizations in charge of this study, who believed that the obesity epidemic was largely to blame when it comes to rising health care costs in the United States.[19] He also questioned how the United States was going to compete with the rest of the world if our economy and workforce were weighed down by bad health. While the US government had set a target for cutting obesity rates in all fifty states to 15 percent by 2010, the news report signaled that this target was fairly impractical considering the way things were going.[20]

The current economic crisis could exacerbate the obesity epidemic amid the swelling food prices of nutritious foods. The problem gets even worse when the impact of the job losses and uncertainty—raises the rates of depression, anxiety, and stress—are factored in, which fuels even more unhealthy habits and lifestyles.

Another analysis found that the aging baby boomer generation was more obese compared to all previous generations.[21] Hence, the number of obese adults in the population is expected to rise undoubtedly at a faster rate and drain our already-stretched health care system.

Therefore, the information in this book should serve as no more than just the tip of the obesity iceberg hiding the deeper, hidden consequences of this disease. The need to find a cure is greater than one could imagine, but the unprecedented levels of this disease everywhere is yet to be completely investigated. It's all about discovering bit by bit both the obvious and the hidden upshots of obesity. A little research and reading can go a long ways to allow us to grasp the short and long-term costs of skyrocketing obesity numbers in the population and the personal health effects of this disease. While the upcoming chapters are segmented into various subtopics, the overall objective here is to lead everyone to join the effort to stop obesity in unison. That said, I sincerely hope the following pages will bring us all a few steps closer to finding an absolute, one-way cure for this growing problem.

I

THE BIG PICTURE

1

UNDERSTANDING OBESITY

One of the world's leading causes of death from preventable diseases is obesity, widely considered one of the most dangerous and threatening public health dilemmas of the century. The disease has reached global epidemic proportions and affected over 300 million adults who suffer from its clinical form.[1] It is currently viewed as the major culprit of the worldwide burden of chronic disease and disability. It spares no age group, race, gender, religious, or socioeconomic group, and is even found in developing nations with malnutrition and undernutrition in high numbers.

The current obesity epidemic shows the major changes that society has gone through in the past few decades. Although genetics is known to play an important role in defining someone's propensity for obesity, in the end, it could be just an energy imbalance determined by caloric intake and lack of exercise.[2] It is still important to note that changes in nutrition and social transition are driving forces of this epidemic, as are globalization and economic growth. In a world where nations boast a higher number of cars than people, fast food chains rapidly expand to reach even the poorest regions. Jobs go from being highly physical and manual to sedentary. That said, obesity is a dangerous reality at your doorstep.

Obesity levels differ from region to region, with a level of under 5 percent in Japan and some parts of Africa, to a little over 75 percent in Samoa. Even in countries with low nationwide prevalence, such as in China, a few cities like Beijing report that over 20 percent of their population is obese.[3]

Childhood obesity is also reaching epidemic levels in some parts of the world and is on the rise. Estimates show that there are approximately 22 million children around the world below the age of five are overweight.[4] This is observed in Thailand, a country that felt a recent increase in obesity in children between five and twelve years old. The rates spiked from around 12 percent to 16 percent in a two-year period.[5] The circumstances appear to show that not a single region of the world escapes the shadow of obesity.

With the discovery of appetite controlling hormones such as leptin and adiponectin and neurotransmitters such as neuropeptide Y, interest in this disease has grown and, as a result, scientists and pharmaceutical companies developed drugs such as orlistat and sibutramine. Although obesity could have previously been accepted as a sign of good health and wealth, it's now looked upon as a warning sign for many other potentially fatal medical conditions. Global cognizance of the obesity problem is also rising, in hopes of controlling this disease and its catastrophic consequences.

PLANTING THE SEEDS OF OBESITY

The way in which people have looked at obese populations varies by culture over time. In the past, obesity was considered a sign of prosperity, health, fertility, and happiness. However, texts from as far back as the days of Hippocrates describe sudden deaths and horrible ailments in obese people. The thought of obesity being equivalent to wealth and high social class is an older assessment that is antiquated in most cultures today.

For around 95 percent of their existence on Earth, humans have survived as hunter-gatherers and have had to deal with frequent periods of food deprivation. The hunter-gatherer system led to a natural selection process where individuals with a genetic makeup that allowed for energy storage in the form of fat were the ones to survive. Overweightness and obesity were desirable in prehistoric times, since those who survived periods of famine were undoubtedly the ones with greater amounts of body fat. This allowed for the continuance of both tribe and species.[6]

Shaping Obesity into Existence

Signs of obesity have been identified in artifacts from the Stone Age. In the Neolithic Age, artisans made a point of sculpting robust female figurines to symbolize fertility and good health. The earliest evidence of the existence of obesity is the prehistoric statue known as the Venus of Willendorf. Thought to be around 25,000 years old, this statue is exhibited at the Museum of Natural History in Vienna, Austria. It is basically a female figurine with a massive belly and large, pendulous breasts. This was probably meant to represent motherhood and fertility.[7]

Two other known maternal obese figures include the ivory statuette of Lespugue and the limestone statue of Laussel. These figures represent morbid obesity not as a symbol, but a reminder of obesity's theoretical significance in preserving the species.

The Pharaoh's Creed   Ancient Egyptian paintings show obesity as a disease, and some archaeologists have discovered Egyptian mummies of persons who were obese when living. The mummified bodies were of people who had died from complications related to obesity, such as diabetes and heart disease. The four-thousand-year-old mummies of wealthy Egyptians also showed striking signs of atherosclerosis and myocardial infarctions (heart attacks). However, statues and depictions of the pharaohs and Egyptian courtesans are almost always "athletic" and designed to inspire admiration. These portrayals differ drastically from the reality of the time, since many famous pharaohs were renowned for their obesity. Amenhotep III and Ramses III were among those topping the list.[8]

China's Output   The ancient Chinese were attentive to the early onset of obesity and were aware of its varied consequences. They were among the first to encourage the prevention of fatness as a way to prolong their life expectancy. However, the first Europeans to visit China and the Far East depict the rulers and high officials of the court as being obese.[9]

Indian Roots   In Hindu mythology, overweightness was regarded as a symbol of inner happiness. Many ancient Hindu and Buddhist sculptures depict obese, abdominally large, smiling gods.[10]

The Greco Effect The Greco-Roman medical writers Celsus, Pedanius, and Ephesus are widely accepted pioneers in the description of obesity as an illness and seconded the Hippocratic line of thought that the same could in fact be treated. Oribasius, the Roman emperor Julian the Apostate's personal physician, clarifies the basic treatment options such as exercise, dieting, baths, and massages, while all the writers of that era described the importance of emotions and temperament in the onset of obesity. The ancient Greeks and Romans are considered the original experts of diet therapy, and Hippocrates ranks among the first of the great physicians interested in the topic of nutrition. He initially described some of the factors leading up to obesity as well as ways to combat the illness, including adequate amounts of exercise and sleep and diet plans.[11]

Also noteworthy are the Spartans, who lined up their young men at the beginning of each week and enrolled anyone who looked like they had gained weight in a rigorous exercise program. If the results weren't up to par by the beginning of the following week, any young man who didn't fit the bill was banished from Sparta as he was deemed worthless for battle. The health-conscious Spartans considered obesity an unforgiveable sin and shame to their nation.[12]

Britain During the Middle Ages and the peak of the European monarchies, obesity stood for power and influence in high circles of society. Due to favorable views on obesity, great wealth and prosperity accompanied those who survived the famines and plagues, and monarchs were frowned upon if they lacked huge appetites and were thin.

The Church The Catholic Church's position on obesity was that it was a punishment for gorgers. Being obese was a deadly sin. Whereas the church frowned upon obesity, most artists of the time ignored conventional standards and painted obese individuals as the primary subjects of many portraits. This attitude was also adopted by monks, among whom obesity was common at the time. During the thirteenth century, however, Pope Innocent III centered his attention on gluttony and condemned all clergymen who were obese and overweight. Researchers discovered that Benedictine monks living in a monastery in Edinburgh, Scotland, during the twelfth century developed a natural potion to reduce appetite so they would be able to fast without feeling hungry. According to historians and anthropologists, the monks of the

Sutra Aisle monastery and hospital made this concoction using a bitter plant centuries ago.[13]

The Tribal Sense Since ancient times, in some parts of Mauritania, women who are not obese are unlikely to marry. Larger brides-to-be are revered, celebrated, and sought out for marriage due to the belief that their weight ensures good health and betters the odds for childbearing. Mothers dedicate much time, effort, and wealth to feeding (and sometimes force-feeding) their young daughters to ensure they will be attractive to future suitors. In exchange, men offer their riches and proposals of marriage only to the most overweight girls.[14]

Many African tribes look at obesity as a requirement for having children, and great care is taken to "plump up" girls until they reach an acceptable weight before the marriage is allowed to take place. Family conflict ensues since mothers take great care in giving the future bride the best food (and in most cases the only food) the family has, potentially leaving others to starve.[15]

Is Obesity Part of a Lost Custom?

In the sixteenth and seventeenth centuries, overweightness and obesity were considered symbols of sexual attractiveness and well-being. Scholarly theses on the subject of obesity date back to as early as the end of the sixteenth century, and medical monographs describing the illness first appeared in the eighteenth. Most of these texts blamed the obese person for being morally weak—for allowing themselves to reach such a state of apparently unacceptable health. Although these texts were still influenced by the thinking of Hippocrates and Galen, they introduced some new ideas about chemical and physical aspects that made a theoretical basis for understanding the functions of the body.[16]

One of the greatest proponents of these ideas was the Italian named Giovanni Alfonso Borelli. His ideas about the origins of obesity took some of the fault away from the person and put more blame on the functioning of the body.[17] Obesity may be part of a lost custom after all, partially proven by this time period, which also depicted obesity in the form of art, for example, in paintings by Peter Paul Rubens, who required that his models be overweight. The term *rubenesque* is named after him and refers primarily to overweight women.

WATERING OUR KNOWLEDGE THROUGH RESEARCH

During the eighteenth and nineteenth centuries, medical research brought forth many important findings that were related to obesity and its causes, beginning with the identification of the human cell. Many human cell types were described, including the "fat cells" known today as adipocytes. The possibility that obesity was due to an excess of this cell began to be widely accepted by doctors and researchers.

Lavoisier's calorimeter, the first device to successfully measure calories, unearthed the idea that calories are involved with obesity. Known as the creator of the caloric theory and as the "father of modern chemistry," Lavoisier is credited with conceptualizing both direct and indirect calorimetry.[18] His theories have been tested and proven.

The body mass index (BMI) as a standard for measuring body weight was developed in the nineteenth century, and remains an important but nonexclusive part of obesity diagnosis today. The role of hereditary factors in the onset of obesity was also described in detail in the past when it comes to obesity research.

With the Declaration of Milan, countries outside the European Union acknowledged obesity as a multifactorial problem associated with numerous comorbidities, including cardiac, rheumatologic, digestive, and endocrine problems. In 2002, the World Health Organization, through its resolution WHA 55.23, developed the Global Strategy on Diet, Physical Activity, and Health. This manifest was adopted by member states in May 2004.[19]

Initiatives to fend off worldwide obesity should apply not only to research professionals, but also to sectors of the population encompassing all levels of government, public health services, the food industry, and the general public. Sectors such as catering, education, and technology should focus on plans to provide information and encourage athletics and physical activity. The World Health Organization has classified obesity as a worldwide epidemic and several countries now have nationwide research programs dedicated to obesity prevention and awareness. This is especially true in industrialized nations.

New hopes in the twenty-first century should lead to more scientific discoveries, especially in genetic research. Another hopeful insight, perhaps more realistic, is the better understanding of how regulating body weight may contribute to the future advancement of more effective medications for obesity treatment.

THE DEFINING MOMENT

Unfortunately, present day culture scoffs at obesity victims and promotes thinness, sometimes to the extreme. This is defined by European fashion runways, as young models strive to be "beautiful," which tortuously means "thinnest."[20] Research also shows a massive increase in incidence rates of anorexia and bulimia in both young females and males. However, these statistics are small in comparison to the obesity numbers and its many severe complications.[21] Research suggests that more than 30 percent of all adults living in the United States are obese, and difficulties from obesity are the number one cause of death in the country.[22] This may unhappily turn characteristic of many other countries in the years to come.

Regrettably, people occasionally associate the term "morbid obesity" with massive, deformed, bed-ridden bodies, unable to move and weighing hundreds of pounds. The medical disease known as "obesity" generally refers to an excess of total body fat that may lead to adverse effects on your health. The word has its origins in Latin, where the *obesus* is a contraction of two Latin words: *ob*, which means "toward," and *edere*, which means "to eat."[23]

The body is comprised of different substances including a high percentage of water, protein, and fat, among other things. The normal functioning of the human body depends on a careful balance of these percentages. Adequate percentages of fat are required for the storage of body energy, shock absorption, and heat insulation, as well as other essential body functions. When these percentages are distributed inaccurately, along with the excess of fat, obesity develops.

Being obese and being "overweight" isn't the same. BMI compares your weight and height and is used to determine when you are overweight or obese. BMI is calculated by dividing your weight, measured in kilograms, by your height, measured in meters squared (m^2). When in generally good health, you reach a BMI between 18.5 and 24.9. A BMI above 25 may indicate too much fat unless excessive muscle weight is responsible. A BMI greater than 30 delineates you as obese. So, fatness is not limited to what is called morbid obesity, but to anyone with a BMI greater than 30. This is very common, with some capital cities having a 25 percent prevalence of overweightness in their adult population.

WHEN ONE LEADS TO THE OTHER

There are quite a few physical, social, and psychological consequences associated with obesity. Being obese is a serious risk factor for many life-threatening medical conditions and symptoms including: cardio-vascular diseases such as coronary heart disease (CHD) and hypertension; Type 2 diabetes; elevated cholesterol; gallstones; gout; osteoarthritis; lower back pain; and pulmonary diseases such as sleep apnea.[24] Some studies point out that at least 80 percent of people diagnosed with Type 2 diabetes mellitus are either obese or overweight.[25] This correlation is very important because being overweight puts extra stress on your body, bringing down your ability to maintain adequate blood sugar levels.

Obesity-Related Conditions

Diabetes-Related Obesity   Obesity can turn into diabetes, and with it, the series of health risks that the latter brings. In several cases, obesity will make the body resistant to insulin, thereby affecting the way you use insulin and transform energy. For people with diabetes, it will mean that a higher dose of insulin will be required for treatment. For people *without* diabetes, getting obese substantially bumps up the risk of having the former.[26]

High Blood Pressure   One of the most common obesity-related heart conditions is hypertension. Studies confirm that hypertension is three times more common in obese people than in people who maintain a normal range of weight. Hypertension in obesity is linked to a size increase of the left area of the heart, an enlargement called left ventricular hypertrophy (LVH). This increase in size can at length lead to coronary artery disease, heart attacks, heart failure, and other problems.[27]

Obesity and Sleep   Sleep apnea is more than likely in the obese because of excess fat in the chest and throat area. This excess fat won't allow for movements of the chest, which are necessary for correct breathing, including movements of the respiratory muscles and the diaphragm. Sleep apnea in obese people is sometimes referred to as obesity hypoventilation syndrome.[28]

Gallstones   Obesity victims are more likely to suffer from gallstones than those who maintain a normal weight. This is especially true for obese women. Additionally, several studies have found that obese people are more likely to produce more cholesterol. This upturn in the amount of cholesterol will show up in your bile, a yellowish digestive fluid, which won't dissolve correctly and may lead to the formation of cholesterol gallstones.[29]

Osteoarthritis   Obesity victims also suffer from chronic illness of the joints. The most affected joints are the knees, hips, and lower back. This can explain the presence of lower back pain. The extra weight exerts a greater amount of pressure on your hips and knees and begins to wear the cartilage down. This cartilage normally protects the joints and makes body movements smooth, but with the extra weight and pressure, the cartilage is worn and torn, leading to long-term joint pain and other serious implications.[30]

Gout   This is yet another problem that may arise after some time. Gout is an illness due to very high levels of uric acid in the bloodstream. The excess uric acid can form small masses or stones that get lodged inside different bone joints. The more overweight you are, the more likely you are to have gout.[31]

Cancer   Obesity has also been associated with many forms of cancer, such as that of the breast, cervix, and colon. Among the causes of obesity, discussed further in chapter 3, is a lifestyle that consists of poor eating habits and is void of any physical activity. The excess of body fat leads to problems with oxygen circulation within the blood, inflammation, and blockages in the bloodstream. These ramifications are also evident in many cancer sufferers, making the connection between cancer and obesity undeniable.[32] Obesity and lack of exercise are directly linked to colon, pancreatic, kidney, breast, and esophageal cancers. Moderate levels of exercise, like brisk walks and swimming, lower the risk of cancer. Obesity not only has higher cancer risks for its sufferers, but makes cancer treatment and maintenance more problematic.[33]

Pregnancy and Infertility   Female obesity is responsible for re-duced fertility rates, which means the more you weigh, the lesser the chances of getting or staying pregnant. Obesity can also lead to serious problems during pregnancy, such as preeclampsia, a disease in which high blood pressure puts the pregnancy in danger of not reaching term. Preeclampsia can also result in premature birth. In more serious cases, obesity during pregnancy can indirectly result in the death of the mother or child.[34]

Mental Health   Psychological consequences of obesity can include discrimination, low self-esteem, bulimia and its related eating disorders, and depression. Across the world, millions of people deal with obesity every day. Obesity is not just a physical condition, but one that is closely related to your mental health. Research indicates that people who are obese and overweight tend to eat and snack more when they feel bored or depressed.[35] Some experts relate this condition with the security that one would have gained from oral stimulation as an infant. Snacking on junk food that is high in fats, salt, or sugar seems to placate a person when they feel upset or lonely. People who suffer from mood disorders and depression have a tendency for obesity. The connection between mental health and obesity is a vicious circle, as obesity is observed to lead to depression and mood swings.[36]

Problems with Fat Distribution in the Body   Generally speak-ing, the higher the BMI, the greater the possibility of suffering from fat distribution problems. The increased risk associated with obesity doesn't depend exclusively on the level of obesity, but also on *where* the weight is lodged. In other words, weight distribution in obese people will help determine the potential health risks awaiting them if the obesity persists. Body fat that is concentrated around the waist means an increased risk of metabolic problems such as Syndrome X, described later in further detail, and Type 2 diabetes. This type of weight distribution also places you at a much higher risk for breast cancer and heart disease.

Simply put, obesity is also responsible for shortening your life span.[37] Obese men twenty-five and older will live for roughly thirteen years less than those who maintain a weight within the normal range.[38] Approxi-mately 300,000 people die each year from conditions that are associated with obesity.[39]

THE FACTORS WITHIN

Obesity's most common causes include any or all of the following factors: excessive calorie intake (by eating too much of the wrong foods), lack of exercise or physical activity, and hereditary or genetic factors. A small number of people are obese due to other medical or psychiatric conditions, including chronic depression. Obesity is a complex issue to address when considering the many factors that play a role in its onset. While these factors will be described more extensively in the next few chapters, it's important to get introduced to energy imbalances, genetics, and cultural and environmental issues of obesity right now.

Energy Imbalance

An energy imbalance results from increased caloric intake and insufficient physical activity. This is one of the most important factors that lead to obesity in the general population due to countless types of "fast food" with high-caloric value and the busy lifestyle that leaves little or no time for physical activity. The combination of high-calorie diets and the comfort of automobiles, in addition to heavy workloads in sedentary environments, lead to rapid weight gain and obesity.[40]

Genes

In a way, your genes help to determine your weight. Genes can directly cause obesity, such as in ailments like Bardet-Biedl syndrome and Prader-Willi syndrome. Others that may lead to weight gain, and in some cases obesity, include Cushing's disease, polycystic ovarian syndrome, and chronic clinical depression. The amount of cases per family may suggest a genetic origin, but it is difficult to decide just how to blame genetic predisposition for obesity.[41]

DISEASE OR VICTIM: WHO IS RESPONSIBLE?

For the most part, an individual's lifestyle choices regarding diet and exercise can greatly influence the development of obesity. Personal behavior and the environment are therefore key factors of prevention. These factors are currently the focus of global strategies seeking to decrease the rate of obesity and preserve adolescent and childhood clinical normality.

One of the main determinants of eating behavior is the person's family and social environment. Families with a tradition of huge eaters can pass down eating behaviors. Social pressure can induce high-energy consumption in exposed individuals such as salespeople, executives, and other attendees of social gatherings where food serves as an essential lead-in.

A society's culture also plays a substantial role in the development of obesity. There are many cultures where food is a key part of every special occasion, from birthdays to weddings to funerals. Tables laden with all kinds of food are found at every major event, inviting attendees to overeat.

Clinical studies of obesity suggest that personality disorders can trigger obesity in some individuals. Personality issues lead to greater consumption of food in times of anxiety, stress, loneliness, and boredom. Prolonged exposure to these situations can result in binge eating situations like bulimia.[42]

Another thing to keep in mind is the availability of food. Societies where food is readily available at large supermarkets and fast food restaurants on every street corner are more likely to have more obese inhabitants than those with food shortages. This normally goes hand-in-hand with the sedentary lifestyle common to industrialized nations where (1) people travel even the shortest distances in vehicles instead of walking and (2) most jobs don't require much physical activity.

FUELING THE FIGHT

To better understand what's gone wrong in obesity, it is vital to comprehend how the human body really works. Your body is like a machine, and the first thing any machine needs is a source of energy. In this case, the machine's "fuel" is food, which contains calories. Therefore, energy enters the human body through our food.

Calories as Fuel

Calories are like pockets of energy contained in food. They are the unit of energy measurement and a key factor in defining the energy balance of a human body. A calorie, by medical standards, is the amount of heat needed for raising the temperature of a milliliter of water by 1 degree Celsius. Your energy balance will be determined by the difference between the energy intake (food) and energy expenditure (level of activity). In other words, the calories you eat minus the calories used will result in a base amount of energy stored. The stored energy is commonly found in the form of fat cells in different parts of the body and can eventually lead to overweightness and obesity.[43]

Foods tend to vary in the amount of heat produced. This is the basis for the wide scope of diets available on the market which promise weight loss. Carbohydrates, protein, and fats each have their own thermogenesis (heat producing effects) on the body, raising the body's basal metabolic rate (BMR) by 4 percent, 30 percent, and 6 percent, respectively. BMR is also known as the resting metabolic rate. Changing the amount and type of food eaten will greatly determine how the metabolism works and how much energy will be spent. This is also known as diet-induced thermogenesis.[44]

Heat production can be achieved through activities like caffeine, nicotine, and alcohol consumption—leading to what is called drug-induced thermogenesis. Other nontraditional methods include (1) shivering in response to cold weather or a cold environment, (2) thermogenesis in response to physical and psychological stress, and (3) daily activities that are not considered full-blown exercise.

Sometimes, certain foods may not seem too rich in fat, and thus may lead people to build up and store excess amounts of it. People gain weight and fat as they eat more calories than their body burns off even in a day. They way you fuel yourself by eating is really like putting gas in a car, so you need the energy to get through the day. Activity is going to burn off a certain amount of energy, measured in calories. If there is any energy left over, the body stores it in fat cells, and thus one way you accumulate fat is through excess intake of calories.[45]

Without this constant intake of food, production, storage, and expenditure of energy, you wouldn't be able to move or breathe. Energy is needed in varying amounts to accomplish basic tasks such as blinking, as well as complex forms of thinking. Even if you appear to be resting, your cells are working relentlessly to keep your heart beating, lungs breathing, and even making your hair and nails grow.

Metabolism

Metabolism is the collection of chemical processes and reactions that cells undergo. It turns the fuel ingested (food) into the energy needed for the body to continue working. There are basically two types of interactive paths that the human metabolism can take. The first is called catabolism. Catabolism denotes the process by which food is broken down into its most basic components. Once this occurs, the body can use these substances to produce energy. Catabolism is sometimes called destructive metabolism because it breaks and splits bigger molecules into smaller ones that are useful for energy purposes.

The second type of metabolic pathway is anabolism. Anabolism is also known as constructive metabolism because it is through this process that the body repairs and regenerates itself. Anabolic reactions help new cells grow, heal damaged tissue, contract muscles, heat the body, maintain and repair organs, and store energy for future use.

TIME IS MONEY, BUT SO IS ENERGY

As you can see, energy comes from the calories found in food. Once food is ingested, it goes through the entire digestive process and breaks down food into different products and nutrients that pass into the bloodstream. Body cells retrieve the nutrients they need from the blood so that energy production occurs. The molecules retrieved are given to enzymes found in each body cell. An enzyme is a chemical that works to transform these molecules of food and nutrients into different types of fuel and products of biochemical reactions. This allows your organs to function right. Some of the products are used immediately, while others are stored for later.

Getting Energy

There are two basic fuel sources: animal and vegetable. Foods from animal sources provide most of the human body's needs for protein. Vegetable foods give the body most of the fiber and carbohydrates needed to function. Both sources will also supply some of the fat required for adequate body function. These are the three basic types of "fuel" the human body needs: protein, carbohydrates, and fat.

The intake of such fuels will result in a series of complex signals moving to and from every cell in the human body. These signals are vital for the production of energy and function of the body. In the end, interconnections and messages moving around inside you do require the expenditure of energy. Any condition that affects this complex topic of digestion and energy production will lead to an energy imbalance that could result in obesity. This is true when there's a problem with the thyroid, hypothalamus, or pituitary. Hormonal imbalances can also be responsible for altering the signals needed for adequate energy use and storage, later giving way to obesity.[46]

Spending Energy

The way energy is used or spent will also determine your weight. This is because the more energy spent, the less energy stored. In other words, energy expenditure will allow less energy to be stored as fat in the body, thereby decreasing the general amount of fat and controlling your weight. Energy can be spent in three ways: thermogenesis, metabolism, and physical activity. Thermogenesis refers to the production of heat to use up energy. Conventional physics dictate that energy cannot be created nor destroyed, but the latter can certainly get transported, changed, transformed, and stored.

The same is true for energy within the human body. When food is eaten, energy is required for the entire digestive process. From the moment food enters the mouth, different chemicals are released into the bloodstream to begin the whole process of breaking down the food into nutrients for the production of energy in mitochondria. Mitochondria will be discussed further in the section titled "Wonders of the Cell."

The release of chemicals requires energy to be utilized correctly. In short, the modest act of eating will activate your metabolism and lead to energy expenditure and energy production. This explains why many modern diets demand that you eat many times a day, but in smaller amounts. Splitting meals into smaller portions will keep your metabolism right since it leads to the continuous use of energy throughout the day.

Physical Activity and Energy

Physical activity is the most easily modifiable method of energy expenditure, and it not only refers to exercising at the gym or strenuous workout regimes, but also includes a wide range of activities that will allow your basal metabolic rate to rise and boost the amount of energy you spend. This will lead to less energy storage, and, in due course, less stored energy in the form of fat. Energy expenditure is contingent on the intensity and duration of the exercises performed.

The third way to expend energy is directly through your BMR. You use up energy even when at rest, and according to a medical research report, the metabolic rate during this time is responsible for 50 to 80 percent of all energy used.[47] However, this percentage will vary depending on the total amount of muscle mass of each person. The more muscle mass you have, the higher the basal metabolic rate, and finally, the more energy spent. This is why it's important to preserve muscle mass when attempting to lose weight. It also explains why body builders have a higher basal metabolic rate than people who only do aerobics.

Remember, energy balance is vital in your quest against obesity. This "balance" is scientifically defined by the amount of energy introduced into the body minus the amount of energy spent. Energy imbalances will result in different conditions that affect health. When stored fat is converted into energy due to increased physical activity or dietary changes, the fat storage cells become smaller as they empty out. Fat cells don't exactly increase or decrease in number, though there are a few very rare exceptions. The only thing that changes is their size. When the amount of fat is too much for all available adipocytes, free fatty acids will roam free in the bloodstream, basking in different areas of the body and incidentally diminishing your energy levels.

WONDERS OF THE CELL

All body cells have several energy generators which dedicate themselves to processing everything you eat. These generators are called mitochondria. The term originates from ancient Greek, where *mito* meant "thread" and *chondro* meant "grain." This definition stems from the fact that early scientists saw the mitochondria as a tiny threadlike structure resembling a grain with thread wrapped around it.

Cells Are Like Little Factories

Different types of body cells will always have varying numbers of mitochondria, which are parts of the cell essential for our survival. Mitochondria give birth to the basic molecule of cell energy: adenosine triphosphate (ATP). They also produce waste in the form of water and carbon dioxide. These mitochondria are essential to a cell's life in that they repair and regenerate each cell permanently. Their function and survival depend on your food intake and therefore rely on a properly balanced diet.

A single muscle fiber may possess up to 1,000 of these important "energy factories," while an unfertilized egg in a woman's ovaries may have around 500,000 mitochondria.[48] The sheer amount of these microscopic organelles shows how much energy in any given cell type will need to function. Without mitochondria and their ATP, people wouldn't be alive.

Fat is digested primarily in the small intestine, though it's emulsified by a liver substance called bile. A lot of enzymes join in the breakdown of fat into other products that will be used as energy or stored in fat cells. An enzyme called lipase is secreted in the mouth to start the digestive process and other enzymes present in the stomach continue to work on the fat found in the ingested material. Eventually, the food turns into chyme once it enters your small intestine. Chyme is the result of the mixing of the food with all the substances secreted by the cells of the stomach wall. However, the real work begins in the small intestine, specifically in a part known as the duodenum.

The pancreas gives off enzymes into the duodenum to allow the fat molecules found in chyme to be broken down into smaller products for energy expenditure and storage. One of the most important enzymes at this level is lipase. Lipase splits the fat molecules into smaller substances such as fatty acids and glycerol. This is an important task, and basically all the lipase can accomplish since it can only affect fat molecules on the surface. For further breakdown of these fat products, the digestive system uses bile. Bile is produced in the liver but stored in the gallbladder.[49]

The gallbladder, like the pancreas, has a duct that leads into the duodenum. This duct, the bile duct, takes bile from the gallbladder to the duodenum to continue the digestion and breakdown of fat. Bile is necessary to emulsify fat, and it separates the molecules and blends them with the rest of the contents in the duodenum.[50] Since the molecules are now smaller and suspended in the watery chyme, the lipase can once again attack and continue breaking the molecules down for use by the body as energy.

Enzymes and Lymph Vessels

Lipase, along with other digestive enzymes, will break down the molecules into free fatty acids and glycerol. This whole process takes around ten to fifteen minutes. The absorption of these broken-down fat molecules is performed by the walls of the small intestine. These intestine walls are lined with millions of villi. These are microscopic finger-like projections that cover intestinal walls and contain blood and lymph vessels.[51]

Lymph vessels absorb the free fatty acids and glycerol via the lymphatic system. The free fatty acids and glycerol is later released into your circulatory system. The absorbed fatty acids travel through the bloodstream to adipocytes (fat cells) where the acids are stored. These fatty acids are also taken to muscle cells for energy expenditure. The absorbed glycerol is carried via the bloodstream to the liver so it can morph into glucose (sugar) for energy production.

When you eat foods with too much fat and subject your digestive system to this process for too long, the amount of stored fat in adipocytes could spike and eventually lead to obesity and related conditions.[52]

STASHING AWAY THE "BAD" GOODS

Unused energy is stored for later use in the form of fat. This fat is found in special cells called adipocytes, found in several different locations throughout the body and lodged in two places: under the skin (subcutaneous fat) or around the organs of the digestive system (visceral fat). Adipocytes have the ability to change shape and size to hold a greater amount of fat. In extreme cases, adipocytes clamp more than forty times the amount of fat they are supposed to.

Fat is found mostly in the form of triglycerides, the molecular form of fat when it is absorbed by the intestines. Triglycerides are later taken to the liver.[53] The liver can store fat in such a form or break it down into smaller particles for use by different cells in the body. When there is an excess of stored fat, the adipocytes will produce other substances that can basically harm organs and upset energy balance. These substances can later lead to serious conditions such as Syndrome X and insulin resistance. An excess of stored fat can eventually exceed the capacity of fat storage cells and overflow into other tissues and organs like the muscles and liver. When this happens, fat flows in the form of free fatty acids. These free fatty acids are commonly found in overweight and obese people and are believed to be the main culprits of decreased insulin sensitivity. Free fatty acids also play a role in increased blood pressure and other heart problems.

THE WRAP UP

There are many who don't understand why understanding everything possible about obesity is important. Although there are several reasons why everyone should try to learn the most about obesity, there are two very important ones that are worthy of mention here: (1) understanding your health risks and (2) correcting the problem. If a person does not understand how serious obesity is, he or she will likely not care anything about it. However, if a person understands the health risk, he or she will feel compelled to take better care of himself or herself. This includes maintaining a healthy body weight or losing weight if needed.

You were introduced in this chapter to a broader overview of obesity. As you may know, getting "the big picture" of a huge problem before diving into additional details usually helps. Discussing the overall nature of a problem like obesity is essential for addressing any major epidemic—not just obesity. Obesity victims know they need to lose weight, but some don't know how or where to begin. Simply put, understanding the basics of obesity will make things go a lot easier as a patient.

2

THE DIAGNOSIS

DIAGNOSING OBESITY

When learning how obesity is diagnosed, remember that it is a disease as well as a sign of other medical conditions. The diagnosis of obesity as a condition leading to other diseases can be made by not only determining the causes of obesity, but also by diagnosing other related illnesses. Clinical examination and a series of lab tests are also often involved.

A Struggling Past

One of the first things your doctor could ask you is, "How old were you when you started to gain weight? When did it really set in?" Your doctor might show some interest in knowing whether your weight gain spanned many years or if it grew rapidly over just a few months. Several studies have shown that people who are diagnosed as obese before reaching the age of forty are more likely to suffer less severe consequences than those who begin to gain weight during or after their forties.[1] When you gain more weight over a shorter period of time, you are more likely to present with cardiovascular illnesses and complications than if you gained weight over many years at a stable pace.[2]

Obesity sufferers are often asked about possible causes they have found for their weight gain and obesity. There will be circumstances that serve as possible triggers or partial explanations for obesity and type of weight gain. The following will always have some effect on weight and could be partly to blame:

- Quitting sports
- Getting married
- Pregnancy
- Starting or leaving a job
- Family quarrels or other problems
- Quitting alcohol or tobacco

A history of sickness, in conjunction with past medical treatment for other disease, will help determine factors that may be worsening weight gain and increasing risk for serious complications of obesity.[3] When you talk to your physician, ask about this, especially if you suffer from one or more of the following: high blood pressure (hypertension), high blood sugar (diabetes mellitus), irregular levels of fat in the bloodstream (dyslipidemia), gout, coronary heart disease, sleep apnea, or complications from past surgeries. The presence of any of these problems will change the way your doctor will handle your obesity treatment plan. The same is true of your family history.[4]

In other words, treatment protocols can vary immensely if someone in your family suffers from or has a history of any of the above conditions, or if there are other members of the family who are obese.[5] Along with considering any other illness or condition you have, ask about your past and current medications. There are several drugs connected to weight gain, such as antidepressants and certain types of oral contraceptives. If you are getting medications, be sure to take the drugs at their proper dosage and assigned time. Medicinal obesity treatments will be discussed further in chapter 4.

THE CONVERSATION SPARK

The Past Can Lead the Way to the Future

Mention any previous treatments and medications to your doctor. Perhaps you used diet pills or treatments in the past or were trying to adhere to a very low calorie diet. Either way, this is vital information to share because some treatments have a rebound effect when followed incorrectly. Medical research shows that some people who don't change their lifestyle and eating habits permanently after undergoing surgery for weight loss will actually *gain back* much more weight than they initially lost.[6] Such reversals have been observed in people who have undergone liposuction and tummy tuck surgery.

Eating Habits

Your eating habits may determine the amount of weight you gain. This is due to the way energy and metabolism works, as discussed in chapter 1. By knowing your eating habits, the attending physician will be able to design the best treatment plan for each individual. They may ask you about the number of meals you eat per day, meal times, which meal is your largest, and which foods are the most consumed. You should also think about *where* you eat, whether at home, at the office, or a diner. Do you eat alone or with others? Do you eat while reading, listening to music, or watching television? Divulging small details to your doctor will help with the diagnosis of obesity.

The Psychological State

The myriad mental pressures you can fall under as an obesity sufferer can also affect your eating habits and weight gain. This pressure can come from your occupation or social environment, including family problems, relationship problems, feelings of anxiety, boredom, anger, despair, or loneliness.[7] Your psychological stability is of key value for studying the development and progression of your obesity. Approach your healthcare provider if you think you are suffering from any psychological issues.

Your doctor could ask about your mood and general state of mind to determine if you will need extra support to successfully lose weight with any given treatment plan. It's important that your treatment plan for obesity include a support group, whether it's based in your own family or in others.[8]

Discuss Your Physical Activity Level

Your physical activity level is a key indicator of your past and future clinical status. Telling your doctor about the kind of physical activity you engage in is also important because it will allow the attending physician to decide the best type of exercise regime. If you are a victim of obesity but already enjoy things such as walking or riding a bicycle, you can simply adapt to a stricter exercise plan.

Your lifestyle and daily habits are equally necessary when diagnosing obesity. Obesity and weight gain are greatly influenced by your lifestyle, which includes smoking and the consumption of alcohol. It is well documented in professional experiments that drinking and smoking play an important role in weight-gain patterns and the onset of obesity. [9]

THINGS DONE RIGHT: DIAGNOSES DEMAND SYMPTOMS

At some point in the conversation, the doctor will ask you about the reason for your visit. People usually go to a doctor when they are already going through obesity-related consequences. Though the symptoms of obesity will be covered extensively in chapter 3, it's important to know from the get-go that some symptoms may not be so obvious. These symptoms can help your doctor create the "bigger picture" pointed out before, to identify obesity as the uniting cause of all your problems. Aside from the aesthetic and sociocultural problems an obese person may experience, most seek medical attention prior to diagnosis and are concerned about one or more of the following:

- Difficulty in the movement of some body parts when performing otherwise simple tasks, such as putting on their shoes
- Getting tired too quickly when stepping up the stairs
- Sleeping difficulties, including interrupted sleep, frequent awakening, and snoring
- Hardships with concentrating that are usually associated with poor sleep and lack of oxygen flow to the brain
- Joint pain occurring mostly in the knees and backaches in the lumbar region
- Problems with the veins, such as varicose

Collateral symptoms include the following:

- Headaches, which in males are mostly due to hypertension, while in females are usually linked to cervical arthritis (cervical spondylitis).[10]
- Menstrual disorders, reduced fertility, pregnancy problems, and difficulties during childbirth are possible complaints in females.
- Miscarriages (spontaneous abortions) and newborns with high birth weight are problems that are sometimes associated with gestational diabetes, a condition that is common in obese females.
- Polyuria and polydipsia (increased urination and excessive thirst, respectively) are usually (but not necessarily) linked to diabetes and normally absent in obese people who don't suffer from this illness.[11]
- Dyspnea is a common symptom without any relation to illnesses of the respiratory symptom or of the heart. Dyspnea pertains to difficulties with breathing. It is due to fatigue, which is brought on by the extra effort it takes for some people to accomplish the simplest tasks, such as walking or bending over to pick up an object.
- Urinary calculi may be present in obese people with high levels of uric acid. For people with urinary calculi, it is important to rule out the possibility of gout.[12]
- Gallstones may be present in obese people that lost weight and later gained it back. This is especially true if you lost and gained weight several times and had a low-calorie diet.[13]

Diseases Often Diagnosed Conjointly

To avoid any misapprehensions during your obesity diagnosis, your doctor will most probably be able to rule out many other conditions leading to obesity and its risk factors, such as the following: [14]

- Hypothalamic obesity: may present with vision problems, impotence, headache, polyuria (frequent urination), and symptoms of increased intracranial pressure.
- Hypothyroidism: associated with chronic constipation, fatigue, dry skin, hair loss, feeling of cold, slower heart rate, and lack of mental agility.

- Cushing's syndrome (hypercortisolism): red stretch marks around the abdomen, thighs, and buttocks. This disease is due to the improper function of the adrenal glands which produce a crucial substance named cortisol.[15]
- Hyperinsulinemia: low blood sugar levels, acanthosis nigricans, which are patches of darkened skin in different parts of the body, especially where there are skin folds such as armpits and under the breasts.
- Stein-Leventhal syndrome: obesity caused by ovarian problems.[16]
- Obesity due to drugs: people who take tricyclic antidepressants, lithium, benzodiazepines, steroids, and some other drugs that lead to weight gain and obesity.
- Obesity that is prompted by alcoholism.

Once all these questions have been asked and taken note of by the doctor, it is time to get a physical examination. All obese people should undergo a complete physical inspection and examination to make sure nothing is left out. Everything from body measurements to nervous system evaluations must be performed to uncover other underlying illnesses and help determine the cause of your weight gain. This is also essential for classifying the specific type of obesity and looking for imminent health risks.[17]

GETTING SKIN CLOSE

When examining the skin, it is important to look for *cyanosis*, the blue coloring of the skin that appears in the absence of adequate blood supply. Cyanosis will show up in heart or respiratory people that don't have proper blood flow throughout the body. Other skin problems found in the obese include *acanthosis nigricans*.[18] These conditions are frequently seen in obese diabetics or people with metabolic syndrome.[19] Swelling of the leg and the presence of varicose veins or varicose ulcers are also common findings in obese people due to poor blood flow to the legs.

Using Your Skin as a Diagnostic Test for Obesity

The skinfold test is a very well-known procedure widely used to measure body fat. A technician or doctor uses body calipers to pinch your skin at several locations to measure the thickness of underlying fat, properly called subcutaneous fat. After these measurements are taken, they become part of a mathematical equation and converted into a percentage. This percentage refers to an estimate of your total body fat. Several mathematical equations exist to measure body fat, and each uses a different amount of skinfold points ranging from three to seven.

The skinfold test is accurate, but must be performed by a well-trained individual who uses the same technique for each point measured. If carried out correctly, the test will give a precise reading of your body composition and physical changes over a period of time. It is important to keep in mind however, that this procedure only measures subcutaneous fat tissue. It may be possible to find two people with very similar skinfold measurements but different body fat percentages if other sources of fat were to be measured, such as the fat deposits around some major abdominal organs. Taking this phenomenon into account, some formulas include your age as a variable for calculation of total body fat.

A simple way to perform this procedure is the Yuhasz skinfold test.[20] This is a skinfold test involving small calipers to measure several different regions of your body. These regions include:

- The triceps muscle region
- The *subscapula* muscle region
- The *suprailiac crest*: an area found just along the back of the hip and continuing at a certain angle
- The abdomen: this measurement is usually taken just to the left of your belly button
- The front part of the thigh: this measure is taken midway up the thigh from the knee cap
- The chest: this measurement caters solely to men and is taken from the right side of the right nipple, at a 45 degree angle
- The rear part of the thigh: this measurement is only for women and is taken midway up the thigh, placed centrally

You would normally take each measurement three to four times and then compute the averages. Then you plug in the averages into one of the mathematical formulas that are used to determine body fat percentage.

WHEN SEEING ISN'T BELIEVING

At present, it is agreed upon that body fat percentages vary depending on age and gender.[21] That's why normal ranges of body fat percentages resulting from measurements of skinfolds will vary. Skinfolds are commonly overlooked as a crucial part of diagnosing obesity.

Another factor to keep in mind is your gender, since a US-based experiment found that more women present with extreme obesity than do men.[22] This is mainly due to the difference in how fat is distributed between the sexes. Cultural and ethnic variables are also involved. Some body fat percentages have higher cultural values in some countries and some have been linked to better performance in athletes.

Total body fat percentage is determined by taking your total fat weight and dividing it by your total weight. Research concludes that the normal body fat percentages for men and women with a BMI of greater than or equal to twenty-five are around 20 percent and 30 percent, respectively.[23] When you calculate your body fat percentage, the result will show how much of the body's weight is fat in either of its two forms: essential fat and storage fat. *Essential fat* refers to the amount you need for staying alive and functioning the right way. It's also the fat that is necessary to carry out reproductive functions. *Storage fat* is the fat found in adipose tissue. This fat is found under the skin and is widely considered the subcutaneous fat that is (1) measured with calipers for the skinfold test and (2) covering important abdominal organs. The fat surrounds abdominal organs and protects them inside of the abdominal cavity.

Researchers agree that the skinfold test and the measurement of your body fat percentage is a much more effective way to diagnose obesity.[24] Body fat percentage is the only measurement that devotes itself to the calculation of your body composition without regard to height and weight. This is better than the more commonly used body mass index (BMI) because the BMI merely assumes that every individual's height and weight should be within its normal values regardless of body composition. Researchers who use body fat percentage as a measurement of obesity argue that the BMI gives inaccurate diagnosis in many cases where you have more lean muscle mass, but are still classified as overweight or even obese. Sometimes when a person boasts a perfect percent body fat composition, he or she supposes that they are in great health. In reality, they are not. Waist-to-hip ratios may provide for a better understanding of percent body fat composition than BMI.

The Invisible Hula Loop

One of the most important measurements a doctor will use to diagnose obesity is the waist-to-hip ratio. Several studies have shown that people with more weight stored around the waist, those considered "apple shaped," are more likely to present health risks than those with more weight around the hips, those referred to as "pear shaped." This measurement is used on both female and male people, and normal values will vary depending on other factors. However, research dictates that a normal waist-to-hip ratio for women is 0.7 and for men is 0.9.[25]

The waist-to-hip ratio is calculated by using a measuring tape to measure the circumference of hips followed by the waist. The measuring tape is placed at the widest part of the buttocks to measure hip circumference. To measure waist circumference, the tape is placed at the narrowest part of your natural waist, which is usually found just a few centimeters above your navel (belly button). Once the doctor obtains both values, the waist measurement is divided by the hip circumference to obtain the waist-to-hip ratio.

Normal waist-to-hip ratios of 0.7 in women and 0.9 in men have been linked through clinical research to good overall health and fertility.[26] Women within the normal waist-to-hip ratio range show normal ranges of *estrogen* levels and are much less likely to develop serious illnesses linked to obesity including diabetes, heart disease, and cancer of the reproductive organs (ovaries and cervix). Furthermore, serious weight gain has been noted in women diagnosed with breast cancer.[27] Men within the normal range of waist-to-hip ratio of 0.9 have proven to be healthy and have optimal fertility. These people are also far less likely to develop prostate or testicular cancer.[28]

Recent studies have recommended the use of the waist-to-hip ratio as the first determinant of health risks linked to obesity. The ratio has proven to be a much better and more efficient predictor of death than BMI or waist circumference alone. Researchers claim that using waist-to-hip ratio for determining the risk for heart disease and stroke would triple the number of people at risk around the world. Of the measurements used for diagnosing obesity, only the waist-to-hip ratio takes into account each person's body structure. It is possible to observe two people with varying body mass indices but similar waist-to-hip ratios.[29]

Wear the Belt and Braces

The National Heart, Lung, and Blood Institute reports that a high waist circumference is linked to many serious illnesses and conditions including Type 2 diabetes mellitus, high cholesterol, and dyslipidemia (irregular lipid amounts in the blood), high blood pressure, and other heart diseases.[30] This is especially true when the waist circumference is compared to the BMI and the latter is between 25 and 35. It's important to keep in mind that a BMI over 25 is typical for people diagnosed as being overweight. People with a BMI of over 30 are commonly diagnosed as being obese.

Several classifications of obesity stand today. Table 2.1, based on a 2000 World Health Organization Technical Report, shows several classifications of obesity as it stands today.[31]

Class III obesity is commonly referred to as *morbid obesity*. This type of obesity is responsible for the most serious health risks. For people diagnosed as being in the normal range of the BMI or slightly overweight, the measurement of their waist circumference is very important. This is because in many cases, athletic people are classified as overweight when only their BMI is measured. Once their waist circumference is taken however, this diagnosis can be adjusted.

Table 2.1. Classifications of Obesity

WHO Classification	Body Mass Index (kg/m²)
Underweight	Less than 18.5
Normal range	18.5–24.9
Overweight	Over 25.0
Preobese	25.0–29.9
Obese class I	30.0–34.9
Obese class II	34.9–39.9
Obese class III	Over 40.0

Source: "Obesity: Preventing and Managing the Global Epidemic," *World Health Organization Technical Report Series* 894 (2000): 9.

Waist circumference can be measured at every visit to the doctor so the results may be compared over time. Changes in waist circumference will show how much abdominal fat is lost or gained. The more abdominal fat there is, the higher the chances of suffering heart problems. Many recent studies have shown that waist circumference is an important indicator of risk for heart problems, which includes hypertension, and for diabetes. Researchers who prefer the waist circumference technique say it is more efficient than the waist-to-hip ratio.

The measurement of the waist circumference is a very simple procedure where a doctor or other health professional locates the upper part of your hipbone and places the measuring tape around you at this level. The tape measure must be placed horizontally and as straightly as possible. It has to touch your skin, but not too tightly. Make sure the tape measure is in good shape and not overstretched as this could distort the results. Once the waist circumference is measured, the doctor or health professional compares the result with a measurement chart to determine your level of obesity.

Why Mass Should Not Be Chosen over Matter

The BMI is the most common system for measuring the risk for, but not officially diagnosing, obesity. It is inexpensive and very easy to measure. The BMI is also quite reliable for the diagnosis of obesity when accompanied by other body measurements and a thorough physical examination.

Calculating your BMI is one of the best ways of diagnosis and quantification of overweightness and obesity in the general population. Since the calculation requires knowledge of your weight and height, it is cheap and simple to use for doctors and other health professionals as well as for the general public. The use of BMI lets people compare their weight and body status to that of the rest of the population.

Although BMI fails to physically account for all the fat (solid matter), it is a good way to tip off an obesity diagnosis. The BMI shouldn't be the only measurement for determining your level of overweightness (mass), but research has shown that the BMI correlates to other measurements in determining the amount of fat, including underwater weighing and a procedure known as "DXA" or dual energy X-ray absorptiometry. The scan used to be known by its full abbreviation, DEXA. These procedures are not as widely used for determining overweightness as the BMI.[32]

BMI in people over twenty years of age is interpreted with standard weight and height categories that are the same for any age and gender. When it comes to teens and children, BMI has definite interpretations that will vary among genders and age groups. The connection between BMI and the amount of fat in your body (body fat percentage) is direct but will vary depending on age, sex, and your race and racial background. Therefore, it has been determined that when a man and a woman have the same BMI, it is usually the women who tend to have a higher body fat percentage than their male counterparts. When two people of the same sex have the same BMI, it is usually the older one who has a higher body fat percentage than the younger one.

BMI is very useful for identifying potential weight problems and health risks in adults. However, the index is not meant to be a sole justification for the diagnosis of obesity. BMI simply uses your height and body weight to estimate the amount of fat you have. This method is somewhat limited as a sole procedure for diagnosis because it doesn't take into consideration your body type or composition. For example, if you are reasonably fit and have a high muscle mass, you will probably have a high BMI, which unofficially means obesity. A fit person who is actually healthy and has a very low risk for heart disease or other conditions related to obesity would be misdiagnosed.[33] While many doctors and health professionals use the BMI as the first and main measurement for diagnosing obesity, your body fat percentage is better determined by a direct evaluation such as a skinfold measurement.

BMI calculation is done in a likewise manner for both adults and children. Reiterating what you read earlier, BMI is computed as weight (kg)/[height (m)]^2. However, the interpretation of BMI data among children is really different because some of the criteria are not the same. For children and teens, body fat percentages fluctuates with age and differs among boys and girls.[34] Using BMI results, you can get an overview of how to properly identify obesity among children in the general population.

However, BMI alone is not a desirable screening tool for obesity since it doesn't diferentiate between muscle weight and the weight provided by fat.[35] This shows that a high BMI in an American may not suggest the same degree of obesity as in other populations. People of varying cultures inevitably differ in lifestyle and therefore may also differ in the amount of muscle weight they have versus the weight provided by fat. Polynesians, for example, may have a slightly lower fat percentage of body fat mass compared to Caucasian Australians at an identical BMI.[36] Moreover, the percentage of body fat mass increases with age and is higher in women than in men. Thus, caution is needed when using BMI as a universal tool to identify obesity, even on a population level. BMI is still the popular method used to survey the crude population for obesity prevalence because weight and height are so easily calculable. Other recommended characteristics for diagnosing obesity fat are as follows:

- Body composition: waist circumference, underwater weighing, dual-energy X-ray absorptiometry (DXA), skinfold thickness[37]
- Anatomical distribution of fat: waistline circumference, computer tomography, ultrasound, MRI
- Nutrient storage tests: palmitic acid, extended overfeeding challenge
- Energy intake: total dietary record, macronutrient composition
- Energy expenditure: indirect calorimetry, physical activity level (PAL), heart-rate monitor

CAT SCANS EXPLAINED

For diagnosing a wide variety of illnesses, the widely known CAT scan refers to computerized axial tomography. It is a type of imaging procedure that uses a computer to mix together a series of X-ray images to show your body in "slices" or cross-sections. It implicates the use of a large X-ray machine that comes in the shape of a donut. This round X-ray machine allows several X-ray images to be taken from different angles. The pictures are then processed by the computer to produce additional images showing horizontal slices of tissue. These images are then recorded onto an X-ray film also known as a tomogram.

How does this all tie in to obesity? CAT scans are effective in showing cross-sectional images of fat distribution, so the doctor can see the body fat underneath your skin and the visceral fat surrounding your internal organs. The preceding methods are all used at some point to help diagnose obesity and other illnesses that accompany it. Most are also beneficial to the diagnosis of health risks that come with the onset of obesity, such as cardiovascular disease, diabetes, and kidney disease.

TESTING THE WATERS A BIT FURTHER

After all of these measurements have been taken and calculated, you may receive a full physical examination from head to toe. The shape of your face will help diagnose hypertension, gout, and abdominal obesity. Try to look out for Cushing's syndrome and hypothyroidism if your face is round or bloated. Other things to look for in the head and neck are xanthelasmas, which are small fat deposits under the skin. These are present in people with high cholesterol levels. If you have any problems sleeping, get a rhinoscopy to rule out any possibility of other respiratory problems. A rhinoscopy is when a doctor uses an instrument resembling a telescope to look up your nostrils and into the nasal cavity.[38] It is also necessary to listen for heart murmurs or any uncommon sounds in the lungs and respiratory tract because respiratory diseases such as asthma have been clinically linked to high BMI in adults.[39]

Other Related Effects

Hirsutism and Gynecomastia   Besides hair loss, some obese females will have hirsutism, represented by an excess of body hair.[40] This is mostly found on the chin and upper lip and sometimes on the chest. Hirsutism is a sign of a hormonal disorder. If accompanied by menstrual disorders and infertility, the most probable diagnosis is polycystic ovarian syndrome (POS).

Gynecomastia is demonstrated by the excess of breast tissue in men and is not uncommon in obese males. Heart rate and rhythm are two important things to examine, as is respiratory rate.

The Abdomen   Physical examination of an obese person's abdomen is very significant. Besides helping to determine the way fat gets distributed in your body ("apple-" or "pear-shaped" obesity), it can help the attending physician rule out other illnesses of the abdominal organs. When performing a physical examination of the abdomen, remember to check the right upper quadrant of the abdomen where the liver and gallbladder are located. Any pain or mass found in this region will make the doctor suspect gallstones or other liver problems that could be due to obesity-related physique. The attending physician may also feel or touch the lower abdomen, also called the hypogastric (below the belly button) region. This is done particularly in women to feel for the uterus and any possible masses or abnormalities.

Kidneys   A key phase of a physical exam of an obese person is the examination of the kidneys and urinary tract. The attending physician will need to perform a special technique known as fist percussion. This is done by gently hammering the area of the lower back where the kidneys are located using the softer end of a closed hand. Fist percussion should normally be painless. If you move away from the percussion as a reaction to the pain, you are likely to have a kidney issue. It is important to rule out kidney failure in obese people with hypertension, diabetes, or both.

Visual Inspection of Fat and Tophi   Next up is the physical examination of upper and lower extremities (arms and legs). What doctors are mostly looking for in your arms and legs are xanthomas and tophi. A xanthoma is similar to a xanthelasma in that the former is a small accumulation of fat found directly under the skin. "Tophi" is the plural form of the word "tophus," which means "stone" in Latin. *Tophi* are chalky deposits of uric acid commonly found in people with gout. Both xanthomas and tophi are usually found near joints.

Varicose Veins   A research report tells that obesity is a major predisposing factor for varicose veins.[41] Physicians are always on the lookout for varicose veins in the lower extremities, varicose ulcers, and edema or swelling and may want to pursue official diagnosis. Varicose veins are veins that have changed shaped and have been stretched out due to an excess of blood. When things get a little more complicated, varicose ulcers may soon follow. This is due to the fact that the veins in your legs must work more to push blood back up toward the heart, and being overweight or obese makes this job a lot harder. Therefore, obese people will have varicose veins because their weight makes it really difficult for their veins to push blood up against gravity. The same explanation remains for edema and varicose veins, since edema is also due to difficulty in blood flow and substance transport in leg veins and lymph vessels.

Joint Problems   Other things to look for in your lower extremities include joint deformities posing as osteoarthritis as well as the presence and severity of cellulite tissue. Keep an eye on your joints and feel the pulses in your arms and legs. Have your doctor test each arm and each leg for sensitivity, deep tendon reflexes and muscle tone, and generalized movement.

Holters: The Rain Checks for Doctor Visits   A Holter test is performed with a Holter system. A Holter system is really a machine similar to a tape recorder that records your electrocardiogram for a period of twenty-four hours. It is a machine that is put on you for a whole day to measure changes in your heart function while you perform your daily activities. The Holter test is a very good way to efficiently diagnose heart problems in obese people.[42]

LAB TESTS: A TRIED AND TESTED AFFAIR

To improve on the diagnosis of obesity and its related conditions, the following tests should be included:

- Cholesterol levels
- Tests for liver function
- Tests for thyroid function
- Cortisol levels in twenty-four hours
- Fasting blood glucose levels
- Insulin levels
- Blood sample and red cell sedimentation rate
- Impedancemetry (predicts your body composition)
- Indirect calorimetric test
- Electrocardiogram
- Holter test
- CAT scan or MRI
- Electrolyte levels

Cholesterol Tests

Cholesterol levels are measured by taking a blood sample. Your body uses this molecule to protect nerves and help manufacture cell tissues and selected hormones. Cholesterol is a necessity for the human body. It is produced by the liver. When you consume too much high-cholesterol food, such as eggs, meat, and dairy products, health problems may strike.

Variations of cholesterol traveling through the bloodstream are called lipoproteins. There are low-density lipoproteins (LDLs) transporting your cholesterol to different places of the body, and there are high-density lipoproteins (HDLs) that are in charge of removing cholesterol from the blood flow. Doctors worry about your low-density lipoprotein levels because this type of lipoprotein is considered harmful in larger amounts.

For people who have a high risk of heart disease, a low-density lipoprotein level of 100 is great. Values between 100 and 129 are considered very good, while 130 to 159 is considered the range for medium risk of heart disease. LDL above 160 puts you at very high risk for cardiovascular disease. When measuring high-density lipoprotein levels, keep in mind that the lower the value, the higher the risk for cardiovascular disease. HDL levels below forty put you at greatest risk, while having a number over sixty lowers the chances of heart disease.

When measuring the level of total cholesterol, the ideal value is under 200. Values between 200 and 239 are considered borderline. Total cholesterol above 240 is found in people with very high risk for cardiovascular disease.

Liver Tests

Tests for confirming liver function include a group of screenings done to measure several substances in your liver, such as liver enzymes. Get your liver tests done regularly, especially since the most common liver ailments don't exactly present with physical symptoms until push comes to shove. There are several functions that can be tested with these labs, such as general functionality, cell integrity, and the state of the biliary tract. Table 2.2 shows the different liver enzymes recorded for obese people and their normal values and significance.[43]

Table 2.2.   Liver Tests

Measurement	Significance	Normal Range
Alanine transaminase (ALT)	Alanine transaminase is an enzyme in every cell of the liver. This enzyme leaks into the bloodstream when there is damage to the liver cell. This may happen when you have viral hepatitis or some form of liver damage.	About 4 to 35 International Units per liter (IU/L)
Aspartate transaminase (AST)	Aspartate transaminase is also called serum glutamic oxaloacetic transaminase (SGOT) and is located in cells all over the liver parenchyma. Its values rise when there is liver damage but is also used when looking for heart damage.	Approximately 10 to 40 IU/L
Alkaline phosphatase (ALP)	This is an enzyme in cells that line the walls of the biliary ducts in our liver. When these ducts are blocked, the value of this enzyme will increase. Other causes of increase in ALP are intrahepatic cholestasis and other infiltrative liver diseases. It is also used to diagnose Paget's disease in older adults.	Around 30 to 120 IU/L

Total bilirubin (TBIL)	Bilirubin comes from the breakdown of *heme*. Heme is a part of hemoglobin found in red blood cells. Removing bilirubin from the bloodstream is an important liver function. This is accomplished by hepatocytes, liver cells that breakdown the bilirubin and secrete it into bile.
	
	  When the levels of total bilirubin are too high, you get jaundice. Jaundice is the yellowish coloring of your skin. Jaundice can be a warning sign of many problems at different levels of the liver:
	  • Prehepatic (in front of the liver) jaundice is associated with overproduction of bilirubin. This can be caused by many different situations including very severe bleeding and some types of anemia.
	  • Hepatic jaundice gets more problematic as it interferes with bilirubin metabolism. This is normally the case in people with cirrhosis or viral hepatitis.
	  • Posthepatic (behind the liver) jaundice involves abnormal excretion of bilirubin. This is mostly due to blocking of the bile ducts.
		Approximately 2 to 14 micromoles per liter (μmol/L)

Direct bilirubin	There is a separate lab test measuring the level of direct bilirubin. This will help in some diagnoses.
	  • If the level of direct bilirubin is normal, then the problem is definitely bilirubin metabolism. This is a cue for your doctor to rule out such illnesses as viral hepatitis, cirrhosis, or hemolysis (destruction of red blood cells).
	  • If the level of direct bilirubin is above normal values, then the liver is blocked and unable to secrete bilirubin normally. The doctor may consider gallstones, cancer, or other causes for bile duct obstruction.
		0 to 4 μmol/L

Gamma Glutamyl Transpeptidase (GGT)	This enzyme is very sensitive and may increase with even the slightest degree of liver dysfunction. It is mostly measured in acute and chronic alcohol toxicity.	0 to around 50 IU/L

Thyroid Tests

Thyroid function is determined by measuring the levels of thyroid stimulating hormone (TSH), triiodothyronine (T3), and thyroxine (T4), in your bloodstream. The initial test should be the measurement of TSH. An elevated TSH level means the thyroid gland is malfunctioning due to a direct problem, but if the TSH level is too low, you could be diagnosed with hyperthyroidism, suggesting that your thyroid is working too hard. Low levels of TSH are sometimes due to a problem in the brain, particularly in the pituitary gland.[44]

Cortisol

Cortisol is a hormone that is activated by your physical stress levels. Its quantity is measured to detect problems with the adrenal glands or the pituitary glands. This substance has many functions such as participating in the body's response to stress and helping the body transform sugar and fat into energy metabolism. A high level of cortisol might mean you have Cushing's syndrome.[45] It can also mean you have other types of illnesses including kidney disease, liver disease, hyperthyroidism, major depression, and obesity.[46]

Sugar and Insulin

Fasting blood glucose tests measure the level of sugar in the form of glucose found in your bloodstream after fasting for a minimum of eight hours. An interesting fact to consider is that this procedure is usually the first lab test ordered to preclude diabetes in the obese. Normal values may vary, but for the most part, diabetes can be diagnosed when your fasting glucose level is over 120 mg/dl.

Insulin levels are also important to rule out diabetes and metabolic syndrome,[47] which frequently involves insulin resistance. Insulin is a very important substance and its functions are many. An ideal insulin level is achieved when you have less than ten international units per milliliter (IU/ml). If your insulin levels are over this number, then you have eating habits that are stimulating an overproduction of insulin in your pancreas. This is very serious and can lead to really negative health consequences. It has been shown in several studies that an excess of insulin in your body can lead to weight gain, since one of the functions of insulin is to help store fat in the body. Having too much insulin can lower your magnesium levels.[48] Magnesium is an essential mineral for the body since it is responsible for efficient blood flow all throughout. Excess insulin leads to high blood pressure because it causes the retention of sodium, which in turn leads to water retention.

Complete Blood Count

Blood sampling procedures such as complete blood count (CBC) tests are standard procedures for many people, not just the obese. Erythro-sedimentation rate (ESR) is a standard lab test for almost all people and is useful to diagnose inflammatory or infectious episodes, but it's not so great for specific diagnoses. This test measures the rate at which your red blood cells collect at the bottom of a test tube.[49]

ELECTROLYTES DO THE TRICK

Blood electrolytes are measured through a blood sample taken from you. Electrolytes are the minerals and substances that help keep the body in a chemical balance. From a scientific standpoint, electrolytes are electrically charged atoms or molecules (ions) found in your bloodstream. These substances help the muscles, heart, lungs, and other vital organs to function suitably. The most common electrolytes your doctor could measure include sodium, potassium, chloride, and bicarbonate.

Sodium

Sodium is the electrolyte responsible for regulating water in the human body. The transportation of sodium to, from, and within each cell is fundamental for the right functioning of many organs. It is a key determinant for the transmission of signals to and from the brain, and most muscle tissues have it.

Potassium

This is the main electrolyte responsible for your heartbeat. A very low level of potassium will lead to abnormal heartbeat as well as weakness of the muscle tissue in general. Chloride also helps regulate the amount of water in the human body, while bicarbonate controls acid balance.

SUMMARY

Obesity is clearly unhealthy, so diagnosing it before it gets worse is very important. *Unhealthy*, in this case, would mean a higher risk for high blood pressure, cholesterol, diabetes, and heart attacks. Obese people often tend to have more problems functioning in day-to-day life as a result of such conditions.

The sooner doctors diagnose the growing problem of obesity, the faster it can be defeated. As you will read in the upcoming chapters, obese people also suffer from a lack of confidence or may have self-esteem issues. Obesity can be a problem, not only physically, but emotionally and psychologically as well. Obesity is something many people struggle with, but with proper recognition and awareness, this disease can be dealt with. In its broadest terms, obesity is sometimes uncovered by a thorough clinical examination, which includes taking a detailed personal history and a complete physical exam. Every detail of your past and present medical history, coupled with the right diagnoses, helps your healthcare provider to reach an appreciable goal for diagnosing your obesity from a realistic angle.

3

CAUSES AND SYMPTOMS

When studying obesity as a medical illness, remember to take every aspect of your existence into consideration. Every snippet of information can be valuable in order for your health care provider to figure out what's causing all the extra fat and to come up with an adequate treatment plan for you. There are *several* causes of obesity, and the signs and symptoms will also vary from one person to the next.

As you learned in chapter 2, evaluating someone for obesity as comprehensively as possible is important because it is so difficult to pinpoint a single cause. Your doctor will do a complete physical exam as well as a personal medical history evaluation. All the information obtained from your health care professionals will contribute to correctly identifying the causes and symptoms of obesity.

WHO'S THE CULPRIT?

Almost all obesity cases have more than one cause. It has been well established that this disease is a result of the presence of many risk factors.[1] There are several classifications for all the risk factors causing obesity, albeit it comes down to three major groups:

- Lifestyle
- Genetic
- Other medical conditions

The most probable cause of obesity is therefore a combination of the three groups above. Obesity is usually a mix of genetic or hereditary causes and physical and psychological factors. Cultural and environmental influences are also often involved. All of these factors work together to bring about an imbalance of your nutritional state, unfortunately causing obesity.

Living the High Life

Obesity is not only the result of eating too much and exercising too little, but is partially the result of modern-day living. Obesity is a price people pay for the sedentary lifestyle[2] and technological advancements[3] happening over time for many years. The majority of overweight or obese people suffer from unavoidable weight gain due to the technological revolution that began in the twentieth century, continuing even today. This is because technology affects your way of life and indirectly forces your body out of its intended purpose.

Looking back on the evolution of man, cavemen in prehistoric times stocked up on food for the winter to survive harsh weather conditions. Prehistoric people weren't obese and had plenty of physical activity. These hunters/gatherers looked for food to *eat*, not to *overindulge* all day and night. Looking for food meant walking very long distances to hunt down wild animals with primitive weapons or gathering fruits and vegetables with one's bare hands.

Obesity began to surge when customs started to change. That's why, in ancient times, obesity was associated almost exclusively with the wealthy. People of high society didn't lack any food, nor did they have to work hard for it. The rich spent their days lounging in their gardens or playing cards at tea time while their slaves or hired help worked the fields to plant, grow, and harvest nothing but food. Physical activity in high society was mostly limited to horseback riding and ballroom dancing.

The Real Effects of the Industrial Revolution

The first Industrial Revolution gave way to early technological break-throughs, such as steam-powered ships. This saved people an immense amount of travel time and effort. The assembly line developed by Ford Motors was also an important breakthrough of the early twentieth century. It allowed for plenty of work by large machinery and relegated people to function more as an observer. Workers no longer had long hours of hard labor, and instead were devoted to tasks completed at desks or alongside the machinery. Then came the beginning of an obesity explosion in the adult working-class population.

The effects of the second Industrial Revolution continue today. The revolution brought the rise of service-based jobs instead of goods-based or production jobs. Current statistics show that over 80 percent of all jobs are in the service industry, while only 20 percent are in farming and the goods production sector. The revolution paved the way for an even greater increase in the number of overweight people around the world.

The way people live nowadays opens a lot of doors for obesity. People drive to work in cars or hitch rides in subway trains. They travel in different types of vehicles to all destinations near and far. Cars have become such a vital part of human lives that in some cities, people will go to the convenience store in their vehicle instead of walking two or three blocks to get there on foot. Trains, boats, and airplanes take people anywhere they want to go at a much faster speed than walking. With the hectic lives most people endure in metropolitan areas, walking for the purpose of exercise is simply out of the question and considered a waste of time by many.

WORK THE SYSTEM

Is the "working world" to blame for our hectic and stressed lifestyle? In a globalized society where "time is money," work hours have increased and physical activity has ironically decreased. Most jobs are stationary, and people spend countless hours at their desks, working with computers. This leads to obesity brought on by a lack of physical activity.[4] It also leads to those hurried lunch breaks where workers will buy the first thing they find, normally on-the-go food from a popular fast food chain.

A typical workday begins by getting out of bed in a hurry, jumping in the shower, and rushing out to get to work. Most people will skip breakfast or have it on the go, in the car or on the train. This is a huge mistake that will be discussed later.

Getting To and From Work

Taking any means of mechanical transport to work means no walking or exercising. Once at the workplace, people pour a cup of coffee and sit at a desk for the rest of the day. Lunch break is, as mentioned earlier, mostly comprised of junk or fast food. After work hours are over, whoever doesn't stay overtime takes the car or train back home. At home, people sit on the couch and watch television while devouring food from a random take-out restaurant. Because many work long hours, they sometimes go to bed without the slightest bit of physical activity.

Stress at Work

Job-related stress is also related to obesity. Several medical studies[5] have shown that there is a direct relationship between the amount of stress you go through at work and the amount of weight gained. Obesity has been found in workers with high stress levels and with very low support from coworkers and superiors. This form of stress and the obesity it causes results in unmotivated, underproductive employees. It also leads to more sick days taken by these workers due to stress-related illnesses or work injuries related to obesity.[6]

Schooling

This is a similar occurrence for teens attending school.[7] Stress, when coupled with peer pressure, can lead to either end of the weight scale, from anorexia and bulimia to obesity in both male and female teenagers. Obesity is also at large among the approximately 1 to 5 percent of teens who spend over twenty hours a week in front of a computer. It's also prevalent among the other 2 or 3 percent who spend over forty hours a week doing the same. Emotional "ups and downs" inherent to our teenage years make things worse. It is clear that obesity is a problem which can severely affect the world's adolescent population.[8]

FOOD AND DRINKS: THE COMMONSENSE CAUSE FOR OBESITY

Metropolitan areas are crowded with fast food chains in shopping mall food courts and are even in subway stations "waiting" to greet people and tease their appetites as they step onto the platform. These restaurants try as best they can to live up to their name by offering food quickly and at affordable prices. Many people, including those who are not obese, resort to fast food to save time that would be otherwise spent in the supermarket and in the kitchen. The result is the consumption of high-calorie and high-fat foods as well as less time spent on physical activity. People order fast food from the comfort of our cars or on our way out of the train station, no longer preoccupied with cooking a meal or cleaning up afterwards. The increase in "drive-thrus" and "take-outs" affects the way people live and eat.

Paradoxically, food always goes hand-in-hand with major athletic events and weekend activities. NFL football games may end in a barbecue at one of the players' houses. In Latin American culture, almost all Sunday afternoon soccer games end in several rounds of beer. For women, a day at the spa or the tennis court turns into a shopping date where the food court is an inevitable stop along the way.

Food and Culture

In general, food can be found at every major event in life, no matter the culture. Birthdays, weddings, funerals, office get-togethers, study group sessions, dates, and even church bake sales all have something to do with food. For some Caribbean diets, consuming large amounts of food is the same thing as saying, "My compliments to the chef."

In other words, the hostess/chef will feel very offended if all guests do not compliment her cooking by helping themselves to several platefuls. This is also true of some Central and South American cultures. In the United States and other countries, the "super-size" concept is growing more popular by the minute.[9] The idea of getting extra-large fries, extra-large soda, and just about extra-large *anything* for just a few extra cents tempts you to eat more. Once again, obesity is as real as it gets.

Comfort Food

Comfort food allows for the use of emotion that makes you overeat. Grandmothers make hearty bowls of chicken soup for their sick grandkids. Tuna casseroles that are designed to cheer up an unhappy friend, and an apple pie welcomes a new neighbor. The term *comfort food* itself is partly due to the fact that these foods are not only rich in flavor but also in calories from fat. In the case of comfort foods such as pudding, chocolate, and ice cream, there is often a lot of sugar involved. Carbohydrate-dense foods often increase levels of serotonin, the feel-good hormone that can help assuage feelings of stress or sadness.[10]

Why Drink When You Can Eat?

Alcohol consumption also serves as one of the causes of obesity.[11] When you abuse alcohol, you are more likely to suffer from heart disease and other cardiovascular conditions that may result in serious obesity.[12] High blood pressure is far more likely in people who smoke and drink alcohol. The condition can lead to liver problems. That in turn will affect your digestion and ultimately lead to more fat storage and weight gain. A study found that only 80 percent of consumable alcohol is really "metabolizable."[13] Alcohol is also very high in calories, so the more alcohol a person consumes, the more calories he consumes.

Fry the Fat Away from Your Diet

Fried foods and sugar-rich delicacies will only contribute to increased cholesterol and fatty deposits in the blood that could later clog blood vessels, leading to noncommunicable diseases like heart attack, diabetes, and other coronary heart diseases.[14] Other nonfatal but debilitating medical conditions such as respiratory difficulties, chronic muscle pain, skin problems, and infertility deprives obese individuals of the optimum quality of life.[15] Such disorders restrict movements and affect one's body image.

Women who turn obese as a result of eating fried foods often find it difficult to conceive. Hormones associated with the menstrual cycle and the ability of the ovaries to conceive is related to cholesterol. More fat cell deposits can convert these hormones, particularly androstenedione, which is produced by the adrenal glands into an estrogen hormone called estrone. The steady influx of estrone disrupts the normal ovarian cycle, and this can make an obese person infertile.[16]

GENES MAY TELL IT ALL

Once thought to be unrelated to obesity, genetic makeup is now considered to have an important role in the development of this condition. Several lab experiments and research studies have shown that genes do indeed influence size and shape.[17]

Your genes are really like your personal map. You could also think of it as an instruction manual or your biography that is held secretly inside your body. Genes hold all the hereditary information about you, including anything ranging from what you will look like in the future, to what diseases you are more likely to suffer. Some researchers believe the answers to all human diseases, even till death, lie in your genetic makeup.

Lab Research

Extensive research using lab animals has shown a strong relationship between a living specimen's genes and its body shape.[18] There are many scientists who explain heredity's role in the definition of your body shape. They also argue that specific genes are responsible for the tendency to develop obesity. Studies with a limited sample size have shown that up to 80 percent of children whose parents are obese will develop the condition at some point in their lives.

To further demonstrate the role of genetic makeup in the development of obesity, scientists have conducted a study with identical twins.[19] They took the pairs and separated them at birth. These twins' biological parents were both obese. The twins were then each raised in totally different environments and family settings. At the end of the study, experts noticed that there was no significant difference between raising the child in a family of genetically thin people with healthy lifestyles and raising him or her in an obese family. Both twins were approximately the same size and weight, regardless of the fact that one grew up eating a healthy diet and the other was accustomed to fast food.

Metabolism and the Genetics of Obesity

Another study showed that youngsters with a normal height and weight—but born to obese parents—had lower metabolic rates.[20] Obese children born to normal-weight parents can have ideal metabolic rates from otherwise inexplicable causes. This further proves that genetics do in fact play an important role in the onset of obesity and *can* be considered a contributing factor.

So what does all this mean? These interesting studies provide firm evidence that your genes are important factors for shaping your present and future weight. Experts claim that genes are 25 to 40 percent to blame for your weight. The exact way this works is still not fully understood, but many scientists believe genes are responsible for determining your metabolic rate as well. Your metabolism is responsible for processing the food you consume. If genes are responsible for making a certain part of your metabolism slow down or go bad, then obesity can develop.

Introducing Mr. Ob

In recent years, research looking into the genetic causes of obesity has shown that there is a "fat gene" to blame for obesity.[21] Scientists refer to this gene as the *Ob* gene, with *Ob* for obese. The gene is also known as the *Ob* (*Lep*) gene, with *Lep* meaning leptin, a hormone that you will read about later in the chapter. Researchers believe this *Ob* gene hampers your brain's capacity to determine satiety. If the brain doesn't get this signal, then it will continue to think "I am hungry," and you will continue to eat.

A study done on the Pima Indians proves the existence of *Ob* as if since the beginning of time. Most of the members of this tribe are overweight and they are, on average, obese.[22] It is believed that the Pima Indians are "designed" this way, thanks to their ancestors' genes. The people possess a slower metabolic rate than the average person. This is thought to be due to their hunter/gatherer lifestyle. By having a slower metabolic rate back in those days, tribesmen were better able to store body fat for a better chance of survival. Researchers believe the gene has passed down through all generations of the tribe and is the reason for why they have lower metabolic features. It also explains why they are more likely to develop obesity.[23]

Ob can be produced in a laboratory. Scientists have discovered that they can make an *Ob* gene in mice, which inevitably makes these animals fat and diabetic. Researchers are sure there is a human equivalent to this gene, partially due to experiments with mice. Along with the *Ob* gene, biochemical research has pinpointed a gene called the *beta-3 adrenergic receptor* gene.[24] This gene is found in both humans and mice, and, when physically altered, hinders your ability to break down and burn fats.

Following the *Ob* gene's discovery in 1994, researchers began to study its role in the onset of obesity. Further research uncovered *Ob*'s role in the production of a protein hormone labeled leptin.[25] Scientists also discovered a *leptin receptor* in the human brain. They turned their attention to it right after leptin was discovered. According to their findings, leptin sends the signal to your brain when it is time to stop eating.[26] These studies showed that people who are obese do indeed have leptin in their bodies as well as a good number of leptin receptors.[27] However, what if the mechanism ceases to work properly? Scientists compare this malfunction to the physiopathology (the study of normal and abnormal functions) of the diabetic who has enough insulin but is unable to efficiently use it.[28]

Another group of researchers disregards the presence of this so-called *Ob* gene and maintains that leptin does not have a role in the development of obesity.[29] They isolated a protein which they labeled *GLP-I*. This protein appears to have a more important part in the way leptin suppresses appetite. Scientists found that the protein is responsible for lessening the velocity or rhythm of peristaltic movements of the bowel, thus slowing the passage of the food so more nutrients can be absorbed in the process. Peristalsis refers to the contraction of your gut muscles. Hunger simply ceased in rats whose brains were injected with GLP-I, even though they went for days without food. When presented with food and water, the rats refused the food. It seems GLP-I is powerful enough to make rodents stop eating immediately.[30]

Is it safe to say that genetics is partly to blame for your weight and the onset of obesity? Well, *it is* safe to say that scientists who are working to alter the genes responsible for this illness will probably get a lot of approval from the rising global obesity population. However, there currently isn't a way to physically change your whole genetic makeup, so you have to resort to other types of treatments to battle obesity.

OBESITY AS IT WORSENS

There are a number of diseases and conditions that can lead to weight gain and even obesity. Many of these diseases affect the metabolic system or the digestive system directly, making it difficult for the body to absorb the right nutrients or store only the necessary fat. There are also some medications and drugs that will increase the chances of weight gain.

Among the most frequent diseases that can cause overweightness and obesity are:

- Hypothyroidism
- Cushing's syndrome
- Depression
- Syndrome X, better known as metabolic syndrome
- Polycystic ovarian syndrome
- Hypertension
- Liver disease

Hypothyroidism

This is a disease where the thyroid gland is performing at less-than-normal capacity. The thyroid gland is located at the anterior (front) part of the neck and is partly responsible for regulating your metabolism. The gland produces two hormones which control your rate of metabolism. These hormones are known as *T3* and *T4*. Remember that the prefix *hypo* actually means "less." Therefore, hypothyroidism is really when the thyroid gland isn't producing enough thyroid hormones.

Hypothyroidism can be due to different factors from autoimmune diseases to iodine-deficiency. Iodine is needed to make thyroid hormone and its deficiency can likewise relate to the brain, and more specifically, the pituitary gland. This gland produces a hormone which signals the thyroid to produce its own hormones. When the normal cycle here is broken, your metabolism slows down.[31]

Hypothyroidism symptoms include fatigue, depression, constipation, paleness, muscle problems, and goiter. If you present with any of these symptoms, see a physician right away. Your doctor could order tests to determine thyroid hormone levels and will prescribe the conventional treatment.

Hypothyroidism slackens your metabolism,[32] which is responsible for breaking down your food into different nutrients. These nutrients are stored in the body as fat. If the metabolic rate is slower than normal, then more of the nutrients will be passed on to be stored as fat cells. This will result in weight gain that leads to full-blown obesity.[33]

Cushing's Syndrome

Cushing's syndrome is a medical condition affecting your adrenal glands. The adrenal glands are two small, triangular glands sitting atop each of your kidneys. This syndrome is also known as hypercortisolism because the person is overexposed to cortisol. Cortisol is an extremely important hormone for the human body since it performs such vital functions as:

- Regulating your blood pressure and heart function
- Controlling the immune system's response to inflammation
- Controlling the action of insulin
- Regulating metabolism

Cortisol is part of the human metabolic system because it correlates with your insulin levels. Cortisol may control insulin so the latter does what it is supposed to: tone down your sugar levels. Cortisol also helps regulate the metabolic process by overseeing the breakdown of proteins, fats, and carbohydrates. Therefore, in Cushing's syndrome, the body has more cortisol than it is supposed to. This will ruin the whole process and change the way the body processes the food it receives. By altering your metabolism, Cushing's syndrome can lead to weight gain, water retention, and eventually, obesity. To diagnose this condition, physicians order blood tests to look for cortisol. It is important to detect this illness as soon as possible because treatment options are limited.[34]

Depression

Depression is another medical condition that can lead to obesity.[35] The type of depression people are used to seeing usually goes hand-in-hand with overeating. Depression sadly becomes a part of both and illness and our modern-day way of life. Movies and television shows often depict the depressed ex-girlfriend crying over a huge bowl of ice cream or talking to a friend over the phone while downing a new box of chocolates.

Clinical depression, a more severe case, can also lead to obesity and extensive weight gain, especially around the abdominal area.[36] People who suffer from clinical depression will usually have a very limited amount of physical activity.[37] This is evident when the person stays in bed all day. Reduced levels of activity will lead to weight gain no matter what.[38]

As with standard depression, clinical depression gives way to what is also known as "emotional eating." This happens when your mind tricks you into thinking that when you eat something, you will have all of your depleted energy somehow restored. Emotional eating is also the body's way of looking for the two neurotransmitters that clinically depressed people require: *serotonin* and dopamine. It's like your body is trying to fix itself.

Syndrome X

Syndrome X is a group of signs and symptoms that revolve around weight gain and insulin resistance. It's also called metabolic syndrome. In syndrome X, the body's tissues and cells do not really respond that well to insulin and the metabolic process is then altered.[39] The way foods are broken down and stored will also be affected. Again, this change in your metabolism will lead to weight gain and, over the course of time, obesity.

Metabolic syndrome is a very common diagnosis nowadays. Your doctor might take all factors into account before deciding on this diagnosis, as the treatment is complex. Metabolic syndrome can be treated by anything from a minor diet to surgery. It's a very difficult condition to handle and calls for endocrinologists and similar medical specialists.

Polycystic Ovarian Syndrome

Polycystic ovarian syndrome (POS) is a medical condition involving a hormone imbalance in women that can eventually lead to obesity. In such a disease, a woman's ovaries have cysts on or adjacent to them.

These cysts do not allow the ovaries to function properly or produce the hormones they need to ovulate and be fertile.

By altering the production of these hormones, POS starts a chain of events which will affect the production of other hormones. Symptoms of these imbalances will include altered menstrual cycles and *androgenic* hormone increase. When levels of androgenic hormones such as testosterone rise, you can get irregular menstrual cycles and increased facial and body hair, followed by a male growth pattern. By regulating your reproductive hormone levels, POS will also end up affecting your metabolism and ultimately make you gain a lot of weight.

Hypertension

If you are suffering from obesity, chances are that you are also a victim of hypertension. Hypertension is more commonly known as high blood pressure. It is one of the more serious health problems that dampen any efforts to get rid of your obesity. Complications that arise from hypertension range from minor to life threatening. Hypertension can affect your ability to concentrate and think the right way. A study has confirmed that hypertension can also cause obesity when the former disease is induced by resistance to leptin.[40] This could lead to deterioration of other aspects of one's life. It can also affect your memory, but that is the least serious complication. Hypertension can cause the metabolic syndrome discussed earlier, which hosts a whole set of complications but essentially means your body can't correctly metabolize food. This makes you gain weight, period. You also get higher cholesterol and triglyceride levels.

You can see that extra complications may cause overweightness, making it nearly impossible for many to break free from the yoke of obesity. More seriously, hypertension can lead to blindness through the thickening, narrowing, or tearing of blood vessels in the eyes. It can also lead to serious organ problems or even organ failure if blood vessels traveling through the kidneys are weakened and narrowed. Organ failure is very serious because it puts you in a situation where you must be in the hospital constantly on regulatory machines—all while you wait for a very expensive transplant.

Hypertension can lead to other serious issues that have to do with arteries. Someone who has high blood pressure is at a greater risk to have an early onset of atherosclerosis, of which the complications have been noted above. Furthermore, it can cause an aneurysm. An aneurysm is a place in the artery where the blood vessels have weakened or bulged. If an aneurysm were to explode, it could be life threatening and the victim might have to be hospitalized. High blood pressure can lead to blood vessels rupturing in the brain—a medical emergency at the very least. Interrupted blood flow to the brain is really considered a stroke. A ruptured vessel in the brain and a stroke can be related. Strokes can be considered a terminal illness because the affected individual most often passes away.

Severe hypertension leads to heart and kidney failure.[41] Because of increased blood pressure the heart must now pump more blood at a higher speed to satisfy your organs' various needs. That in turn will cause the heart muscle to grow and the body and the heart compete for a limited amount of blood. As a final outcome, the heart (or another organ) fails since there isn't enough blood in circulation to fulfill its needs.

Liver Disease

The most common organ that is affected by obesity is the liver. The liver is, for our daily survival, one of the most important glands. (The liver is both an organ and a gland. It is the largest gland, as well as the largest solid organ in the body.) It helps digest foods, absorbs nutrients, and removes toxic waste from other organs. You cannot survive without the proper function of the liver. If the liver fails all the way, you'll need painful dialysis treatments, in which a machine performs the vital functions of a liver. If you suffer from liver failure, you can expect other organs to start failing. Among the first to give up is the kidney, since molecules created from digestion enter the liver and any waste travels out of it and into the kidneys. If the liver isn't breaking down the digested food, a lot of substances are passing into the kidney that the kidney cannot handle all at once. Every organ starts to fail after the liver dies. Having liver failure suggests that you're going to be more susceptible to infections all throughout your body, with the infections occurring frequently in the blood, respiratory, and urinary tracts.

The liver manufactures chemicals needed to make your blood clot. However, if the liver ceases to work correctly or malfunctions completely, your blood won't clot with safe timing. The inability to clot may not be a problem for minor injuries or wounds where you can stanch the bleeding. When it comes to internal ulcers and other similar manifestations, you need to watch out. It is common to see an obesity victim with stomach ulcers. These ulcers eat away at the stomach lining and eventually cause bleeding. It is very important that this bleeding stops quickly because when the person gets too much blood in their digestive system and peritoneal cavity, he or she could die from all the infection.

Cerebral Edema

Did you know that cerebral edema is yet another symptom of obesity? Obesity can cause cerebral edema if the person suffers from heart failure. Heart failure is highly associated with the buildup of water all around the body. Cerebral edema is when too much liquid builds up pressure in the brain. This can make it so the brain doesn't receive enough blood or oxygen. Not getting enough oxygen in the brain can have disastrous effects. This essentially equates to a stroke and can deprive you of certain brain functions and capabilities. Oxygen deprivation causes the brain to stop maturing properly.

Worthy of Mention

Other problems that may be caused or that may take place concurrently with obesity are: Down's syndrome, Cohen's syndrome, Beckwith-Wiedermann syndrome, Lawrence-Moon-Biedl syndrome, and Prader-Willi syndrome. Most of these conditions are detected at birth or shortly afterwards. A small group of researchers also showed that children who had their tonsils and/or adenoid glands removed had greater chances of gaining weight as well.

A HEART OF GLASS AND A HEART OF STEEL

The most notorious illness that can arise from obesity is heart disease, widely accepted as the deadliest medical issue facing America today. It accounts for forty percent of all deaths in the United States, which is more than the amount of deaths from all types of cancer combined.

Complications stemming from heart disease are similar to those linked to obesity. If you have heart disease, you are more likely to get atherosclerosis, which could lead to peripheral artery disease (PAD). Peripheral artery disease is a condition where the extremities don't receive enough blood. This can cause pain in your legs, and a very dangerous *aneurysm* can form as well. The aneurysm may burst and put you through a lot of pain or travel down arteries and get lodged. This would be somewhat similar to blood clotting. This may result in multiple health issues that almost always end in death. It can also cause an ischemic stroke when your carotid arteries are blocked and too little blood reaches your brain. A stroke ensues and brain tissue begins to die within just a few minutes.

In the event of a heart attack, or myocardial infarction, obesity victims usually have a blood clot in one of the coronary arteries, thus interrupting blood flow. This will cause damage and even destroy part of your heart muscle. Sudden cardiac arrest happens when the heart suddenly loses function and you lose consciousness and the ability to breathe. A cardiac arrest is really an electrical malfunction that stops your heartbeat. This is a medical emergency that can be fatal. Anyone with sudden cardiac arrest won't survive if he or she does not get treated right away.

These are just a few of the health problems that arise from being obese. If someone is obese for long periods of time, the question may not be *whether* he or she will get a complication, but *when* it will happen to them. Obesity-related diseases make it nearly impossible to break out of the cycle of obesity itself. The by-product of these complications is obesity, if not a loss of the energy necessary for an obesity sufferer to lose weight. Therefore, someone who becomes obese isn't simply risking having an uncomfortable life; they are risking a probable drop in life expectancy.

CLUES FROM PILLS

Corticosteroids

There are common medications responsible for obesity-causing weight gain. Corticosteroids can greatly affect the adrenal glands. These glands, as previously mentioned, are responsible for the production of cortisol. When there is too much cortisol or corticosteroids, your metabolism is altered. This means nutrient production processes change and there is a lot of fat stored in the body. All this stored fat can lead to obesity as well as fat buildup around or on vital organs. It can be dangerous and potentially fatal.

Antipsychotics

Drugs used for treating mental illnesses associated with obesity have an obvious effect on the way you feel. With antipsychotic medication, you feel like the world around you is slowing down (or the other way around) and your metabolism is very relaxed. The slower metabolism makes for a higher amount of fat, ultimately leading to obesity.

Antidepressants

Studies show that antidepressants also have an effect on your metabolism and make you gain weight.[42] They take charge of your behavior and can make you binge eat from an emotional standpoint. This will make it more likely to gain weight. While it seems counterintuitive, antidepressants can have a role in treating obesity, provided the obesity is confined to the abdomen. How this works is not well-known. Antidepressants can suppress the production of your cortisol, a stress-related hormone that is known to aid in the production of fat cells. However, most cases of obesity cannot be treated exclusively by antidepressants. Reducing a person's caloric intake and increasing the amount of exercise a person gets are still the best ways to combat obesity in most people. Use of antidepressants may lead to an elevation in mood and provide motivation for obese people to exercise, but keep in mind that many antidepressants cause weight gain in the absence of physical activity.

Birth Control Pills

This is a controversial topic as there are research groups that claim birth control pills do in fact aid the onset of obesity, while some studies suggest the contrary. A 2005 investigation at the Fred Hutchinson

Cancer Research Center uncovered evidence that overweight and obese women are more apt to become pregnant while using birth control pills.[43] This new study has looked at women taking the newer types of estrogen medications, those with only thirty to thirty-five micrograms of that hormone. The investigators found that a heavier woman is more likely to face the consequences of a missed pill. In light of those findings, physicians have decided to have those patients who are carrying a large number of pounds receive a larger dose of the pill's effective ingredient. Doctors have refrained from counseling their clients about ways to burn off any excess fat. As a result, birth control pills are actually leading to more cases of obesity.

SYMPTOMS ARE RESILIENT AND DECEITFUL

An accurate understanding of the causes of obesity cannot be made without foregoing a thorough medical history, physical exam, and of course, a full review of your symptoms. Your doctor will jot down your full clinical history to help him or her detect possible symptoms. Each of your symptoms will vary depending on the variety of causes mentioned earlier. However, it is of extreme importance that your doctor listen to everything you have to say when describing your symptoms.

Body Fat

Clearly, the main symptom present in the obese person is an excess of body fat. This can be quickly determined by calculating the body mass index (BMI). If you are obese, you will present with a very high percentage of fat tissue versus muscle tissue. Excess body fat distribution is often nicknamed either "apple-shaped" or "pear-shaped" obesity.

If you do not show obvious signs of excess fat or disproportion of the body, your physician will take certain body measurements such as waist-to-hip ratio and waist circumference. A large amount of abdominal fat can lead to the diagnosis of obesity even if the rest of your body is within normal measurements.[44] Waist circumference is a very central concept to note.

The Energy Reality

The most common physical symptom of obesity is the lack of energy. People will complain of constantly feeling tired. Lack of energy makes it hard for the person to go about their normal activities. This is because the thick layer of fat around their body makes it difficult for them to move around. Whenever they try to do something that requires physical effort, they will quickly have shortness of breath.

For obvious reasons, a sudden lack of energy will also lead to less physical activity, and eventually, to depression.[45] This depression will give way to emotional eating. Be careful, because the cycle could just go on forever and your weight could keep increasing. The lack of energy in an obesity victim can be explained by many other symptoms as well, especially heart problems that show up as early complications.

Breathing Problems

Shortness of breath may ensue because the fat in your abdomen forces the diaphragm to move higher than its normal place. The diaphragm is the muscle that separates the thorax (chest) from the abdomen. It is very important in the breathing process because it helps the air enter and exit the lungs. When forced up, it doesn't let you breathe right and you end up taking in a lot less air.

Difficulty breathing can also mean a person has heart problems. With so much extra weight to carry around, the heart must work tirelessly to pump blood to all the regions of the body. This can lead to hypertension and, eventually, to heart failure because the heart expands to take in larger amounts of blood it needs to pump to the fattened area. This is especially true of fat tissue that has numerous blood vessels.

Sleep and Obesity

An obese person will also present with complaints about sleeping issues. This is because the excess amount of fat affects their breathing and may even interrupt it for short moments during the night. This condition is also known as obstructive sleep apnea and is a major concern for obesity victims.[46]

Symptoms Run Skin Deep

Obese people tend to feel warm all the time. The extended, thick layer of fat traps body heat naturally. All this heat tries to escape through profuse sweating—a sign of your body's intent to cool down. Heavy sweating from the sweat glands located deep in your skin is often accompanied by large rashes. These rashes will mostly appear in skinfolds where sweat does not evaporate as easily. You might have rashes under the breasts, behind the knees, and in other places where excess fat and skin are present.

Other skin problems in obese people include cyanosis, when the skin turns bluish. This is when a particular patch of skin isn't receiving enough oxygen. Cyanosis is common in severely obese people and can ultimately lead to skin ulcers. These skin ulcers are very dangerous as they tend to be easily infected. Once you are infected, it is very important to get to a hospital right away so you may receive immediate antibiotic treatment. Complications of these skin ulcers can lead to septicemia, which is a generalized infection throughout your bloodstream. Septicemia can lead to other complications and death.

The Joint Effect

Joint pain is a prime physical symptom of obesity. The extra weight put onto these joints can strain the entire musculoskeletal system. Joints may buckle under the added pressure of those extra pounds. The affected person will most often complain of pain in the knees and lower back. If the obesity is very severe, you will no longer be able to walk and could permanently damage your knee and the cartilage that forms around it.

Muscle Problems

Muscles are also damaged from lack of use. The excess fat stored in the human body will eventually invade muscle tissue and damage it. Muscles lose their tone and you may have a lot of difficulty moving around from place to place. Being severely obese wouldn't make things any easier.

Varicose Veins

Varicose veins are another important physical symptom of obesity. These veins are blood vessels that have been harmed and stretched out of shape due to the large amount of blood trapped inside them. This blood is essentially having a hard time getting back up to the heart due to the excess weight you're carrying around. Varicose veins can be very painful and lead to perplexed circulation. Problems include atherosclerosis, where it's almost like fat cells are *invading* the bloodstream. It is potentially fatal and can lead to thrombosis (spontaneous blood clots) and even heart attacks.

Reproductive Issues

Obese women will frequently present with reproductive disorders, mostly in the form of abnormal menstrual cycles. It's often the hormone imbalances that make women less fertile and more likely to have spontaneous abortions, also known as miscarriages. Obese women are also much more likely to develop gestational diabetes and have problems during childbirth. Abnormal menstrual cycles can be in the form of prolonged or even complete absence of bleeding. It's vital to have a regular checkup with your gynecologist to detect or rule out hormone problems. This is even more important if you're trying to get pregnant.[47]

In men, obesity can lead to erectile dysfunctions or problems with sperm count. This again is due to hormone imbalances. These irregularities can also be seen with the development of gynecomastia, the enlargement of breasts in males. Surgery may be needed.

Other physical signs and symptoms related to obesity include urinary calculi, gallstones, gout, diabetes, hypertension, and scoliosis, the abnormal curvature of your spine. These symptoms are due to the general imbalance in your body that leads to hormone problems, excess production of one body chemical or another, or simply, consequences of all the extra fat. It is important to rule out other diseases that come with these symptoms when looking to determine the exact cause of your obesity.

NO HARD "FEELINGS"

Any statement suggesting that obesity victims are always happy is a far-fetch from reality. A person with obesity could very well be unsatisfied with his or her body image. He or she might feel like there's no way to fix the way they look and everything seems hopeless. This leads to frustration, depression, as well as other psychological and emotional difficulties.

Obesity is linked to selective cases of low self-esteem and lack of self-confidence. The obesity victim may be a genius or at least very skilled at something, but won't necessarily show it. In general, obese people, regardless of gender or age, may consider themselves a burden for their families and a clown to their friends and social circle. Flirting and dating is reportedly rare among the morbidly obese, who will occasionally feel that anyone approaching them does so simply because the latter feels sorry or intends to ridicule.

Women are more vulnerable to psychological symptoms that are related to obesity. Research has shown that obese women have poorer psychological adjustment skills than their male counterparts.[48] Women suffer more from low self-esteem and clinical depression. This is partly due to our society's unrealistic goals of ideal personal beauty. Some obese women are especially hurt by social standards and are quick to avoid being seen in public places. Obese females can be extremely sensitive and may easily misinterpret what one says to them.

Obese subjects in general have been found to suffer from depression and anxiety over three times more often than nonobese people. Obesity victims have reported severe impairment of social interaction three to four times more often than people within normal weight ranges. Studies have shown difficulties with normal psychological functions more often in obese people than their nonobese counterparts. Anxiety can stem from an unsuccessful diet. Your anxiety can quickly become frustrating, and you may stop dieting altogether. You need to know what is going on in your body and how your diet program will actually help you get better.

Social Perspectives

There are several comparative studies demonstrating the relationship between obesity and social aspects of life. For instance, one study describes the association of high waist-to-hip ratios with work problems, unemployment, and low socioeconomic class. Another group of investigators also describes the association between high waist-to-hip ratio and the use of antidepressants. High waist-to-hip ratios have also been associated with low self-confidence and poorer quality of life, especially in female obesity sufferers.[49] Economic hardship has been found to be, via professional research, a direct lead-in to obesity.[50] This correlation is characteristic of different cultures, some due to a long-running history of poverty and scarcity of food.

As an obese person, it can be difficult for you to really feel good about yourself. You might seem frustrated when you look for new clothes, as stores that carry plus sizes are rare. Plus size stores still lack a large selection of clothing with noticeable differences in size. Don't feel uncomfortable for being too large for the chairs when you go out to eat. You could get very depressed and eventually stop leaving home. If this is the case for someone you care about, you must watch over them because emotional eating and weight gain comes with depression which spirals out of control.

Self-Confidence

Obese people can sometimes lack self-confidence and feel they have nothing to offer to a partner or to their friends or employers. They start to fade into their own version of reality and never go out to social events. They prefer to stay at home on their couch watching TV. Again, this leads to less physical activity and more overeating. It is a vicious cycle that can ultimately lead to death.

The Worst-Case Scenario versus Hopeful Add-Ons

When an obese person starts to think they have nothing to offer, that they are for whatever reason a burden to society, the people around them must be extra careful. Experts make it clear that obese people can become suicidal due to the high levels of depression and frustration.[51] Both doctors and the general public should *collectively* warn everyone of this possibility. Let them know that they have a lot of support from friends *before* the violence escalates and morphs into suicidal behavior.

Suicidal thoughts and behaviors are more common in obese men than in women.[52] This is contrary to popular belief since women are usually more worried about their physical appearance than are men.

There are also a small number of obese people who turn to violent behavior as a form of psychological venting. This is evidently a result of the frustration they feel when they don't seem to lose weight or when they give in to hunger pangs.

Without support, obese people would give in to feelings of depression and low self-esteem and would never make it out from the clutches of obesity. Support groups and psychological therapy are fundamental in getting people to commit to diet plans and weight loss therapies. Not to mention that your circle of friends and family are necessary to work toward your weight loss goals. In the upcoming chapters, you will explore the *many* different ways by which the worldwide obesity problem can be tackled. These hopeful techniques range from broader, medicinal methods, to deeper understandings of personal psychology, and motivational factors.

As you can see, the commonest psychological symptoms in obese people are low self-esteem and depression. Get a decent amount of counseling and psychological treatment. Don't be afraid to ask your doctor about the causes and symptoms of your obesity. Keep in mind that every obese person is different, so at the end of the day, everyone has a distinct combination of signs and symptoms to address. Your doctor can provide the positive and supportive environments that *everyone*, obese or not, really need.

It is important to consider not only your health, but all areas of your life when studying the causes of obesity. In order for your health care provider to issue an adequate treatment plan that is best suited for you, it is imperative that you share as much information about yourself as possible. There are various causes for obesity that differ from one person to another. In the previous chapter, you learned the importance of a complete and comprehensive exam. This is done to evaluate the patient and to discover the core cause for all the extra fat. Your physician will have an understanding of your medical background as well as undergo a thorough physical exam. All areas of your health and lifestyle, and the information provided by all of your specialty doctors will help to determine the causes and symptoms of your obesity.

（4）

TREATMENT

It is time to start searching for the best treatment option for your obesity once you confirm that you are in fact suffering from the disease. Treatments range from diet plans to herbal remedies to surgical procedures. It is important that people are fully informed of the pros and cons of every treatment method because many available options pose several health risks and can even prove to be fatal.

Treatment options for obesity are diverse and plenty, but they can be classified into four basic groups:[1]

- Lifestyle changes
- Nonmedical or alternative treatments
- Medical treatments with medications
- Surgical procedures

Simply put, the aim of treatment is to lose excessive fat and remain lean to improve the quality of life both emotionally and physically. When someone looks good aesthetically, he or she may also *feel* good. Moreover, the best way to ditch the fat and lose weight is to reduce the amount of calories[2] in your diet and to increase physical activities such as exercise. Obesity treatment should be viewed as a lifestyle change and not just a fad for maintaining ideal body weight. Careful assessment of an individual's diet, lifestyle, and physical activity should be taken.

Work and home environments are included in the assessment to enhance a weight loss program that fits your lifestyle. You cannot impose a serious weightlifting workout to someone who has never gone to the gym or on a jog for even a block or two in his or her life. The individual could fail due to lack of motivation and confidence that he or she could have used for achieving ideal weight. The key is to gradually make lifestyle changes from watching what you eat, and planning and preparing your meals in the best way possible.

CALORIES AND OBESITY

Chapter 1 discussed how calories provide fuel for the body. However, there's more to the role of calories in relation to obesity treatment. The first thing that comes to mind when dealing with obesity is to go on a strictly low-calorie diet. The logical reasoning is that you will start burning all the stored calories. While this all makes sense, your metabolism systems have a way of slowing down and self-protecting when they realize you are not eating enough. This is why "fad diets" don't really work beyond a few days.

Science[3] has proven that once you shed the pounds and continue to *keep* them off, you follow a diet that slowly changes the way you eat. Abruptly giving up on fast food won't exactly make your life easier. It won't really make sense for someone who is used to eating between 3,000 to 7,000 calories a day to suddenly find themselves on a 1,200-calorie-a-day diet. Things just don't work that way in the world of dieting. Your diet must be designed so the caloric intake gradually decreases. Also, since many obesity victims might be depressed or have very low self-esteem as discussed earlier, it is important to plan a *realistic* calorie plan and set short-term goals that will surely be reached. Your doctor may want to know whether you can count on your family and friends for support.

Before you commit to a rigorous diet plan, make sure you have the right motivation to make it a long-term commitment. You have to be optimistic and realistic when it comes to dieting. Changing your attitude and setting short-term goals for progressive weight loss are the best ways to start losing weight. It is important to let you know that you shouldn't try to lose too much weight too fast, as this can be more dangerous than obesity itself.

Once the mood is set and the goals are agreed upon, it's time to start. The first step toward healthy weight loss is to learn about the types of foods which should be consumed the most. Obesity victims should read about nutrient content and recommended daily allowances (RDA) of different food types.

CONTROLLING YOUR APPETITE FROM HOME

Another step you can take is starting a food journal where you make a note of everything you eat. This gives a fairly good representation of what you are doing to yourself and allows you to figure out your eating patterns. A journal will help you take note of your progress as the diet continues. It also serves as a meal planner where you can write down everything you plan to eat for the day or week. By having these prepared menus, it will be more difficult for you to have an excuse to cheat.

Once you begin your diet, be sure to eat fresh fruits, vegetables, meats, and grains since studies[4] have shown that these items reduce your level of obesity. When shopping for food, it is advised that you go to the supermarket on a full stomach. This way, you're less likely to be tempted to buy the wrong types of foods. Overeating or eating the types of food that are detrimental to the human body are the two most important reasons why people become overweight and obese. By hawking for nutritional foods, an individual may be able to lose weight while still providing their body with the nutrients needed to function properly.

There are a variety of foods that can be used to help control your appetite. These foods are normally used to help curb your hunger because of certain properties they possess.

Let's go ahead and list a few of them below.

Appetite-Controlling Foods

Apples   Have you ever heard the saying, "An apple a day keeps the doctor away"? Munching on an apple is very healthy for an obese person.

Clinical evidence suggests that eating three apples daily will make you lose weight.[5] Apples are high in fiber, and given that they must be chewed a long time before swallowing, they seem very filling when they really are not. Additionally, apples serve as a natural anti-inflammatory substance.[6]

Vegetable Salad before the Main Course   People who have a bowl of salad before a meal eat less of the main course. This doesn't necessarily mean they have a huge bowl of vegetables. Just a little plate of leafy green vegetables will be enough to control your appetite and stop you from overeating other less healthy foods. Try to include cabbage and spinach in these bowls of salad with the understanding that these two vegetables have thylakoids, which are confirmed to suppress appetite.[7] Thylakoids are sac-like structures that house other important structures involved in a plant's energy production process.

Nuts   Pine nuts are the best nuts to use for limiting your appetite. They have a high amount of protein and also contain pinolenic acid. This acid is an important suppressant of your appetite.

Peanuts are among nuts that contain a high amount of protein.[8] This important nutrient is a basic building block of muscle matter, and you require at least fifty grams of protein per day in order to maintain *homeostasis*. What's more, you can counter weight gain by consuming more protein, as your body processes it as muscle mass. No other activity requires more energy than the rebuilding of muscle cells: not even aerobic exercise requires as much energy. On a pound-for-pound basis, few food items have more protein than nuts. Consuming more nuts, whether peanuts or Brazil nuts, keeps your digestive system funneling protein into your body and burns fat to sustain new muscle growth. Owing to their high-fat and high-calorie content, caution is advised when consuming nuts.

Flaxseed   Flaxseed is also growing more and more popular as studies are showing that flaxseed oil is a significant source of omega-3 acids. This highly ignored source of fiber provides eight grams per one-ounce serving. Fiber works as an exceptional appetite suppressant and is also very helpful in keeping your bowel movements regular. Fiber and flaxseed can put off cancer and bring your cholesterol levels down.[9]

Fluids   Eight or so glasses of water a day are required by virtually every diet on the planet. If you are very reluctant to drink plain water, try soups. As appetite suppressants,[10] soups control excess hunger because the warm consommé or chowder gives you a nice feeling of being full and satisfied. More importantly, they fill up your digestive system faster than solid meals do. Soups also tend to have very few calories, but keep in mind that soups do have high sodium content.

Meal Replacements Meal replacement packets that include lique-fied protein powder will help keep your appetite in check.[11] Liquefied or solid protein powder, which meal replacement packets usually include as an ingredient, are outstanding alternatives when trying to find some-thing that really suppresses your appetite since it provides your body with a false feeling of satiety. Whey protein powder also has additional benefits, such as the development of muscle tissue.

Oatmeal If you start your day with a large bowl of homemade oatmeal, you may find that you can avoid eating or snacking for a few hours. Oatmeal is a great appetite suppressant.[12] It is important that you avoid fried foods and foods that contain too much fat and salt. It is also fundamental that you avoid complex sugars and switch to sweeteners for your oatmeal.

DON'T WALK THE GREEN MILE

Here's a little more about the other side: The bottom-line lifestyle change for obese people is physical activity. Increased physical activity is essential to obese people looking to really lose weight and feel bet-ter. This physical activity ranges from simple walks to heavy workouts using gym weights and other tools. The goal of increasing your physical activity is not only to burn off the extra calories but also to help maintain muscle tone and bone strength.

Once you have your mind bent on increasing physical activity, you can focus on starting a healthy and balanced diet to go with a really good exercise plan. It is very important to find your most effective diet and adjust to it at your own pace. Your doctor will assure you that these dietary changes should be permanent. It is of no use to go on a diet and lose weight if you go back to binge eating later down the road.

Walking, Swimming, and Sports

One of the best ways to start losing weight is simply to start walking.[13] Most obese people are usually very sedentary and any other type of exercise will usually discourage them. Thirty minutes of walking per day can be the initial exercise program for the obese person as this will get him or her accustomed to being in motion again. Before embarking on a new exercise program, however, consult your doctor to be sure you do it in the right fashion. Starting an exercise regimen from scratch without medical consultation can result in some complications.

After a few weeks of walking at a normal pace, you can decide whether to move on to the next level. In fact, medical research has proven that you can achieve different levels of weight loss by walking at different speeds.[14] In the presence of supervision, you can start jogging or running. If you are severely obese, it's enough to just speed up the pace a bit. You will feel better and notice that this small change has them losing the first of many extra pounds.

Some people prefer to take up swimming as their exercise routine. This is partly due to the fact that swimming is much softer on bone joints that are not accustomed to that much movement. Mild to moderate swimming exercises are better for anyone with complications from obesity (such as heart failure or hypertension).[15] It also provides relaxation and decreases your resting heart rate over time.[16]

Others will prefer enrolling in aerobics classes or dancing lessons. This is their way of forcing themselves to exercise. They will usually go in pairs or with a group of friends for support and company. Dance and aerobics, like swimming, will make every part of the body "awaken" and get in motion. You may prefer sports to be your primary exercise plan. Whether it's a couple of football games a week, or a few tennis matches, sports help keep you motivated and active. You will be around other people supporting you and are also more likely to stick to your diet and weight loss plan. Nature sports such as kayaking and hiking are also respectable choices for the general population because of the psychological benefits involved.

Recommendations

A medical report recommends at least 150 minutes per week of the desired physical activity or a combination of different exercises.[17] Again, it's critical to set realistic goals so you don't give up as soon as you get too tired or bored. Fifty minutes per weekday[18] is a good amount to get the ball rolling. However, to achieve a substantial amount of weight loss, an obese person may require as much as one hour of physical activity per day.

Besides the planned exercise routine or sport of choice, it is important to encourage the obese person to do any extra movements they can. This means that you should try to park your vehicle at least fifty feet away from the entrance to the store, the mall, or your office. It also helps if you take the normal stairs and not the escalators. Avoid elevators when possible and walk to every part of the shopping center. These extra little walks will help you lose those extra pounds a lot faster.

Get some more exercise in by doing household chores when possible. Set up a day when you empty out all the stuff that's piled up in the garage. You can also try washing window curtains by hand or change the living room furniture around—anything that will keep you busy and moving to help lose the weight. Chapter 11 will cover the topic of exercise even further.

NONPRESCRIPTION TREATMENTS: THE PRIMERS OF OBESITY THERAPY

The three basic nonmedical weight loss supplements in wide use nowadays are hoodia, açaí berry, and Proactol. Each of these herbal or natural remedies help fight obesity in a relatively safe way because they don't possess any synthetic ingredients. Keep in mind that these over-the-counter remedies are not for everyone.

Hoodia

Hoodia (Latin name *Hoodia gordonii*), is a plant species recognized for its ability to curb your appetite.[19] It usually grows in the Kalahari Desert in South Africa and Botswana, but can be seen in parts of Namibia and southern Angola, too. A South African group identified as the Bushmen, members of the San and Khoe tribes, have been consuming this odd plant for hundreds of years.

Its particular use by members of these tribes was to repress hunger throughout the exceedingly long hikes involved in the hunting and gathering they had to endure. They would remove the plant's stem and eat this bitter-tasting cactus. Experts allege that the plant has aphrodisiac effects.

There are in fact a lot of types of hoodia; thirteen to be more precise. However, one should note that not every species have the steroidal glycoside called p57, which has become increasingly popular, as the active ingredient. For example, p57 has barely been found in the *Hoodia gordonii* species, based on peer-reviewed research.[20] A steroidal glycoside is a large molecule that gives fruits and flowers their color.

Hoodia gordonii has only recently entered the market of weight loss supplements and is the source of plenty of buzz when it comes to appetite suppressants. This trend began soon after the plant's appetite suppressing qualities were broadcasted on a national current affairs TV show,[21] where the correspondent visited the barren region where hoodia is found. The newswoman affirmed she felt full for the whole day after tasting the plant. She also claimed she felt no side effects. Regardless of its immense popularity, there are not many convincing scientific studies demonstrating hoodia's efficiency. A few of the most widely discussed studies on humans have revealed that people on the supplement lowered their caloric ingestion up to 1,000 calories per day.

When trying to figure out how the active ingredient in hoodia works in the human body, scientists have discovered that its direct effects are felt in the midbrain, particularly the hypothalamus. The active ingredient creates a feeling of satiety much more potent than that set off by the breakdown of complex carbs into glucose. It's no big surprise that people using hoodia insist they experience no hunger at all for hours. Hoodia is obtainable in different forms via mass production. It can be sold as a pill, powder, or liquid. It is available as an over-the-counter natural remedy and can also be acquired at local health stores. There have been no reports of critical or hazardous side effects for obesity victims taking hoodia as an appetite suppressant. This is really due to the fact that it comes from a plant and does not function as a stimulant on the central nervous system.[22]

Hoodia is not a cure-all wonder drug. People thinking of getting treatment with hoodia should seek advice from their physician first. As with all weight loss supplements, it is important that a consumer who suffers from obesity follow a diet and exercise plan and consult his or her doctor before taking any supplements.

Ephedra

Another appetite suppressant once used is ephedra. Also known as squaw tea or Mormon tea, ephedra is a shrub-like plant which can be found in barren regions of central Asia and faraway parts of the planet. The dried green leaves of the plant are used as treatment for several illnesses. Ephedra is a stimulant. It's composed of the herbal form of ephedrine, a very restricted drug found in over-the-counter asthma treatments.

In the United States, the Chinese herb ephedra and ephedrine are available in many local health stores and sold under an assortment of brand names. Ephedrine is sometimes used for weight loss, as an energy enhancement option, or to improve performance in competitive athletes. These goods frequently include other stimulants. For instance, caffeine may provide for heightened awareness but raise the potential for unpleasant aftereffects. Ephedra is frequently referred to as the fen-phen herb.

Ephedra's chief active pharmaceutical ingredients are ephedrine and pseudoephedrine. These include in their composition a variety of tannins and associated chemicals. The stem possesses 1 to 3 percent total of alkaloids, with ephedrine comprising about 30 to 90 percent of this total amount. The concentrations of these alkaloids depend on the specific ephedra species used in the production process. Alkaloids are carbon-containing substances derived from plants. Examples include morphine and caffeine.

Ephedrine alkaloids are compounds which are comparable to amphetamines. They are used for producing many over-the-counter and prescription medications and possess several potentially fatal effects on your central nervous system and cardiovascular system. Sadly, this is all due to their function as a stimulant. Since 1994, The US Food and Drug Administration (FDA) reported receiving over 800 complaints of adverse effects that were associated with the use of products having alkaloids of ephedrine. A study has concluded that alkaloids have mostly negative effects and therefore should be used sparingly if possible.[23] Among the potentially lethal side effects,[24] the most common were these:

- Elevated blood pressure (hypertension)
- Rapid heart rate or palpitations
- Serious nerve damage to different areas of the body (neuropathy)
- Damage to muscles or muscle groups (myopathy)
- Psychosis
- Memory loss (amnesia)
- Irregularities in heart rate and rhythm (arrhythmias)
- Sleeplessness or insomnia
- Nervousness and anxiety, sometimes accompanied by tremors
- Seizures and stroke
- Heart attacks

Due to these effects and many others, the FDA limits the manufacture and marketing of any product that contains more than eight milligrams of these harmful ephedrine alkaloids per serving.

Proactol

Another weight loss supplement that works by suppressing your appetite is Proactol. Proactol is a natural and unrefined fat binder that is derived from a cactus-like plant known as *Opuntia ficus-indica*. It is an all-natural and organic fiber complex allowing you to get rid of the extra pounds by not letting the digestive system absorb fat.

Proactol is composed of nonsoluble fibers. These fibers work by coming into contact with the food ingested. Once they bind, they become particles that form a gel-like substance which the digestive tract is unable to absorb or digest. These fat complexes will have no option but to leave your body through the intestines. Proactol is able to bind around 25 percent of the fat you eat each day. The fat is essentially removed from your body and you can lose weight faster. If used together with a balanced diet, Proactol will give some decent results.

Proactol is a 100 percent organic appetite suppressant that is fashioned from herbs. It isn't known for severe side effects. It's one of the few of these types of drugs that can make that claim. This is very important given the history of appetite suppressants in the past. Proactol is one of the most modern medications to enter the natural approach to weight loss and health conditions in general. It is said to be a natural remedy which binds fats ingested in foods and removes them from the digestive system as an alternative to them being absorbed and stored as glucose or body fat. For this reason, weight loss with proactol is likely at a realistic pace with no hazardous or unpleasant effects on your health. Again, however, it is not advisable to take anything without consulting with a doctor first.[25]

Amphetamines

In the 1950s, substantial weight loss could be accomplished mostly by one of two behaviors. The first option has always been to go on a ruthless diet. The other was to take over-the-counter drugs. Amphetamines were a very popular, legal medication at the time, but the reaction to amphetamines was also widely known to be *worse* than simple overweightness. Amphetamine pills cause a person to develop a strong addiction. Aside from losing weight, there were no realistic pros, but only cons. Amphetamines were soon banned for use as weight loss supplements due to the hazardous and serious effects[26] they had on obesity victims, especially during pregnancy. These effects range from insomnia to heart disease. There will be a deeper look into amphetamines later in the book.

An Overview of Appetite Suppressants

Once the smoke cleared, doctors looked for ways to create other medications for over-the-counter vending. Throughout the 1970s and 1980s, a wide selection of appetite suppressants and weight loss supplements began to flood the market. They each claimed to produce immediate weight loss with barely any side effects. Yet again, some led to weight loss but had harsh effects on people's health. People taking these medications later went on to have strokes and ended up dying in an effort to lose weight. In response to these deaths, the pharmaceutical companies removed the dangerous ingredients from the equation, but the product was no longer powerful. When the alternative medicine frenzy came to be, natural herbal medicines started to materialize in almost every local health store. These remedies brought with them the pledge of an all-natural, safer method for weight loss.

An appetite suppressant has one assignment: Curb your appetite. Appetite does not have the same definition as hunger. Hunger is your body's genuine need for food. It's a physiological indication of the body "asking" for food so it can construct nutrients and nourish each cell. When devoid of nutrients, body cells won't work properly, if at all. This leads to grimmer health problems for the obesity sufferer.

Under ordinary conditions, appetite is the psychological incentive for food. It is more about when you *want* to eat, rather than when you *must* eat. As human beings, people eat when they are not hungry at all. This is evident at social events or when you feel a certain way (such as comfort eating during sadness). Consequently, appetite is the most important difficulty when it comes to weight loss. It is one of the key causes of obesity and overweightness.

Appetite suppressants trick you into thinking you are no longer hungry. They do this by raising the levels of two neurotransmitters that help the body choose when it's time to eat. These two chemicals, located in the bloodstream, are called serotonin and catecholamine. They both affect your appetite. Research has shown that serotonergic drugs are effective in suppressing appetite and treating obesity.[27] Whenever you use an appetite suppressant, you sense that you are "full" prior to finishing all the food on your plate. These medicines will also lessen your appetite between mealtimes.

There are essentially two types of appetite suppressants: over-the-counter and prescription. Over-the-counter appetite suppressants are on hand at local health stores and pharmacies. These drugs don't require a medical prescription, and they include medications found in prescription drugs but in quite smaller quantities. They also consist of natural herbal appetite suppressants. Green tea is one example.

Prescription appetite suppressants include medications such as Sibutramine and Orlistat. You can only get them at pharmacies with a doctor's prescription. These drugs have possible side effects requiring your doctor's attention. If you are capable of controlling your appetite with these medications, then your caloric intake will lessen. As a result, you end up eating much less. By eating smaller portions, your stomach will be able to get used to eating a smaller amount and will reduce in size to adjust to the quantity of food you consume.

Since you are eating a smaller amount of food, your stomach will now have a smaller capacity. This means that once the handling of overweight and obesity is over, the stomach will be such a size that eating large amounts of food will no longer be comfortable. This will make it less likely for you to regain the weight and, thus, in favor of your obesity treatment. What's another benefit of appetite suppressants? Well, they can function regardless of the kind of food you eat. This means that you will be more liable to continue using them because it's as if you can cheat every now and then without gaining all the weight back. Hence, appetite suppressants are suggested in people that have a tough time sticking to harsh, restrictive diets.

The Merry-Go-Round Story of Sibutramine

Sibutramine has probably been the most renowned appetite suppressant used for obesity. Although it is unrelated to amphetamines, Sibutramine is a controlled substance in the United States. Sibutramine was the first to receive the approval of the US FDA, being recognized since 1997 as an appetite suppressant for the treatment of obesity. This medication offers three different types of benefits when it comes to treating obesity: (1) it enhances weight loss; (2) it improves weight maintenance; and (3) it helps reduce the comorbidities of obesity.[28]

Subitramine works by increasing the levels of two neurotransmitters in the brain: serotonin and norepinephrine.[29] Neurotransmitters are chemicals produced when one nerve cell tries to communicate with another. The neurotransmitter reaches and enters the adjacent cell, as if it were eaten by the other nerve cell. However, not all the parts of the *neurotransmitter* reach the next cell or are bound to specific receptors. These parts return to the cell that produced them and may reenter it. This is what the concept of "reuptake" entails. Sibutramine disallows the reuptake to take place with serotonin and noradrenalin receptors. This means that there are more neurotransmitters available to keep transmitting the message that your stomach is full. Beware, Sibutramine is no wonder drug. A study has shown that it can have many side effects, including:[30]

- Dry mouth
- Impaired sense of taste
- A larger appetite
- Nausea
- Stomach problems

- Constipation
- Difficulty sleeping
- Drowsiness
- Dizziness
- Menstrual cramps
- Headache
- Joint and muscle pain

The side effects of Sibutramine are so grave that the drug is no longer available in the United States.

Orlistat Anyone?

Orlistat is another over-the-counter supplement used for treating obesity. It works by lessening the production and absorption of fat from your diet. The stomach and intestine have enzymes, known as lipases, in charge of breaking down fat into lesser molecules which are absorbed into your body from the digestive tract. Orlistat binds to these lipases and reduces their action, helping to diminish fat assimilation. Yet, this drug does not work directly on carbohydrates or protein.[31]

Orlistat is a weight loss treatment which is designed to treat weight loss in obese adults, not children. The drug was accepted by the FDA in 1999 for use as a prescription medication, but has since been approved as over-the-counter. Orlistat could be inappropriate if you had an organ transplant, have thyroid disease, or are diabetic. Adverse effects of this drug consist of alterations in bowel movements, in addition to menstrual abnormalities. Some doctors declare that it can even result in behavioral changes and that it also gets in the way of the metabolism of specific vitamins in the body.[32]

Avesil

Avesil is a relatively new thermogenic weight control invention, and it's also currently available over-the-counter. It is interesting to notice that the drug's manufacturers have put a lot of effort into the research and manufacturing of this drug. Avesil is basically a patented form of hydroxycitric acid extract. The benefits of the four key ingredients in this recipe are becoming widely known. The research around Avesil can be traced back to more than 200 published scientific studies. These articles have appeared in valued scientific and medical magazines, and most of them were carried out in university research labs.

Avesil works on the basis of thermogenesis—the heat producing method that can boost the rate at which your fat is burned. At this time, thermogenesis research about the human body has fascinated the diet supplement industry, and several see this procedure as the final solution to weight loss supplements. With this mission, the producers of Avesil have included thermogenic ingredients shown to maintain your optimal metabolic rate. The outcome is a recipe which causes the human body to burn food as energy, instead of storing it as fat. These components also help curb your appetite and break down stored fat, a procedure called lipolysis. Avesil supposedly does all of this while helping to sustain and promote lean muscle mass. While clinical studies have shown the drug to have very few side effects,[33] you should always consult with your doctor before taking it for weight loss.

WHEN WEIGHT LOSS GOES PRESCRIPTION

Prescription treatments are available and should be used with a lot of caution. It is advisable to people who are seeking to lose weight as a "quick fix" to avoid using such drugs.[34] There is always the tendency to put the lost weight back onto the body after the drug regimen is stopped. Careful assessment from a physician is required before a prescription weight loss drug regimen is started. Pharmacological treatment should be linked with lifestyle changes, diet, and exercise to be effective and beneficial to its goal.

Phentermine

Phentermine is a very strong drug used to help speed up weight loss by reducing the hunger hormones and chemicals in the brain. It has been scientifically proven to work by releasing serotonin into the bloodstream.[35] This pharmaceutical method of treating obesity has been met with mixed reactions. Some people claim that popping pills to cure a lifestyle problem will only cause more problems in the long run. Others feel that the jump start phentermine offers in treating obesity helps to move obese people down the road to a healthy lifestyle. Whatever your train of thought, the fact is that phentermine works for obesity victims in different ways. The drug helps to reduce your natural feelings of hunger, causing you to be able to eat less without feeling the need to eat.

Using phentermine alone as your only plan of action isn't always a good idea. While phentermine can give you a head start down your path of weight loss, the drug won't help without a lifestyle adjustment on your part. It is important to use phentermine as a supplement to an active weight loss plan, such as a change in diet. Combined with regular exercise and a healthy diet, the drug can help you lose weight over time but is not a quick fix to an obesity problem. It is definitely not one you would want to get addicted to. Phentermine is a prescription medication, which means you cannot simply pick it up at any pharmacy without a prescription.

Regular use of phentermine can bring on unpleasant side effects.[36] There are risks to taking the drug on a regular basis for weight loss. Because the drug works by stimulating your central nervous system, insomnia is a common outcome. If you are experiencing sleep loss from phentermine pills, contact your doctor right away.

Are Amphetamine Pills a Tall Order?

Amphetamines, in their unadulterated form, are liquids with a strong scent and a burning taste. In essence, they are manmade stimulants. They are marketed in ampoules, capsules, and tablets. They can be manufactured as an unscented crystalline powder, and are taken orally or by injection. Amphetamines have been around since the 1930s. They were used initially as a nasal inhaler to cure common colds and hay fever. They were later found to excite the central nervous system, a purpose they serve even today.

As a stimulant, amphetamines sharpen awareness, control hunger, expel sleepiness, and chase away depression. They produce feelings of improved physical and mental power and create an increase of mood and feeling of well-being. Amphetamines that are commonly abused today include benzedrine or "bennies" and dexedrine or "dexies." These drugs are obtainable not just in their unadulterated forms, but in tranquilizer and barbiturate mixtures. Barbiturates are sedatives.

Amphetamines also stimulate the brain areas linked to watchfulness, humor, and heart action. It's no wonder that these drugs are called "speed." Throughout mental crises, artificial stimulation of brain cells is very important. However, detrimental effects can take place when stimulation is enhanced by amphetamines. When things really get going, amphetamines cause a release of norepinephrine, a material stored in your nerve endings, and bring them up to the brain's nerve centers. This speeds up your heart and affects your metabolism.

These are some of the negative physical and mental effects of amphetamine abuse:

- Side effects and overdose: augmented heartbeat, pulse rate, and blood pressure, occasionally going up to fatal levels.
- Gradual effects: physical breakdown, mental problems, and death.
- Long-term use: Weariness from lack of sleep and undernourishment due to numb appetite, lack of self-balance and self-control, lack of any practically or logic, difficulty in thinking and speaking, devastated emotions, and other sporadic reactions. As you may know, brain damage can lead to a coma. Temper tantrums and episodes of aggressive psychosis are frequent when an addict uses large amounts of amphetamines for a long time. You could suffer from social, emotional, physical, mental, and economic devastation.
- Body harm: brain, heart, and liver problems can diminish an abuser's life expectancy to no more than five to seven years after initial addiction.
- Infections: hepatitis, tetanus, and others from unsterile needles and syringes used for injecting amphetamines.
- Mind damage: apprehensive, raw-nerved, reckless, on occasion, violent conduct, which makes a "speed freak" grouchy and susceptible to violent instincts. This fear-filled lunacy, called "a paranoid psychotic state" in medical lingo, can endure long beyond the drug's activity. It manifests almost like paranoid schizophrenia.
- Disintegration of values: social, family, and moral values decline. Like the heroin addict, an obese person addicted to amphetamines will do anything to obtain their dose of "speed."

- Judgment issues: an obesity victim who is addicted to amphet-amines will have difficulty judging space, time, and distances cor-rectly, as well as mental and physical lack of coordination. The ad-dict tends to go out of control, is very likely to take enormous risks.
- Hygiene neglect: a frequent side-effect, which can show the way to several health problems such as skin infections, dental decay, and undernourishment.

DON'T BRING A KNIFE TO A GUNFIGHT: SURGICAL OPTIONS

In a few cases, weight-loss (bariatric) surgery is a preferred alternative. Weight-loss surgery offers the greatest chance of losing a lot of weight, but keep in mind that it can cause grave risks. Weight-loss surgery limits the quantity of food you can eat or restricts the metabolism of food and its nutrients. While it shouldn't be your first choice, weight-loss surgery may be the way to go if you:

- Have severe obesity, with a BMI of at least 40
- Have a BMI of 35 to 39.9, along with a grave weight-related health issue, including diabetes or high blood pressure
- Really want to make the lifestyle changes required for invasive surgery to give desirable effects

For extreme, life-threatening cases of obesity, the treatment option of-ten advised by physicians is surgery. This is advised only if the benefits outweigh the risks. There are different forms of surgical procedure done on obese people. Bariatric (weight loss) surgery comprises two types: gastric banding and gastric bypass. In the adjustable form of the procedure, there is insertion of a band that limits the width of the opening from the esophagus to the stomach. The band can be taken out when necessary. In contrast with gastric banding, gastric bypass is a complete "redirection" of the stomach. The proximal (closest) portion of your stomach is connected to the small intestine, creating a small pouch where food goes. It is anastomosed (fused) at a location about two feet from the normal insertion point. Surgical treatments don't guarantee weight loss. You need to undergo rehabilitation following surgery and engage in a dietary regimen to achieve the desired results of the procedure in the first place. In gastric bypass, you can basically say good-bye to around 65 percent of excess weight if you stay on track.[37]

Like any other weight loss treatment or medication, surgery is no miracle cure. Obesity surgery isn't a guarantee to lose all the excess weight or keep the weight off forever. Successful weight loss after bariatric surgery depends on willpower and support needed to commit to permanent lifestyle changes.

There are several forms of weight-loss surgery. Some are considered *restrictive*, which means they promote weight loss by restricting the total amount of food your stomach can hold at a given time. Others are *malabsorptive*, a name they receive because they make the body unable to absorb nutrients and calories from your food. A few are a combination of these two types. The most common weight-loss surgeries are laparoscopic adjustable gastric banding and gastric bypass.

Laparoscopic Techniques

Laparoscopic techniques, which warrant the use of a thin telescope-like instrument to look inside your abdomen, and other advanced medical technologies used throughout surgery permit for lesser degrees of scarring and greater accuracy. When malabsorption and food restriction happen at the same time or on the same person, the weight loss results are faster. Individuals going for weight-loss surgery procedures that employ both methods may drop no less than two-thirds of their extra weight in twenty-four months. People drop their weight at distinctive rates. In addition, every obesity sufferer has special requirements and hindrances which may affect the general outcome of surgery.[38]

"Bypassing" Reality

Gastric bypass is in fact a mixed surgical technique. It uses gastric restriction through a section of stomach, allowing you to feel "satisfied with less." This redirects food so it doesn't pass through the first loop of the bowel. You may also experience a decreased absorption of nutrients and calories. Gastric bypass is a weight loss procedure that's highly effective in the long term, keeping you as close as possible to normal weight for many years. Among its main advantages, this surgery produces a rapid initial weight loss and is available as a minimally invasive procedure. Consider that the average total weight loss after bariatric surgery is over 50 percent of the obesity victim's total weight.

Like most surgeries in modern-day society, gastric bypass has its drawbacks. The process can cause some medical complications due to nutritional deficiencies, such as that of iron,[39] if left unchecked. It also has a higher rate of surgical complications and mortality than other surgical procedures. Gastric bypass can be performed as an open surgery or through laparoscopy. However, the laparoscopic approach offers all the benefits of minimally invasive procedures, such as painlessness and faster recovery. The greatest advantage of laparoscopic surgery for obesity is a reduced risk for incision hernias (up to 20 percent in open surgery) and low infections (up to 17 percent in surgery). Gastric bypass is indicated for people with a BMI greater than 40, or who have a BMI of 35 with related diseases such as diabetes mellitus, hypertension, and sleep apnea, among others. To serve as the best candidate, you would have to be between eighteen and sixty-five years of age, a nonsmoker, and without alcohol or drug dependence. Gastric bypass surgery comes in different forms.[40]

Roux-en-Y Gastric Bypass (RGB)   This method is the most frequent gastric bypass surgery performed in the United States. A small stomach pouch is created by stapling a portion of the stomach together, or through a process known as vertical banding. This restricts the quantity of food that may be easily eaten. Consequently, a Y-shaped piece of the smaller gut is bridged with the pouch to let food pass the *duodenum* and the first section of the jejunum. This successfully causes a smaller amount of caloric and nutrient assimilation in the body. The duodenum is the first section of your small intestine. It is followed by your jejunum.[41]

Biliopancreatic Diversion (Extensive Gastric Bypass)   This technique is more difficult than the RGB process for a few reasons. First, the lower portion of the stomach is removed in totality, which leaves only around 50 percent of the stomach in your body. The remaining portion is then linked directly to the final part of the small intestine. This leaves both the duodenum and jejunum free of any ingested material. With the RGB method, the stomach is not removed forever, but only the route the ingested food takes is changed and shortened. With the biliopancreatic method, the segment of the stomach left over is a little larger, so a greater amount of food gets through than with RGB. Moreover, biliopancreatic diversion keeps the pylorus, the end part of the stomach, undamaged. It also keeps the contents of your stomach from moving too rapidly through the small intestine, frequently referred to as "dumping."[42]

Laparoscopic Adjustable Gastric Banding (LAGB)

LAGB involves connecting a balloon to a band around the upper fraction of the stomach. A reservoir is positioned under your skin. Its function is to pump air into the balloon and regulate the gastric band. As the balloon inflates, the gastric band grows tighter and reduces the quantity of food passing through your stomach at any given time. When the balloon deflates, the band loosens its grip around your stomach and food can then pass through with much more ease.

Unlike other restrictive alternatives, LAGB doesn't involve permanently modifying the structure of the stomach or small intestines. LAGB is in fact, a reversible escape route without the risk of harsh nutritional deficiencies. Founded on this principle, LAGB is usually looked upon as a much safer practice than the gastric bypass or malabsorptive surgeries. While weight loss induced by LAGB is usually much less than that of the malabsorptive procedures, research finds that gastric banding procedures help to alleviate depression in obesity victims.[43]

The Surgery Verdict

Keep in mind that there is always a danger of having nutritional deficiencies with weight loss surgeries used to eliminate areas of the stomach or modify the course of ingested food. Weight-loss surgery involves dedication and an understanding of daily dietary needs that can require you to take extra vitamins and minerals. You have to be increasingly attentive to your nutritional state in order to stay within your normal weight range and be healthy.

Every weight loss procedure has its severe risks and potential complications. Numerous complications have been accredited to weight loss surgeries, such as stretching of the stomach pouch, which can make the stomach grow back to its standard size. Band erosion reinstates parts of the stomach and makes the stomach return to its original size. Other complications include movement of the staples during surgery, thus backfiring on the whole procedure.

Weight loss on overweight participants in a study revealed reduced red blood cell aggregation and improved *fibrinolytic capacity*,[44] which decreases the possibility of heart attacks and thrombosis or blood clots. Rapid weight loss, such as that gained from weight-loss surgery, in noninsulin dependent diabetes mellitus (NIDDM) consistently shows marked improvements in glycemic control and insulin sensitivity. Improvements can last from one to three years even if the weight is regained. In 75 percent of NIDDM-diagnosed obesity victims, a 15 to 30 percent weight loss reverses the elevated mortality risk of NIDDM.[45] Furthermore, exercise training improves glucose tolerance and helps increase insulin sensitivity. In some obese women, weight loss of 5 percent or more improves insulin sensitivity and ovarian function. For others suffering from amenorrhea (absent periods) or irregular menstrual cycles, normal menstruation may be restored after weight loss.[46]

Stomach seepage is a very serious surgical reality that causes injuries to other internal organs and tissue. The untimely passage of stomach contents in the small intestine may present with nausea, sweating, dizziness, and diarrhea right after eating, in addition to a loss of physical strength and the failure to digest sweet foods. Changes in food choice and nutritional supplements, in addition to the amounts and daily allowances may influence your digestive system and your standard of living.

A detailed discussion with a knowledgeable bariatric surgeon is an excellent way to decide which measures are best for each situation. Every obesity victim is unique, so discussing the best weight loss methods with your wishes and goals in mind is the first step to completely understanding the pros and cons of virtually any weight loss treatment you choose.

ANALYSIS

The most powerful approach to treating obesity from a realistic standpoint is making healthy lifestyle adjustments. This begins with eliminating all harmful ways of life, such as the use of tobacco and overconsumption of alcohol. These are two of the most detrimental things an obese person—or anyone for that matter—can do. Treating obesity is indeed a global challenge, but the benefits which treatment provides will improve the quality of life on both sides of the Atlantic from a physical, mental, and emotional standpoint.

Your true challenge is maintaining the new weight after a successful weight loss program, either naturally or through surgical intervention. The influence of weight loss on the risk of suffering from epidemics such as hypertension is always a positive one. Dieting commonly brings negative psychological effects including depression, nervousness, and irritability. In spite of all this, studies have shown that weight loss is associated with a decrease in depression levels, thus bringing a positive effect on self-esteem and body image as well.

5

OBESITY IN AMERICA

Obesity has been an ongoing issue that plagues many Americans. Two-thirds of American adults are overweight and about half are now considered to have full-blown obesity.[1] Advertised weight loss regimens, diet pills, and fitness programs are made available almost everywhere you look. This is an alarming signal that obesity in the United States has spiraled out of control, but nothing is really being done about it. In America the prevalence of obesity is undoubtedly high. Data from the National Health and Nutrition Examination Survey III (NHANES III) showed that around 20 percent of all men and 25 percent of all women in the United Statse are obese.[2] More recent data suggests a dramatic increase.[3] In 2010, thirty-two states in the United States had obesity prevalence equal to or greater than 25 percent. Six of these states are equal to or greater than 30 percent. With the minimal-activity lifestyle most Americans are adopting and exercise commixed with fast food culture, it's unsurprising that the United States is leading in the increasing trend of obesity. With the countless reminders and health advisories from different health departments and institutes, the number of obese Americans still continues to rise. People can only ask, "Why is this so?"

MASS PROMOTION AND TASTY FOODS

The human body has been made to physiologically adapt to both external and internal changes. It is full of dynamic processes that simultaneously work together to ensure that the body is in tip-top shape. What
you do to your health can either enhance or destroy your anatomy.

The vast majority of Americans have been exposed or will be exposed
to the advancement in technology that most industrialized countries
possess, but even worse, the impact of this achievement takes a toll on
the American society in terms of living a healthy lifestyle. Technological
gains have made it easy to remove physical exercise from conventional
American lifestyle. These gains have also promoted the mass production
of cheap, great-tasting food that is high in calories. Along with technology comes the advancement in advertising wherein the media has managed to influence what the American population sees with commercials
encouraging everyone to eat these sumptuously unhealthy foods. Imagine this same scenario as it was decades ago: If you have a sugar craving
or a cookie addiction, you have to mix the dough to be able to prepare
the ingredients to home-bake the cookies. These days, you can simply
head over to a convenience store to get a pack of cookies for less than
a dollar. If that's still too much effort on your part, you can just hit the
dial button on your phone to have it delivered right at your doorstep.
It's that easy.[4]

The wide selection of tasty yet very fattening foods such as baked
goods, sweets, and high-calorie drinks that people tend to crave—not to
mention that commercial "mocha" coffee drinks are smothered with so
many calories (equivalent to that of a full meal), that the average American consumes three to four servings of these high-calorie, sugar-rich
foods on a daily basis. People now eat 19 percent more carbohydrate
additives in our basic diet than they did in the early 1970s. This is based
on recent figures from the US Department of Agriculture.[5]

A HOLE IN YOUR WALLET

The impact of the growing population of obese and overweight individuals in the United States raises medical costs on a national level.

Economic costs related to obesity and overweight people are becoming increasingly synonymous with the growing rate of obesity. According to the *British Journal of Clinical Pharmacology*, direct medical costs in the United States are estimated to surpass $93 billion.[6]

Obese Americans are predisposed to numerous health risks such as diabetes, cardiovascular diseases, cancer, metabolic disorders, and other chronic health conditions. For this reason, excess medical expenditures for treatment of these associated health risks prove to be significant. At least 5 percent of medical spending from the US adult population is attributable to obesity.[7] Diseases included in the cost estimates from the first national study conducted on the economic outcomes of obesity in the United States were NIDDM (non-insulin diabetes mellitus), cardiovascular disease, hypertension, gallbladder disease, and colon and post-menopausal breast cancer.[8]

The World Health Organization reports that total obesity-related expenses were estimated to be around $39 billion, representing 5.5 percent of the overall cost of illness in 1986. In a revised estimate in 1990, it was estimated that the total medical cost of obesity was $68.8 billion in which $45.8 billion were direct costs of obesity associated health conditions.[9] It is noted that indirect costs of the disease relates to the loss in productivity due to the worker's absenteeism, staff turnover, and reduced worker productivity resulting from obesity-related sickness. Potential cost savings associated with the decrease in obesity prevalence shows that average savings in prescription costs per subject, over the course of a year, was approximately $440.[10]

The global economic costs of obesity will be discussed further in chapter 10, but as one can see, the situation is critical enough in the United States alone.

THE LAND OF MODERATION AND NORMAL BODY WEIGHT VERSUS OVERWEIGHTNESS

In the last twenty years, there has been an increase in obesity in the United States, as shown in information available from CDC (Centers for Disease Control and Prevention). It reveals that only one state, Colorado, had a prevalence rate for obesity of less than 20 percent. Thirty-two states have an obesity rate equal to or greater than 25 percent. Five of these states, South Carolina, Mississippi, Oklahoma, Alabama, and West Virginia, have equal to or greater than 30 percent obesity.[11]

It seems Colorado is the land of moderation and normal body weight, but in spite of widespread campaigning from health sectors, media, and the public regarding advantages of healthier diets and exercise, the overall prevalence of obesity and overweightness in America has doubled significantly over the past four decades.[12] It's an alarming find that Americans, having been the backbone of the most influential country in the world, have succumbed to fat. People have adopted the practice of consuming more than enough by "super sizing" meals and making unhealthy, yet affordable and delicious foods available everywhere, including grocery stores, malls, gas stations, and shopping centers. They don't even have to go anywhere to get foods rich in transfat, sugar, and calories. It can be made available by delivery at your doorstep by a single click on the Internet or by pushing a few buttons on your phone.

Things would have been great if it were second nature for most Americans to go through some exercise and increase physical activity. In retrospect, everyone knows this is not the case; *all* of us are guilty of the so-called sedentary lifestyle to a certain extent. Watching a late night movie while munching on a bag of chips topped with a can of beer is not an uncommon scenario in the lives of many Americans. Looking back at the time where people had to hunt for foods such as high-protein meat or gather high-grain crops, one can realize the full potential of healthy foods. Back then, foods were a lot richer with natural minerals than they are today, and people ate heartily and stored the fats as adipose tissue to be converted to energy during their next hunt.

People now have the convenience of acquiring and consuming abundant amounts of food to store as adipose tissue but a lower amount of activities on which to spend our energy. Food is available everywhere, and you are overwhelmed by the ads anywhere you turn, whether it's on television, print ads, billboards, or on the Web. There are fewer opportunities to increase physical activities. The country does not have enough parks for walking, sidewalks and bike paths, or accessible stairways.[13]

An American usually burns around 2,000 calories per day with normal activities.[14] In the meantime, approximately 2 pounds of fat in human body stores 9,000 calories of energy.[15] Therefore, a person has to take in

9,000 calories to put on 2 pounds of weight, he or she has to burn 9,000 calories to lose that same weight. It's very easy to put on weight—all you have to do eat. However, it is very difficult to take away 9,000 calories. From simple calculations, a study found that in 2007 that the average person in the United States consumed around 800 to 1,000 calories per fast food meal.[16] If you share a meal with someone at a restaurant in the United States, fast food or not, you will consume half the normal caloric intake. This will also go easier on your wallet.

FREEING A CHILD FROM OBESITY IN THE UNITED STATES

An estimated 22 million children under five years old are over-weight. Obesity in US preschool children two to five years old went from 5 to 10 percent between 1976 and 1980 and 2007 to 2008 and from 6.5 to almost 20 percent among six- to eleven-year-old children. Among adolescents twelve to nineteen years old, obesity increased from 5 to 18 percent during the same period.[17]

Obese and overweight children are most likely to become obese adults.[18] One study[19] has noted that 25 percent of obese adults had a BMI greater than or equal to 30 when they were children. It was also noted in the study that if overweightness begins at or before eight years of age, the likelihood of adult obesity is severe. Indicators for obesity in children between two and nineteen years old are slightly different from adult BMI. The children's BMI values are plotted on the CDC growth chart to determine the BMI for age percentile. Overweightness is characterized by BMI at or above the 85th percentile and lower than the 95th percentile. Obesity is attained when the value is above the 95th percentile. Childhood overweightness is determined based on age- and gender-specific BMI percentiles rather than by adult BMI categories, since a child's body composition varies more with age and gender.[20]

True Pressure

Environmental factors of childhood in the United States are unlike that of any other country, due to advancing technologies and growing eco-nomic and familial independence of kids these days. Caution is advised in promoting discipline in your child to avoid weight gain. The child may perceive this gesture as a restrictive thing and can develop eating disorders in the future if expressed incorrectly. You have to communicate clearly that the importance of maintaining a healthy body is not for aesthetic purposes only and that health benefits should be a priority. This will prevent additional pressure to the youngster to meet the weight standards which are implicated by the general public. Influences of media, particularly in the world of fashion, contribute to the pressure of keeping up a thin and lean body. Most American teenagers, especially girls, experience extreme peer pressure to blend into a society where "model thin" is "in." They don't realize that it isn't really the big picture for health by medical standards.

Overcoming the stress and pressure of peer acceptance in the adolescent years is difficult for any teenager. Obese adolescents can experience psychological pressure twice that of their slim counterparts. The pressure to get accepted and "fit in" is almost always present. An overweight and obese teenager may experience episodes of depression and isolation. In the United States, discrimination against obese individuals is prevalent especially in educational institutions and in the neighborhood. This places the child at a very high risk for decreased self-esteem and negative body image. Rejection from peers is a challenge for every obese student in school. A study conducted in the 1960s in a public school and summer camp asked six hundred subjects to view six different pictures of kids varying in appearance, physique, and disability.[21] They were then asked who they would like to have as a friend. The majority of the participants ranked an obese child last among those with disabilities and disfigurement. Bias and negative stereotyping against obese children are reported to happen as early as eight years of age. One study assessed descriptions of perceived stigmatization among adolescent girls.[22] The study showed that 99 percent of them had negative experiences like teasing, jokes, hurtful comments, and name-calling. Such discrimination continues at the secondary and tertiary level. That's why correcting and preventing obesity early in the childhood years can benefit a child's social development as he or she grows into adulthood. Prevention of overweightness and obesity must be initiated early in life and should include the continuous healthy eating and physical exercise patterns to avoid obesity in adults.

"GROWING UP" AS A GROWNUP: ADULT OBESITY IN AMERICA

For the US adult population, the prevalence of obesity is often incorrectly determined through the BMI, represented by the measured weight in kilograms divided by the square of the height in meters (kg/m^2). While this method does not provide accurate results to defining obesity as compared to fat distribution in the body, it's widely used for population screening because it only requires two easily available quantitative data values: height and weight. Other methods of measuring body fat and body fat distribution are measurements of skinfold thickness, waist circumference, waist-to-hip circumference ratio, and medical assessment tools such as computed tomography, ultrasound, and magnetic resonance imaging.

WHY US?

Reasons for America's growing problem with obesity lies in the lifestyle changes it has undergone since the early roots of our modernization. Serving portions are now twice as much as they were twenty years ago. Servings of fast food items like hamburgers, chips, and fries are available not only in large sizes, but in colossal servings. It seems difficult for an average person to eat one of these in one sitting, but he or she manages to "gobble up" these foods in a short period of time while watching television or working at a computer.

An innate desire to eat flavorful, rich-tasting, deep fried, and salt laden food is so enticing that willpower alone isn't enough. The influence is literally broadcast everywhere in the United States. Anyone within reach of a television, cell phone, or print magazine ad would be encouraged to grab a bite and eat. The love for sugar-filled foods fuels an unwinnable battle, and it seems only a few can resist eating moist cakes, creamy cheesecakes, delicious ice creams, pastries, and "divine" chocolates. With more people keeping up with the fast-paced environment almost everyone lives in, people view the act of eating as a form of stress relief. This wouldn't have been an unruly problem in the United States if everyone knew that moderation is the key to maintaining the right waistline.

Is the American Diet Enough?

In the United States there are numerous weight-loss programs and exercise regimens released every day to combat weight gain along with the highest prevalence of obesity among industrialized countries. The effort to cure rather than to prevent the growing epidemic is what's hindering us from obtaining a healthy optimum way of life. The saying "Prevention is better than cure" sometimes applies only to the problem at hand. It's one of those things that are better said than done. If people consistently watch what they eat and thoughtfully stay away from high-fat, high-caloric foods, everyone will be able to maintain a clean healthy body with organ systems functioning optimally.

Diet alone cannot guarantee protection from weight gain. Researchers believe that to maintain a given weight, energy from calories consumed should break even with calories burned.[23] Physical inactivity is a relative factor that contributes to weight gain especially if caloric intake is greater than what you burn. Physical inactivity, sometimes called sedentary lifestyle, is when body movement is minimal or absent and energy expenditure approximates the resting metabolic rate. Physical inactivity also involves passive activity like reading, working in front of a computer, talking with friends or on the phone, driving a car, or meditating. If your day-to-day activities involve mostly passive activities such as those mentioned and your caloric intake increases more than your energy expenditure in a prolonged period of time, the higher the risk you'll have for being overweight. Modest weight reductions, according to medical research, can decrease your blood pressure.[24] It can also lower your total cholesterol. For a disease like obesity, even these small changes can be important to the nation's health. The surging social media influence—whether in print or on television, encourages people to patronize nonnutritious foods depleted of vitamins and essential nutrients their body needs to supply the energy they expend with daily activities and work. Many overweight people are inclined to eat high-fat, high-calorie, and sugared foods simply because they taste delicious and they come in at cheap prices. Junk foods are found in virtually every grocery and retail store in the United States. If you eat junk foods while doing passive activities like watching TV, playing computer games, or surfing the Internet, the stored fat will begin to really show signs as you reach fifty years of age. Currently, one can feel the consequences from unhealthy eating and lack of exercise as early as forty years of age. This is a bit frightening since, technically speaking, you are still supposed to be at the prime of your life at this age.

US Obesity and Genes

Several factors contribute to weight gain, like genetic predisposition, race, gender, and cultural background in the United States. There are fifty genes involved in fat accumulation. A few of these genes influence how your body gathers fat and metabolizes energy. Other genes regulate how much you want to eat and how much it would take for you to feel full. They also regulate how likely you will utilize the stored calories by performing physical activities.[25] The FTO (fat-mass and obesity-associated) gene is known to be linked to the risk of increased BMI. This gene is known to be involved in the regulation of energy balance and the body's metabolism.[26]

People carrying two copies of an FTO variant have a 30 percent increased risk of getting obese compared to those without any copies. This explains how sometimes, when two people who eat the same exact foods and have similar physical activity levels, one has to try a lot harder than the other to lose weight.[27]

People Are What They Stem From

Cultural background plays a contributing role in understanding how the problem of obesity began in the United States. The food system today has dramatically changed as technology boosted US agriculture and food production. Most food categories are available during any season, making the supply of any particular food seem as if it never ends. Though this has improved food availability, the nutritional value is the real topic in question. Since the United States is one of the leading industrialized nations in the world, advancement in food processing technology has made food cheap and easily accessible to most people. Unfortunately, these cheap foods are usually mass produced, and nutritional value is little or lost.

In many communities in America, socioeconomic levels give rise to an increase in the prevalence of obesity, possibly because fresh and healthy food is expensive and hard to come by in low socioeconomic communities, while unemployment allows, but may not necessarily lead to, physical inactivity. A report suggests that a single dollar can buy 1,200 calories of cookies or potato chips, but only 250 calories of carrots.[28]

NEIGHBORING ON AMERICAN OBESITY

The above explains why most people belonging to the lower socio-economic bracket are more prone to obesity. It's much cheaper to buy processed foods than fresh foods like fruits and vegetables. These processed foods are compact and contain less water but have more fat, sugar, and salt (preservatives), which makes them delicious, filling, and all the more fattening.

A disease such as obesity doesn't have to stem from eating too much, but rather, from swelling consumption of the wrong foods coupled with poverty. In underprivileged neighborhoods in the United States, a person's neighborhood and community can affect an individual's lifestyle. In poor neighborhoods where houses are cramped and a place to do physical activities such as walking, biking, and jogging is scarce, individuals will normally disregard exercise as part of their daily routine.

Employment loss and the shift of women taking on jobs to sustain families in the lower economic bracket of the US population have changed family dining habits. The mother will normally prepare a meal for the family but due to the lack of "home time" caused by work, the family resorts to eating instant, fast food items, or processed prepared meals that are high in sodium and fat, rather than a well-cooked, balanced meal.

Cultural background and practices, ethnicity, and other lineages are factors that influence the American's dietary patterns and contribute to the increase in the number of individuals suffering from obesity. Religious beliefs can also determine which dietary intake one will need to adapt. As in the case of Islam, religious followers are banned from consuming pork. Thus, their diet has been modified.

UNDIVIDED, YET DIVERSE

Obesity is affected by globalization, the process which integrates regional economies and culture with an international network of communication and trade. However, the trade industry is affected by the distribution of nonnutritious foods by food processing companies and retailers across relatively underdeveloped countries. Acculturation happens when traditional beliefs are changed due to the merging of different groups in a society. This is typical in the United States as many migrants from all over the world are arriving. Differences in dietary practices are still widespread, as evidenced by the personal preference ratings of many international minority groups in the United States. Branding has a great impact on the country's obesity, especially in the vast distribution of affordable American processed foods. This includes anything ranging from chips, chocolates, sweeteners, sodas, and other energy-dense items. Since it is cheaper and convenient, mass-produced foods that are highly caloric and sugar rich sell rapidly. From a nontraditional standpoint, mass-produced foods affect obesity by encouraging the abandonment of cultural characteristics which minimize the risk of obesity. It also promotes the adoption of new beliefs and behaviors that make you more prone to obesity as well as many other health problems.

Other Epidemics in the United States

The increasing risks associated with varying lifestyles among cultures are what everyone really should be concerned about in America. The life threatening, chronic health risks associated with obesity constitutes four areas: (1) cardiovascular problems, including hypertension, stroke, and chronic heart disease; (2) conditions associated with insulin resistance, for example, non–insulin dependent diabetes mellitus (NIDDM); (3) certain types of cancer; and (4) gallbladder disease.[29]

Obesity is predisposing Americans to a number of cardiovascular risk factors, including hypertension, raised cholesterol, and impaired glucose tolerance. This is particularly true for most Americans diagnosed with cardiovascular diseases and BMI greater than 30. Based on the Framingham Heart Study, one can conclude that the degree of overweightness is related to the rate of development of cardiovascular disease (CVD).[30] This is very alarming, since a recent report writes that heart disease is the predominate cause of death in the United States and globally.[31]

The risk is higher in younger Americans and those with abdominal obesity. Spiking blood pressure is a common incidence in obese people and is regularly associated with decreased activity and increased intake of fatty foods that are chiefly responsible for weight gain. The direct link between obesity and elevated blood pressure can be attributed to high circulating levels of insulin. This is due to renal retention of sodium, which results in hypertension.[32] Increasing intra-abdominal fat correlates with triglycerides and cholesterol levels in the blood and subsequently lowers the high-density lipoprotein in the body. This could thicken your blood and predispose you to blood clots. Your arteries can clog, causing impeded blood supply to vital organs, such as the heart and brain, which regulate all bodily functions. Once blood supply is incidentally redirected from these vital organs, irreversible damage may take place and symptoms of neurological imbalance will result. Droopy eyelids, paralysis, slurred speech, decrease tactile sensitivity, and a loss of consciousness can occur.

Getting fat is not only aesthetically unpleasant for many onlookers, but it's also a danger to an American's physical capabilities and normal functioning. Restrictions in our ability to perform well in work and outside of work may be brought by the increased weight. Problems such as gout and osteoarthritis may bring discomfort and prevent us to do the things people need to accomplish. Stress is said to affect obese Americans more than those who are physically fit, and the stress coming from the stigma and prejudice of being fat doesn't make things any better. Emotionally, stress affects our self-esteem since social stigmatization on obesity still occurs in the workplace, subways, shopping centers, and parking lots.

Seceral US studies have found a correlation between obesity and cancer, particularly endocrine and gastrointestinal cancers. This increased incidence in the obese population is greater in those with truncal obesity and is said to be caused by certain hormonal changes.[33]

The risk of acquiring diabetes concurrently with obesity is high in the United States. Diabetes can be life-threatening as it affects various organ systems in the body. There was a study where women between thirty and fifty-five years of age were observed for fourteen years for the risk of developing NIDDM.[34] Obese participants in this study were over four times more likely to get NIDDM than those who were slim. Type 2 diabetes, which is another name for NIDDM, is a progressive disease if not controlled by insulin, diet, and exercise. It will lead to multiple organ failure if it isn't managed effectively. Insulin resistance is often associated with obesity especially in intra-abdominal fat accumulation. Obese individuals are likely to develop insulin resistance as accumulated body fat disrupts the body's normal response to insulin. A lot of people suffering from diabetes have not shown symptoms of the disease and are unaware of the existing condition. As diabetes progresses, it will affect the blood vessels, heart, kidneys, and nervous system. Treatment with proper diet and drug regimen, either by oral glucose treatment or insulin, is needed.

Obese individuals in America are also predisposed to metabolic disturbances such as dyslipidemia, when triglycerides are increased, HDL or "good cholesterol" is reduced, and LDL or the "bad cholesterol" levels are elevated. This is mostly seen in obese individuals with intra-abdominal fat accumulation.[35]

Gallbladder disease is correlated with obesity in the development of gallstones in all age groups and gender. Gallstones occur three to four times more often in the obese as compared to lean individuals. There is greater risk for obese individuals with intra-abdominal fat accumulation. The supersaturation of bile can be induced by cholesterol, so reducing the motility of the gallbladder is considered to be the underlying factors in gallstone formation. Complications in obese individuals, including acute and chronic cholecystitis (gallbladder inflammation), acute pancreatitis, and biliary colic, are likely to develop.[36]

Other medical conditions that impede optimum quality of life in the United States are the debilitating health problems associated with obesity: osteoarthritis, gout, difficulty breathing, and sleep apnea. Osteoarthritis can be uncomfortable and usually affects the joints in the lower extremities due to the excessive strain and the mechanical stress the joints take from the excess fat accumulation concentrated on your abdomen. Increased risk of gout in obese individuals is brought on by hyperuricemia (too much uric acid) particularly in women and may also involve central fat distribution.[37] Pulmonary stress is also evident in obese people who have symptoms of breathing difficulties and episodes of sleep apnea characterized by narrowing of air pathways related to accumulation of fat in the pulmonary area. A study involving 200 woman and 50 men noted sleep apnea in 3 percent and 40 percent in the participants, respectively. In the same study, 77 percent of those with a BMI higher than 40 experienced episodes of sleep apnea. Research suggests that sleep apnea is possibly attributed to central obesity as well as neck size.[38] Although this research was done in China, similar results may exist for obese people in the United States.

Facing the Other Epidemics

Getting yourself to start eating healthy and planning nutritious foods to serve on the table is never an easy task. Since many people really don't have the time to seek out meals with high nutritional value, they are tempted to order and eat out at any one of America's growing fast food chains or to buy processed frozen foods. Facing away from the potential risks that people impose on their bodies, the population has formed this habit of eating "instant" food that's very appealing to taste buds. All of this of course applies to foods containing high sugar, high fats, and high sodium, enough to fill our senses with a natural euphoric sensation. Health risks don't show until one day you realize how large you have become and are feeling a bit tired and fatigued at the end of a normal workday. Activities become limited and before you know it, you're visiting your medical doctor more often for symptoms of stress, cardiovascular diseases, and fatigue. This holds true for most Americans, as reflected by year-long medical expenditures.

OBESITY PREVENTION IN THE UNITED STATES

The American health care industry focuses more on curative strategy than prevention when dealing with health problems. Addressing obesity which is evoked by overeating and other sociocultural differences among Americans is a goal that is far from completion. There are numerous factors responsible for the prevalence of obesity in the United States. Some of these factors include, but are not limited to, physiological and regulatory mechanisms of the body and genetic and biological factors, such as race, gender, and hormonal activity. Modifiable factors that an obese individual can control are diet and physical activity.

Interventions should be carefully planned out and should aim at prevention rather than cure to avoid the incidence of obesity. Principles of prevention and effective management of weight should be simplified for easier understanding and compliance will be ensured. Primary prevention is essentially up to you, the patient, because you are the major driving force in preventing the modifiable risk factors for obesity. Primary prevention strategies should focus on (a) normal-weight individuals on the verge of becoming overweight, (b) people who are already overweight, and (c) previously obese individuals who have successfully shed pounds through an effective weight loss program. In the latter, the goal is to maintain normal weight levels for as long as possible.

Primary Prevention in the United States

Concentrate more on prevention than *curing* obesity, because obesity doesn't happen overnight and the longer the time for fat buildup, the less likely it is for a "miracle" treatment to succeed.[39] Obesity over a long period gives you complications that may not be easily reversed by weight loss. For instance, the problems with diabetes and coronary heart diseases cannot be reversed automatically if you begin to lose weight or if weight loss is greatly achieved.[40] Though prevention may not effectively work for countries that already have too much prevalence of obesity and overweight population, it will still be useful for the population that has just started to adapt a change in lifestyle, like rural areas, for example, and prevention strategies will be helpful for obese and overweight children in preventing continuing obesity as they approach maturity.

Secondary Prevention

Secondary prevention strategies are more about screening for obesity so your doctor can identify your situation before things get really bad. In the United States, obesity prevention objectives can be specified in a health care setting because primary prevention is normally aimed at decreasing the number of new cases. Primary prevention essentially keeps normal-weight individuals in check against obesity. This approach seeks to lower the known cases of obesity by targeting any possible sources.

Tertiary Prevention

This form of obesity prevention attempts to stabilize or reduce the amount of disability and complications resulting from the disease.[41] Preventing obesity and managing the known cases of the disease begins by having a broad knowledge of the disease itself. Like any national disaster, Americans cannot address a problem without fully acknowledging that such a problem exists. Information dissemination is essential to promote awareness of the problem that faces the United States today. It commences with widespread information awareness campaigns that will propose targeted goals and outcomes of prevention and management.

Training health care individuals to help obese individuals get treated is significant for more reasons other than to simply increase the level of knowledge and skills in obesity management. It is crucial for getting rid of negative attitudes against the obese and the disease itself. With this in perspective, social stigmatization must be stopped so people can take one step further toward fully understanding the disease.[42]

NOT JUST A PIECE OF CAKE

Any obesity prevention program should promote a healthy diet that has very low fat, has an adequate amount of calories, and is rich in vitamins and minerals. The importance of a complete and balanced diet should be stressed to avoid unnecessary fat accumulation that can lead to irreversible damage to the body. Shared responsibilities between the US government, educational sectors, media, and local groups concerning the crisis on obesity should be utilized:

- The US government can facilitate provisions in food production and mandate nutrition and fortification of foods with essential vitamins and minerals. The government can also propose programs that will enable workplaces to be conducive to exercise.
- Places for physical activity should be provided in the community not only for the high socioeconomic bracket, but to economically disadvantaged communities as well.
- Regular walks in the park are highly enjoyable and offer sunlight and fresh air, which gym workouts cannot offer; they are also free.

This is where the government's efforts to provide a place where people can do these nonstrenuous everyday activities pose a challenge. Making streets safe for walking so people don't use cars so much helps to promote physical activity while conserving environmental resources such as fuel.

- Encouraging exercise as a fun and enjoyable activity rather than as a vigorous and strenuous one will increase compliance to the goal of promoting and maintaining regular energy expenditure and will avoid sedentary lifestyle.
- Countrywide programs such as marathons, walkathons, and other mass activities not only engage the community in social awareness, but will also instill values of responsibility in taking charge of one's health.
- The media can do more through regulation of food advertisements and releasing educated advocacies focusing on keeping a healthy lifestyle.
- Educational institutions in the United States can help out with information dissemination and implement balance between proper diet and physical activity in schools to prevent childhood obesity.
- The provision of convenient exercise facilities like parks and bike lanes are very helpful when it comes to health promotion. Increasing physical activity to advocate the positive use of physical energy. The emphasis should be placed on long-term, low-impact physical activity rather than vigorous exercise.

The ultimate goal in obesity treatment and management is weight loss. This is a concept that much of the American population must accept in order to defeat obesity within US borders. Various weight loss programs are being advertised in print and media. Most of them use different approaches to dieting such as low-protein and low-fat diets. Exercises like yoga, cardio workouts, and pilates also help. Chapter 11 describes in much more detail how exercise techniques are centralized into a single objective: ditching the extra pounds. Once an obese individual loses a significant amount of weight, these weight loss programs often stop there. There are only a few programs that teach you how to keep your weight suppressed after losing a huge chunk of it.

Follow-Ups, Exams, and Shared Responsibility

Obesity prevention and management in the United States focuses on how to keep a previously obese individual from regaining the weight that he or she lost. Prevention generally requires dieting techniques and physical activity. The majority of the work will come from the individual's self-discipline and willpower. A body weight kept constant over ten years represents a successful outcome. It's an important achievement for anyone belonging to an obese family that is particularly susceptible to worst-case scenarios. People should realize that moderate and sustained weight loss of 5 to 15 percent of initial weight is medically more ideal than abrupt and rapid weight loss stemming from "crash diets." Such a percentage of weight loss is very beneficial, especially if it lasts.

A comprehensive health assessment is a great starting point in obesity treatment that can prove useful in many ways. In the United States, a comprehensive health assessment can take place once (annual exam) or twice a year (biannual exam). These exams serve as benchmarks for identifying potential health risks associated with your current state of obesity. The exams determine if you are predisposed to acquiring illnesses such as diabetes, coronary heart disease (CHD), and other medical conditions as indicated by family history, diet, lifestyle, laboratory tests, and other personal history information. Factors such as dietary patterns, physical activity, anthropometric measurements, and genetic predisposition play important roles in determining your overall health as an American.

Make it a shared responsibility between yourself and your medical provider. Health professionals in the United States usually advise on dietary changes somewhere along the course of treatment. They also talk about exercise, appropriate medical interventions, and social support. Social stigmatization should be eradicated in the health care profession here since doctors are on the frontline in helping obese people feel good physically and emotionally. Though you would like to manage obesity alone if possible, you can't embark on the journey alone. It takes support from the community, guidance of health care providers, and help from government, media, and the right food to address your obesity issues effectively.

Proper identification of the risks that predispose an individual in the United States to obesity is very important for lowering the probability of acquiring such a disease. If awareness is there, intervention and other preventive measures to address the problem will facilitate better health. It's all about gathering available data and planning future strategies that will tackle the underlying causes of this national epidemic.

HOLD YOUR HEAD UP HIGH

In the land of seemingly unlimited opportunity, it's never too late for a change. It begins with awareness, and from there, a lot of hard work and perseverance is needed to succeed in changing how Americans eat. Food choices need to improve and people need to exercise almost daily. Support from the government, media, and community is essential to prove that our projects and advocacies for treatment of obesity are successful. The support from the family in increasing awareness about the disease is mandatory, especially because there is a genetic predisposition to the existing condition.

Lastly, approaching our obesity problem domestically may seem very complex in a mechanized country like the United States. With assistance from international clutches such as the World Health Organization and other obesity support groups, it will be much easier to take down the beast. To address the problem at the national level and to be able to present it in a structured manner, one should also take into account the risk factors that are unearthed by both individual and social assessments of obesity in the United States.

6

WORLDWIDE OBESITY

The problem of obesity affects many individuals across many nations. The increasing prevalence of obesity poses greater health risks than any other health condition. It is a problem of both developed and underdeveloped countries worldwide.

An article in *The Malaysian Journal of Nutrition* points out that obesity is now well into epidemic stages, with an excess of 1 billion adults weighing above normal.[1] More than 300 million of these cases fall into the clinically obese category. This adds to the worldwide issue of long-term obesity. Obesity affects psychological and social breadths of life around the world, traversing among people of almost any age and socioeconomic level.

OBESITY IS NOT THE SAME EVERYWHERE

The extent of this worldwide problem is reflected mostly in children who have become clinically obese. As kids grow older, external influences like peer pressure, media, and environment add up and compel them to get on an unhealthy eating schedule. Foods loaded with sugars and saturated fats and low in fiber greatly contribute to fat deposits in the body, which obstructs the bloodstream. This leads to diseases like hypertension, diabetes, and stroke.

The criterion for obesity and overweightness is not exactly the same everywhere. Globally, overweightness is characterized by a body mass index (BMI) of greater than or equal to 25.[2] BMI isn't a direct measure of fat, but it is an alternative for measuring body fatness.[3] BMI cannot serve as a diagnostic procedure to screen for weight problems for adults everywhere in the world since basic diets vary immensely between countries. To clarify: If a doctor were to make a hypertension (high blood pressure) diagnosis, he or she would have to admit that the idea of "normal blood pressure" remains the same no matter the person or geographic location. If everyone diagnosed all obesity cases in the world equally, then the entire population on the planet would have to perceive "food" the same way, but they don't. Simply put, a health care provider will need to do additional assessments to determine whether someone is at a high risk for weight-related problems in any given country.

The lack of advanced technologies in developing countries could be responsible for the increasing numbers for worldwide obesity. Test and assessments requiring such technologies include diet evaluation, physical activity, extensive family and genetic history, and skinfold measurements, along with other appropriate screening tests. BMI is a helpful tool for worldwide obesity assessments since height and weight data is easily available from participants.

Technologically proficient countries often suffer from medical problems as a consequence of their advancement in technology, despite the long-term modification of health practices in response to the changing environment.[4] Physical activity is neglected and replaced by sedentary activities that occupy your daily activities. A simple climb up the stairs is chosen far less often than a ride in an elevator. Working hours are spent mostly in front of computers confined to a chair. Employees are too tired to work out when they get home. Most are too busy to include exercise in their weekly schedules.

ARE PEOPLE SIMILAR, YET DIFFERENT?

Obese individuals differ not only in the amount of fat they have, but also the regional distribution of fat within the body. The distribution of fat affects the risks to disease linked to obesity or over-weightness. It's helpful to distinguish "abdominal fat distribution," or what is commonly termed android obesity, from the less serious type called gynoid fat distribution. The difference between the two rests primarily on the location of fat in the body. In android obesity, the majority of the fat deposits lies on the trunk of an individual, around his waistline or body. The gynoid type is where fat is mostly distributed throughout the body, including the limbs, face, and extremities. Because food menus differ among world cultures, the rate and other specifics of these two subtypes of obesity also vary depending on where you live.

Paraphrasing what you will be reading in chapter 7, childhood obesity serves as a significant warning sign to the world. Seven percent of boys and 5.5 percent of girls are categorized as morbidly obese. These statistics are cited from a report based on research supported by Kaiser Permanente in California,[5] but childhood obesity results from poor eating habits and lack or inadequate physical activities—irrespective of location. Kids are greatly influenced by what they see on television and in food advertisements that promote fried chicken, sweets, pizza, and other processed foods normally categorized as junk foods.

The Molecular Tides of Globalization

In developed nations, children at school eat hamburgers, nachos, corn-dogs, and other nutritionally deficient foods along with a can of soda. They don't realize that these foods contain deep-fried fats, commonly known as trans fat or unsaturated fat. Trans fat is basically a synthetically produced unnatural fat. Hydrogen is added to liquefied vegetable fat to solidify it and turn it into trans fat. Companies in modernized countries that manufacture foods rich in trans fat choose to utilize the latter be-cause of its affordability.

Trans fat also lasts a long time in the cupboard. That and other forms of unsaturated fat threaten your health by raising your LDL, or low-density lipoprotein. Increased LDL levels will lead to developing heart disease and stroke. Trans fat also lowers your HDL. HDL serves as the lead-in for "good cholesterol" in your body.

How Childhood Obesity Became a Global Issue

In reality, the global shift in children's diet presently consists of increased intake of high-caloric, high-fat, and high-sugar items, but lacks nutrients such as essential minerals and vitamins. Things get worse with less physical activity evidenced by the sedentary lifestyle of watching television all day long, playing video games, and surfing the Internet, using little or no physical activity at all. Parents should consider careful planning and preparation of meals containing a balanced serving of essential vitamins, minerals, and nutrients that can help a child meet his or her ideal energy levels. The food pyramid can serve as a quick reference guide in identifying categories of foods rich with vitamins and minerals that are ideally served to children. Serving proportions are also specified in the food pyramid to determine how much of a particular food group is necessary to supply energy demands for everyday activities.

EXPOSING THE WORLD OF OBESITY

European obesity experiments prove that there is a wide prevalence of obesity and overweightness among children and boys have a higher prevalence than girls in most countries at all ages, except for a few exceptions. In Denmark, France, Ireland, Netherlands, and the United Kingdom, girls aged eleven to thirteen are more overweight and obese than boys in the same age range. The data trends conducted on the research reveals that despite the ongoing national and international effort, satisfactory results haven't been evident. Current data reveals the need for greater commitment for putting into practice the recommendations and tools given by the World Health Organization (WHO) to countries. These commitments call for lifestyle changes, nutrition, and physical activity.[6]

Obesity can be regarded as a form of malnutrition, which is—and always has been—a major issue around the world. Malnutrition results from improper diet, so technically speaking, overweightness and obesity both fall into this category. Malnutrition is commonly viewed as a lack of adequate nutrients in the body which brings diseases such as marasmus, anemia, scurvy, beriberi, and protein energy malnutrition. It's uncommon to regard someone who is overweight or obese as malnourished, but keep in mind that malnutrition is the inadequate intake of nutrients in the body. Although people who suffer from obesity tend to eat a lot, it doesn't necessarily mean that they consume the nutrients specifically needed to treat their disease. It's as if you are consuming too much of the wrong food. Large portions and sizes of unhealthy foods are easily available to the public through grocers and fast food chains.

The alarming prevalence of obesity is causing concern where, in several countries, the numbers are spiking in the adult population, and, possibly worse, are increasing among children. This could lead to an increase in epidemic comorbidities such as Type 2 diabetes mellitus and could eventually result in increased health and economic costs. For the above reasons, WHO has treated obesity as a major problem of the twentieth century and, along with various research institutions and scientific groups, is leading an international call to action against overweightness and obesity. The number of clinically obese people is increasing at a very rapid rate around the world, making the disease the fastest growing public health matter of the century.

The French Connection

For years, France has been testing billboards that use location-sensitive technology to automatically "contact" you with additional product information. Various advertisements, print media, and publications influence you to eat more unhealthy foods, which will only make you less healthy. These foods possibly lack essential nutrients, fatty acids, and protein necessary to support your day-to-day activities.

Obese people often have a diet high in unsaturated fat, sugar, and calorie content. This, coupled with a sedentary lifestyle or physical inactivity, paves the road for excessive body fat that you actually don't need, excessive fat that you accumulate so quickly that it makes it difficult for your organ systems to function well. The resultant stress takes its toll on your body in the next five to ten years if you don't have a healthy lifestyle.

Africa and the Middle East

In Africa, where people focus primarily on *under*nutrition as opposed to the problem of obesity, the data available to study obesity on a continental scale is scarce. However, WHO was still able to measure obesity to a certain extent. A recent Mauritius experiment suggested the same trend as that observed in the additional WHO regions—a large increase in obesity over the course of five years in males and females between twenty-five and seventy-five years old. The proportion of obese males spiked from around 3 percent in the late 1980s to about 5 percent in the early 1990s. However, the number of obese women went from approximately 10 percent to around 15 percent within the same time frame.[7]

The United Arab Emirates (UAE) recognizes obesity as a major public health problem. This is evidenced by a research finding that 38 percent of married women and almost 16 percent of married men there are obese. In Bahrain and Iran, there are a lot more obese women than men.[8]

China

In the 1970s, many of the Chinese celebrated obesity and overweightness because they related it to good fortune and strong health. Chubby-cheeked babies were also smiled upon, their parents congratulated for their good luck. Obesity victims of all ages were the center of most of the country's artwork and religious icons at the time.

During these years, thin members of the population were often psychologically neglected and considered a bad match for marriage due to the false assumption that they won't be able to withstand childbirth or care for their family. Most of these "sick people" would subject themselves to strict, very filling diets. Upon failure, they would go to the local elders in search of a cure or exorcism from their supposed unnatural illness.

Europe and the Southeast

In most areas of Europe, the obesity rate has jumped by around 10 to 40 percent in the past ten years.[9] Obesity is somewhat typical in Europe, especially in eastern and southern European nations. In Southeast Asia, malnutrition is a huge concern, and due to a limited amount of available data, trends in measuring obesity have been difficult. Continuous monitoring and evaluation are needed to watch out for the possible increase in obesity as the region undergoes rapid change in dietary habits and nutrition education.

Pacific Regions

The prevalence of obesity in the general population of Australia and New Zealand ranges from 10 to 15 percent.[10] Of Malaysian adults between eighteen and sixty years old, around 5 percent of men and approximately 8 percent of women were found to have a BMI above 30. Among the Malay population, a higher proportion of men and women had a BMI over 30. Obesity prevalence rates for both men and women are 11 percent and 15 percent in urban and rural areas, respectively.[11]

Rates for overweightness and obesity in adults combined are over 50 percent in at least ten pacific countries that are already economically developed. The increasing obesity epidemic is characterized by urbanization and consumption of high-calorie, high-fat foods that require little or no physical activity to acquire, such as foods in grocery stores and fast food chains, which don't require any outdoor hunting.[12]

A study at the University of Sydney Children's Hospital suggested that there were no substantial links between the prevalence of obesity and age, socioeconomic status, or gender when pertaining to obese children.[13] However, the researchers found that the obesity prevalence in boys was almost 5 percent higher in urban areas. There was no difference in obesity rates between rural and urban girls from a locational standpoint. Students who were studying in Australia were found to have higher obesity rates if they came from the Middle East or Europe.

Influence from other areas, especially Western nations, have greatly affected the way of life in the Pacific. Traditional cooking using earth ovens are replaced by cooking with fats and oil, frying, and roasting. With economic development comes commercialized food, which is often more convenient and cheaper than fresh local produce. Stores overseas don't really vouch for a lifestyle that could potentially help obesity victims to exercise and have moderate consumption of nutritious foods.

A Global Spread Indeed

The international viewpoint of obesity tells you that the disease doesn't only affect economically advanced nations such as the United States. Obesity is also evident in developing countries in Southeast Asia, particularly Malaysia, as well as in Australia. While the disease is relatively uncommon in Africa and Asia, it's more prevalent in urban than rural populations. When speaking of economically advanced areas, the rates match those of developed and highly industrialized countries.[14] Obesity doesn't affect industrialized countries only because of the technology and advancement they have that contributes to their lifestyle change.

Much like improved communication however, technology reduces the effort required for you to move from one place to the other. As a result, the amount of activity and exercise one can get simply diminishes. People now use modern telecommunications to avoid the extra trip or walk to the store. People can just dial a number to have something done or commodities delivered at the doorstep. The convenience of eating at a fast food restaurant as opposed to preparing a healthy and balanced cooked meal at home is very tempting. This is especially true in a fast-paced world where time is of great value and things that are instantly attainable are preferred.

Not only is obesity a disease on its own but it is also one of the key factors for noncommunicable illnesses such as heart disease and diabetes together with smoking, high blood pressure, and hypercholesterolemia.[15] The adverse effects of obesity are influenced by body weight, location of body fat, and sedentary lifestyle. It is also important to take note of the ethnic differences when studying the prevalence of obesity among nations.

Some populations in the United States are at a greater risk of developing obesity-related diseases compared with those in Asian countries. Cultural practices and customs also make a significant impact in the prevalence of obesity. A few countries agree that excessive weight signifies royalty and status in society. Others have healthy eating policies to cleanse the body and soul or to satisfy religious beliefs. Either way, it can contribute to a lesser prevalence of obesity among their population.

No matter where in the world you reside, you get obese when there is excess fat in the food you choose to eat and when total energy intake is more than total energy expenditure. In other words, there is less activity and excessive food intake comprising a sedentary lifestyle mostly associated with "couch potato syndrome." This syndrome typically involves watching television while munching on chips, excessive hours on the computer, and other physically insufficient activity. Research suggests a hormonal dysfunction that causes couch potato syndrome in as many as 10 percent of obesity victims, specifically focusing on individuals suffering from familial morbid obesity.[16] Much like obesity, couch potato syndrome is a global issue.

WORLDWIDE OBESITY AND THE OTHER EPIDEMICS

Complications arising from obesity have been studied for many years as its prevalence continues to increase in children and adults worldwide. Most of the health risks that are associated with obesity have a high impact on the quality of life and life expectancy. Obesity during childhood and adolescence has been linked to a few common health risks such as Type 2 diabetes, hypercholesterolemia, reduced levels of HDL, and hypertension. Worldwide, these diseases are common to the elderly and only predispose adults in their twenties and thirties when diagnosed with obesity in early childhood and teenage years. The rising rate of childhood and adolescent obesity creates a higher risk for adult obesity, thereby leading to other problems such as cardiovascular diseases and diabetes.

Diabetes

Obesity is regarded as the key risk factor for Type 2 diabetes, which is a significant issue since it has been officially diagnosed in more than 100 million people worldwide. In Type 2 diabetes, the body doesn't produce enough insulin or fails to respond to insulin. This is termed insulin resistance. Insulin is necessary for the body to take in glucose into the cell and convert it to energy. When you eat, your body breaks down specific nutrients into glucose, the basic fuel needed by cells to produce energy. Insulin binds to glucose to facilitate passage inside the cell. If there's no insulin available or if enough of it isn't produced, buildup of glucose in the blood develops. This causes hyperglycemia, an unusually high level of sugar accumulating in the bloodstream.

No matter where in the world they live, obese people are likely to suffer from insulin resistance[17] (Type 2 diabetes) because fat impedes the body's ability to utilize insulin. Many who suffer from diabetes don't even know they have it. Diabetes develops gradually and symptoms may not appear until it is already too late. When the glucose accumulates in the blood, it can damage the heart, kidneys, eyes, and nerves. These complications pose the risks involved in the disease and produces symptoms such as blurred vision, weakness, increased appetite, increased thirst, and infections that are slow to heal. If not treated with proper diet, exercise, and insulin supplements, the body may give up and severe complications may set in.

Heart Disease

Remember that obesity-related heart disease is increasing everywhere in the world and not just in the United States. People with excess body fat, especially in the waist area (called truncal obesity), are more predisposed to heart disease and stroke even when other risk factors are present.[18] Excessive body fat increases blood cholesterol and triglyceride levels. It also lessens the good cholesterol called HDL. This process clogs your bloodstream, narrowing the blood vessels through which oxygenated blood passes to get to vital organs. Without oxygenated blood, your cells would die. In stroke victims, the blood supply doesn't reach the brain sufficiently enough to supply the needed oxygen. Parts of the brain soon shut down, resulting in neurological symptoms. In some instances, paralysis sets in. It is known that hypertension and obesity are directly related to each other. Both systolic and diastolic blood pressure increases with body mass index.[19] Obesity victims are more predisposed to hypertension than are lean individuals.

An international news agency reported that obesity has surpassed smoking as the most common cause of premature heart attacks in adults worldwide.[20] The report cites a study that found that overweight people or those with a BMI between 25 and 30 had a heart attack much earlier than individuals with a normal BMI of 18.6 and 25.[21] Obese individuals with a BMI above 30 had an initial heart attack around seven years earlier than normal-weight people and more than ten years earlier for severely obese subjects with a BMI greater than 40. The implications of these findings are disturbing. Life expectancy is shortened due to the prevalence of obesity among adults. The quality of life is compromised as these health risks pose an alarming wake-up call to individuals who are presently or almost obese.

Depression

In a recent study, medical investigators found that severely obese participants, especially obese women with poor self-esteem, are at high risk for depression.[22] These women demonstrated sustained mental improvement from weight loss, but some findings support the hypothesis that severe obesity often causes depression. Symptoms of depression correlate with a certain dissatisfaction of body image. An obese person feels stigmatized, discriminated, and undergoes other psychological disturbances that affect the well-being of a sane person.[23] These psychological disturbances may aggravate a preexisting depressive illness. Failed attempts to lose weight add to a depressive state which an obese individual could be in, along with feelings of shame, hopelessness, and guilt from failure to reach personal weight loss goals. Obesity is associated with a high prevalence of binge eating disorder,[24] a disorder where you eat a large amount of food at one time even when not hungry. The person then feels embarrassed and ashamed of doing so afterwards. This action may lead to a condition called bulimia nervosa, exemplified by binging on food and later purging it from the digestive system. These individuals are often depressed and feel a huge amount of guilt after they eat or binge on food. Binging is not a regional but a worldwide problem among obesity sufferers, though not every person suffering from bulimia is also obese.

In an attempt to lose the weight gained from binging, sometimes obesity victims will engage in rigorous exercise only to arrive in a situation of compulsive eating later.[25] Some reports have showed that there is marked improvement in mental state after losing weight from bariatric surgery. This also happens after nonsurgical weight loss treatments. However, not all studies show positive outcomes, as it was reported that mental status gets better after a gastric bypass surgery in six to twelve months following surgery but returns to its pre-operative level about two years after, with some cases of suicide.[26]

THE COST OF OBESITY IS A GLOBAL DILEMMA

Although you'll read about the *full* economic effects of obesity in chapter 10, it is important to understand now that the problem of obesity doesn't stop at the personal level. The issue extends to the increased costs of health care you incur when suffering with the disease. Medical costs related to obesity and overweightness, including both direct and indirect expenses from clinical complications rose from around 9 percent of total US medical expenditures in 1998 to as high as $78.5 billion in 2002.[27] Most of these costs were paid by health maintenance organizations or health care insurance companies. Since obese people are at a high risk for chronic medical conditions like diabetes and heart attack, they eventually pay more for medical care compared to the nonobese individuals. In other words, obesity relates directly with high mortality and health insurance costs.

Worldwide, long-term obesity victims have chronic complications of diabetes and other heart-related illnesses that originate from a sedentary lifestyle and prolonged unhealthy diets. Companies currently focus on improving copayments and talk about health care savings when what they should really be concentrating on is how to prevent the population from adapting a lifestyle that predisposes people to overweightness and obesity. Food companies (discussed in chapter 9) may not tell you this, but the greatest expenditures of health benefits come from diseases and illnesses brought on by unhealthy lifestyles. Thus it would be better if they could focus on prevention and addressing the root cause of the underlying problem of common medical expenditures today.

IS THE WORLD FREE OF BIAS?

In dealing with obesity, an individual could experience psycho-emotional problems along the way. Social isolation and discrimination induced simply by disproportionate body fat is common and usually begins early on in an obesity sufferer. While social stigma against obesity varies among countries, it's still placed on the obese and overweight individuals in mainly three facets of life: health care, employment, and education. It starts with "fat" jokes in almost any public area, like schools, supermarkets, malls, parking lots, sports fields, restaurants, and shopping areas. In the media, obese people get ridiculed, and sometimes derogatory portrayals are emphasized. You'll hear stories of obese people who are discriminated against in job openings while receiving high grades at school and promotions at work. Many of them are denied the job while slimmer candidates are hired right away. In fact, one book cites that obese people should be put in prison for their own sake.[28]

The Odds at the Office

The preceding examples are isolated cases of discrimination and cannot be considered "alarming" if not taken seriously. Stories of discrimination among the obese will greatly affect the global society now that people suffer from an increasing rate of obesity not only in developed countries, but in other parts of the world as well. Workplaces are highly susceptible to these kinds of discriminatory attitudes and bias against obese people. Sad to say, some infer that an obese job applicant lacks self-discipline, has low potential to move up the professional ladder, and demonstrates poor hygiene—all based solely on his or her weight and appearance. One study had a mock interview and was videotaped with actors playing the role of job applicants for a computer sales job. The actors' weights were manipulated by artificial prostheses.

The experiment revealed that employment bias was greater for obese applicants, and such bias was more directed against women. Obese individuals are employed in analyst positions much more than sales jobs.[29] Obesity stereotyping is also documented in many research studies around the world. Overweight employees are often viewed as less competent, irresponsible, lacking self-discipline, sloppy, and emotionally unstable. They are perceived to be slower, have poorer work and school attendance, and are supposedly last when it comes to being role models.[30] Discrimination may not stop at the hiring level and continues until retirement. An experiment involving 445 obese people showed that out of 50 percent of those above ideal weight range, 26 percent said they were denied health insurance because they are above normal weight. Seventeen percent indicated they were fired or forced to resign.[31]

The Clinical Level

In the medical field, doctors routinely see people firsthand as they are active professionals when it comes to the care of a patient. Any bias or discriminatory attitude that a health care provider feels toward an obese person may greatly affect the quality of care provided. An experiment involving around 320 family physicians revealed that two-thirds of the doctors reported that their obese clients had less self-control, while about 40 percent of doctors stated on anonymous questionnaires that their obese clients were lazy.[32] A similar study involving nurses revealed that 24 out of approximately 110 registered nurses strongly agreed that caring for an obese person is repulsive.[33] Twelve percent indicated that they preferred not to come into contact with an obese person. It's very important to address these negative attitudes against obese people, for this will affect clinical judgment, diagnosis, and quality of care an obese person receives.

From a global perspective, this can be devastating because the reluctance of health care providers to treat the obese may cause obesity sufferers to stop seeking medical care altogether. People may become embarrassed by their weight and appearance. Negative social stigma against obese individuals may discourage them from scheduling a doctor's appointment. Unwillingness to seek medical help is related to fear of a physical exam that requires them to expose the extra fat to the doctor. An obese individual may feel too shy to take off his or her clothes to undergo a physical exam due to negative perceptions of body image.

Traumatic experiences of an obese child include harsh times at school. Childhood obesity is discussed further in the following chapter, but one must acknowledge that social stigmatization against obesity during childhood is a global issue and therefore a contributor to worldwide obesity rates. Social stigmatization is a challenge to overcome early in life. Teasing and peer rejection are the most common problems an obese individual may experience. This will greatly affect a child or an adolescent's self-esteem, which will lead to episodes of depression, anxiety, social isolation, and suicide in the worst-case scenario. A survey of kids aged nine to eleven years showed that clinically overweight children had lower self-esteem than nonoverweight children.[34] Self-esteem was low for obese students who believe it's their fault that they have become overweight, and this leads to the reason why they have fewer friends and are excluded from various activities such as sports and games. Moreover:

- Ninety-one percent of the individuals felt ashamed of being over-weight
- Ninety percent believed that the teasing will stop and friends will accept them if they lose weight
- Sixty-nine percent also feel that they can secure more friends if they lose weight

Discrimination, rejection, and stigmatization of obese children at school should be addressed as an important social problem everywhere.

THE NEXT FLIGHT OUT: MEDICAL TOURISM

For severe cases of obesity that interfere with the health of the individual and greatly endanger the life of a person, a physician may recommend surgery. Medical tourism in India, Brazil, and Argentina provides for surgical procedures like vertical banded gastroplasty (stomach stapling) and gastric banding at somewhat affordable prices. These restrictive procedures prevent the stomach from stretching its size, which leads to the feeling of satiety or fullness. If an individual continues to consume food, he or she will feel nauseated and may develop vomiting and pain. This trains one to eat only until he or she feels full. Another technique that is readily available in the medical tourism industry, called gastrointestinal bypass, involves decreasing the size of the stomach and fastening a portion of the small intestine directly onto the stomach.

If you are thinking of getting this procedure done overseas, know that it can cause significant complications such as mineral and vitamin deficiencies. There is malabsorption occurring as the food immediately enters the small intestine partially digested. Surgical treatment of obesity, whether domestic or through medical tourism, is not a guarantee for successful treatment of the disease. This is especially true in the absence of proper diet, exercise, and lifestyle change. Weight-loss surgery, whether done in the United States or overseas, is believed to be successful only when 50 percent of excess fat is reduced and is sustained for five years. A stern diet, exercise, and a healthy lifestyle are essential for keeping the weight off after getting weight-loss surgery.

WHAT THE WORLD IS DOING ABOUT OBESITY

Exercise and diet has never been more emphasized in reducing weight and maintaining a healthy body. Unhealthy foods and physical inactivity are main risk factors for increased blood pressure, raised blood glucose, and other major chronic diseases. The WHO Global Strategy on Diet, Physical Activity, and Health encourages an effective plan to promote and protect health through healthy eating and physical activity. The major causes of death and disease that are characteristic of wealthy countries are significantly increasing in developing countries as well. Worldwide, noncommunicable diseases account for almost 60 percent of the almost 50 million deaths annually. They also accounts for around 50 percent of all diseases worldwide.[35]

In promoting a healthy diet anywhere in the world, the following recommendations are widely encouraged:

- Avoid consumption of unsaturated fats
- Increase consumption of foods high in vitamins and minerals like fruits and vegetables
- Limit intake of sugars
- Keep your salt levels down and make sure the salt you consume is rich in iodine

As for physical activity, it is recommended that there is constant energy expenditure throughout your life. At least thirty minutes of regular and moderate physical activity such as brisk walking, jogging, or other cardiovascular exercises should be done three times a week.

What does all this mean? It means that no matter where you live, you have to gear yourself up toward a healthy lifestyle. Try to overcome all the propaganda from food advertisements that promote affordable, great-tasting, but unhealthy foods in the market.

Clubs and Organizations

Some organizations, advocates, and groups provide support for the obese and overweight in many of the world's densely populated countries. They help these individuals overcome the anxiety and pressure of being discriminated against, ridiculed, and teased. These organizations also promote widely used weight-loss treatments. International organizations that are funding research for treatment and prevention of obesity cases worldwide are very helpful in creating a way to solve this emerging problem that affects developed and developing countries all over the world. Based on solid research, adult obesity is more common than undernutrition.[36] There are 525 million obese adults. Twice as many are overweight, which means around 1.5 billion adults need to get in shape fast.

The International Association for the Study of Obesity (IASO) launched many projects to help promote a healthy lifestyle. The European based PolMark project aims to protect children from the negative effects of food and beverage marketing. It functions to raise awareness on the health consequences of food advertising to children and how this influences their eating patterns and nutritional intake. In a similar vein, the Health Promotion through Obesity Prevention across Europe (HOPE) project has identified determinants of obesity resulting from proposed food policy recommendations. These projects give systematic views of obesity interventions, thus paving a powerful way to fight the disease head-on from a universal angle.

Raise Public Awareness Wherever You Go

Increasing public awareness about the worldwide obesity crises is the first step in resolving the problem. Obesity is a sensitive issue that appeals to people who have been fat at some point in their lives. A major portion of the public avoids talking about it because it might offend those affected. People shy away at the mention of the words "obese," "fat," or "overweight" because of the stigma it denotes on an individual, irrespective of the language it's spoken in. It is sad that society looks upon obese people as personages who lack discipline and are unhygienic and lazy despite the fact that not all cases of obesity are a result of overeating. Some cases are caused by a genetic disposition or a hormonal imbalance in the body. An example is hypothyroidism, which is known to cause metabolic problems. It is highly prejudicial and discriminatory for obese individuals to be treated badly for something over which they may not have any control.

Why Something Needs to Be Done

Neglect of the problem at hand makes you more vulnerable. What many don't realize is that not addressing the worldwide problem of obesity only makes matters worse. As you may know, the initial step to resolve any kind of problem is to admit and identify the problem as early as possible. Obesity is projected to expand worldwide in the upcoming years if people don't agree to take it seriously. Identification of (1) the factors that contribute to people's present lifestyle of inadequate physical activity, (2) large consumption of fatty foods, and (3) stressful living conditions will all serve as a starting point in creating a realistic platform against worldwide obesity. Various international agencies can use such a platform to execute a health plan to lower the prevalence or eradicate obesity as a disease. They can also increase awareness through education. Dissemination of information on the causes and factors that increase the risk for obesity is helpful for people of all ages, cultures, and races. In addition, supplemental information about proper nutrition and physical activity is relevant to prevent the occurrence of obesity.

The prevalence of obesity worldwide is climbing and will fully affect individuals in years to come because of all the health risks associated with this disease. Further evaluation and comprehensive research will help one determine how he or she can address the growing dilemma of obesity. The problem people are facing is a result of social, economic, and cultural problems arising from developing and industrialized countries. Obesity, diabetes, coronary heart diseases, along with cigarette smoking, decreased physical activity, and a sedentary lifestyle, are frequently by-products of modernization and acculturation. People are gearing toward globalization, and in doing so, taking health for granted by adapting to a lifestyle for the fast-paced person immersed in work.

Aiming for ideal health among all the populations of the world, people need to start by working on their own weight and, in due course, lead others by influence. The world is not a perfect place, but eating healthy, boosting your activity, and avoiding stressors that may induce poor eating habits can in fact lessen many of its problems. If possible, get involved with international groups in the fight for obesity and its consequences, since these gatherings serve as one of the best channels for both information and practice.

II

THE FRONT LINES

7

CHILDHOOD OBESITY

America is a country of bright lights and industry. It is a world super-power, and many foreigners believe life here is perfect, but reality suggests otherwise. How can life be so adverse in a country with such a high standard of living? The United States is among the wealthiest countries in the world and people benefit from it immensely. In spite of all this, childhood obesity remains in and out of the nation's borders.

THE CHILDHOOD OBESITY ENVIRONMENT

Protégés of Fast Food Culture

Americans often take their kids to fast food restaurants as there seems to be one on every corner. Fast food is an inexpensive way to eat, but the meals are far from healthy. Fast food meals vary from 450 to 1,700 calories or more.[1] Currently, an average American eats four meals a week at fast food restaurants.[2] Fast food is very convenient, but its negative effects are continually downplayed by advertising campaigns where food companies prefer to show you how happily your kids will dine if you buy their products. These companies also elaborate on how there's something in it for everyone in the family. This is slowly becoming part of who people are as a society. It seems that soon, fast food might be the only way for children to get anything to eat. The fast food phenomena is taking over children's lives. While the unhealthy side of fast food is devastating, people are willing to choose the worst due to the opportunity to avoid cooking time and convenience.

Since one cannot wholly attribute childhood obesity to fast food culture, one can assume that parents are inadvertently forcing children to assume such a lifestyle. Parents are role models at home and beyond, and kids absorb the grown-ups' characteristics and ways of life. When they see their parents running on full schedules, kids start filling up their own schedule with sedentary activities like those of their parents. They soon learn not to spend any time preparing healthy food and decide to take the easiest and fastest way out.

Children learn from their environment, proven by the fact that everyone is obviously born into this world without really knowing anything about it. This includes not knowing societal values, customs, and ways of life. That's one explanation for why kids pick up their parents' dietary habits. The more society puts an emphasis on academic accomplishments and "reaching the top," the more time one will devote to work. In the end, a person spends less time on things that are not even work-related, such as eating. That in turn teaches children to eat in an unhealthy manner.

Children and adolescents may feel that eating healthy won't get them anywhere. They may also think that spending time eating right will only hinder them because of the amount of time being potentially wasted as a result. People are living more sedentary lifestyles in today's world. With the invention and subsequent boom of the Internet, people are spending less time moving around and exercising. With explosion of technological breakthroughs, millions of jobs were created where people don't have to go out or do manual, physical labor for any major reason. They spend all day working really hard, on the computer, on the Internet, or on the phone. Also partially to blame are Internet games, social networking, and chat programs. Children see their parents spending time on the computer and assume that everyone is supposed to be doing something besides exercising. Also, owing to busy work schedules, children are with their parents less often than they used to be.

Parents and Their Never-Ending Work

Who hasn't had a tough day at work? Normally, work-related stress never ends. It is as if the only time to unwind is during a vacation, which is only two weeks of the year for the average employee. To that end, it's fair to assume that when most people finally come home from work, they just want to unwind and relax. Kids will witness their parents repeatedly sitting on the couch and watching television, which serves as another bad example of how life should be lived.

One of America's strengths is that people live fast lives. Professional working people who have kids don't have time to slow down; it is all about results and how much you can get accomplished in your lifetime. Some may be overwhelmed with work as they try their best to get promoted. People desire to save time in whatever way they can, but they really need to use the time to prepare better meals for themselves *and* for their children.

Parents are usually so tired when they come home from work that they just throw something into the microwave for another quick meal to avoid the hassle of making a full spread. It's that simple. Microwavable dinners are favored even when they don't have ideal nutritional value for kids and don't satisfy all of the food pyramid requirements. The serving sizes are generally bigger, so the label on the back is misleading, and the fat and sodium content is often much higher than it is in freshly prepared meals. Many families don't have dinner together and consume meals on the fly. Moreover, children are normally unaware of the best vegetables and may not be familiar with fat and calorie content. Because of this lack of nutrition education, they resort to processed foods, junk food, and takeout orders when they are adults. This causes obesity and becomes a vicious circle.

Simply put, eating on the go is bad for your health. There are several reasons why you need to take the time to sit down and eat a meal or a snack, rather than have it on the go. Usually, people who eat a snack while they are traveling or moving tend to opt for processed snacks, simply because of the pressure to reach their destination on time. These are high in calories and low in nutrition. This is an important cause of obesity. A meal eaten without distractions offers satiety and satisfaction, but a snack consumed while your mind is focused on work (or play, as applied to children) will leave you hungry.

Kids are taking in a remarkable amount of bad eating habits from this. Most children in the United States live relatively stress-free lives with few responsibilities; most don't often have to worry about where their next meal might come from. They are taught not to worry about what they're eating and to fill up their daily schedule with as many things to do as possible. This involves doing activities that they like, and because some kids are not exposed to many outdoor activities without any parental supervision, they spend most of the day inside. They choose to play video games for hours on end. Teens surf the Web aimlessly, chat, talk on social networks, and play games on the computer. They don't spend enough time running outdoors. When they invite friends over, everyone just stays indoors and watches TV or plays video games. In the end, they are not burning many calories. This becomes a huge problem when added to the fact that they are consuming a massive amount of calories with almost every single meal.

Childhood obesity is a "powder keg" that needs to be stopped by addressing as many of the "little" environmental details as possible. Obesity isn't just about being a few pounds overweight. Overweightness during younger years shows a propensity for gaining weight easily, but it isn't considered obese. To be clinically diagnosed with obesity, one must be more than thirty pounds over the healthy weight for age and body type. One in five children in the United States between five and sixteen years old are in this category,[3] so the question is this: Why does childhood obesity still exist?

WHO'S REALLY LETTING KIDS GET FATTER

America is a place known for its diversity and freedom, and both adults and children will do as they please. That's the beauty of freedom in the first place. It is up to family and society to check on a child's weight problems, since children are not normally the ones making the life-changing decisions at home. Habits essentially trickle down from their parents. If a child has one overweight parent, then they are 50 percent more likely to be obese; if both parents are overweight, they are 80 percent more likely to be so.[4] This shows that children learn from their parents' habits, and before they become aware that they are doing harm to their bodies, it's often too late for them to change their habits.

It's not easy to shed a few pounds. It takes a lot of willpower because results don't come quickly. Furthermore, childhood obesity leads to many emotional problems. It opens the door for ridicule, ostracism, and low self-esteem. Innocently caught in a vicious cycle, many obese teens turn to food as a means to feel better. This exacerbates childhood obesity problems in the long run.

Admittance and Action

Are parents in denial about the fact that their child is clinically diagnosed with obesity? According a study released by the University of Michigan, 56 percent of parents with an obese child thought their child's weight was normal.[5] Parents think that obesity in children is just a phase, and soon, something will change and allow the youngsters to drop the extra weight. These changes may include increased activity levels and better nutritional intake. Conversely, an obese child will most likely grow up to be an obese adult unless something is done about it. Putting an overemphasis on eating or not eating may lead to the development of an eating disorder so they do not intervene when a child is eating too much or not eating the "right" food.[6]

Parents are essential influences when it comes to exercise and nutrition for children. As a parent, you need to encourage your children to eat well and exercise, or else they will risk being obese throughout life. Parents love their children, so it's understandable that they think their child is already perfect. However, when you make it difficult for your kids to understand the importance of healthy eating, major problems arise.

The first step in overcoming childhood obesity lies greatly in the parent's influence over a child's eating patterns. It is society's prime responsibility to sustain kids physically and emotionally to help them become responsible individuals even after they grow up. The food pyramid can be a good reference for parents to identify the foods rich in vitamins and minerals, which kids need for a healthy diet. The pyramid also specifies how big a serving is required to maintain a well-balanced meal throughout the day.

Parents can also promote exercise by encouraging their children to join sport clubs, available all over town. Sports will really make a child physically fit and can foster the value of teamwork and perseverance as well. A child is greatly affected if a parent lacks the ability to prepare and handle the family's nutritional needs.

The Snake's Tail

All across the world, children are collectively being tricked into eating unhealthy foods. Food manufacturers have ad strategies encouraging kids to eat junk food all the time. They get an athlete to endorse a product and say that he or she uses it multiple times a day. Youngsters immediately make a correlation between the "hip," in-shape athlete, and the product. Some companies make online games available and have the user's health "reset" after getting the junk food, sending the ancillary message that you feel as if you are living life at 100 percent if you eat their product. These games include those with the companies' logos displayed throughout the course of play. Companies also use campaigns to encourage children to collect boxes and cans of their product and redeem it for prizes, money, or other rewards. In reality, these kids must spend money and eat foods that result in harm that outweighs the reward.

Parents who genuinely want their kids to eat healthy are fighting an uphill battle against retailers and even society, where apparently it's "cool" to address curiosity by buying the newest gadgets, tasting the latest cuisine, and other adventures.[7] In other words, advertisers and companies are taking advantage of the trusting nature of children. Advertisers try to get to kids before the latter realizes that manufacturers have no concrete emotional attachment to them and are strictly business-oriented.

Serious problems occur when a child finds it difficult to break through a bad eating habit. This is comparable to a snake eating through its own tail. Children are doing something wrong, but once they become aware, it's way too late. If they want to break this cycle, they have to get through a lot of influences encouraging them not to. They may continue to push for the wrong eating behaviors throughout life. Lifestyles and behaviors might make children believe what they are doing is acceptable, if not normal. Kids are now part of a society that pushes them toward eating out of control.

Sometimes people are not aware of the inherent dangers which obesity can really cause in youngsters. Everyone wants to live a happy life where they are free to do what they want and not be judged. One shouldn't judge people simply because they're overweight, but should let the latter know about the damages and potential risks they are taking by eating unhealthily.

PUT THE KIDS TO BED THE RIGHT WAY

Obesity leads to lack of sleep in children due to hormonal imbalances brought on by the extra fat. These hormones include leptin and ghrelin, described in chapter 1. It is possible to survive for a while without any sleep, but at the end of the day, it catches up to you. It has been known since the 1950s that lack of sleep disrupts every physiological function your body carries out.[8] People are not designed to survive without sleep for long periods of time. It makes them more susceptible to illness. Looking back at people's caveman-like instincts, the body is sometimes put on high alert when a person lacks sleep because there would otherwise be some sort of danger to stay awake for long periods of time. This causes the body to release more stress hormones such as cortisol, thus increasing blood pressure. Children are no exception here.

Sleep disruption is just one of the serious problems linked to both adult and childhood obesity. A medical study revealed that lack of sleep led to a heightened tendency for obesity.[9] By surveying more than 6,500 working adults, the researchers found that if you sleep less than seven hours per night, you are much more likely to become obese because insomnia "throws off" the hormones your body releases to regulate appetite. This is one of the harshest realities of obesity. If an adult can be so greatly affected by this, imagine what it would do to an obese child. This shows that once a child become obese, it is almost impossible to crack through an overeating cycle. It is similar to a Ferris wheel that never stops.

Childhood Obesity and Asthma

Obesity is related to asthma, which nearly one-third of obese people have.[10] Asthma is a childhood breathing disorder that normally disappears as you get older. This disease can put children in the hospital and render them unconscious, but rarely kills. It is a lot more difficult for a child with asthma to exercise for long stretches of time. For asthmatics, it's very hard to exercise because they cannot breathe at the level that they want to, but for obese kids, the most common way to lose weight is to just work out. Keep in mind that obese people are five times more likely to be hospitalized from their asthmatic condition than nonobese subjects of the same age range. Hospitalization can lead to other health problems from airborne pathogens, and spending even the smallest amount of time at the hospital is becoming increasingly expensive as the population dives deeper into the millennium.

WHAT OBESE CHILDREN ARE REALLY UP AGAINST

As you may already begin to see, it is difficult to overcome obesity as a child. Once a child is obese, they are likely to suffer from lifelong obesity in the absence of proper intervention. Being obese in early stages of life also leads to more serious health problems than just the lack of sleep and asthma. It can lead to gallstones, diabetes, heart disease, cholesterol and triglyceride problems, high blood pressure, and liver problems. For women, it can even cause menstrual complications.

Gallstones in Obese Children

All of these diseases sound terrible, and it's unsurprising that they are. Gallstones are a major and painful inconvenience. Gallstones in children can lead to a number of terrible symptoms. It starts with pain all throughout the body, and if not treated quickly, can cause serious medical problems. Usually, gallstones work their way out of the gallbladder and get lodged in ducts throughout the child's body. One of the most common ducts that gallstones block is the common bile duct. This causes problems in the digestive system and can lead to jaundice and infection. Another possibility is the gallstone(s) getting stuck in the pancreatic duct. This may lead to pancreatitis, which causes instant and constant pain in the abdomen. Acute (sudden) pancreatitis is the rapid inflammation of the pancreas gland. This condition is considered a medical emergency that demands immediate hospitalization.[11] Imagine the consequences if it happens to a very young obesity victim.

Diabetes

A serious by-product of childhood obesity is diabetes. Type 1 diabetes, formerly known exclusively as juvenile diabetes, is a disease where a child's internal organs are unable to control the amount of sugar in his or her circulatory system. Sugar in the bloodstream gives people the energy it takes to complete daily activities. If an obese child has diabetes, their daily activities are restricted because they don't have the energy to complete many simple, everyday tasks. The chances of a child getting Type 2 diabetes increases dramatically if and when a child is obese.[12] According to the Centers for Disease Control and Prevention, people who are obese are over seven times more likely to have diabetes than their nonobese counterparts.[13]

Furthermore, both Type 1 and Type 2 diabetes in obese children can lead to a whole host of complications. Diabetes can hurt the retina, and is therefore one of the leading causes of blindness later in life. It can also hurt your nerves and cause foot wounds and ulcers. Over time, the story may quickly turn to leg amputations, of which diabetes is the leading cause in the absence of direct trauma. Diabetes with childhood obesity also accelerates the onset of atherosclerosis, which leads to arterial blockage and clots. This is what causes heart attacks. Diabetes weakens the body's ability to fight infections and makes them prone to other diseases. Of further importance is the fact that obese children with diabetes generally have Type 1 diabetes, which is more severe than Type 2. Diabetes is currently a leading cause of kidney failure.[14]

The Cholesterol Dilemma

Childhood obesity leads to elevated cholesterol levels later in life. High cholesterol prescribes its own set of problems such as atherosclerosis. The onset of atherosclerosis is hastened by childhood obesity. Too much cholesterol, along with the formation of plaques, causes hardening and thickening of the arteries resulting in increased clots and blockage. As time passes, this will lead to a heart attack or a stroke. Either can result in death or at least hospitalization and loss of motor nerve skills and brain functions. An obese child can potentially end up in a heap of trouble because they could have high cholesterol and diabetes simultaneously, which would make them twice as susceptible to heart attack and stroke later in life. Also, clots could lead to a loss of leg use because the blood is eventually unable to circulate throughout the body, including the lower extremities.[15]

Giving Heart to Your Thoughts

It is especially important to teach children about obesity at an early age. As young children, they don't learn the decision making processes that are necessary to eat healthy foods. They are at the whim of their impulses since they don't normally think as far ahead about future consequences. A child's personal scope of development, compared to that of an adult, is very limited. They may be thinking about later that night, later that week, next month, maybe even next year. They are not thinking fifteen to twenty years into the future, when physical complications from obesity really sink in.

Childhood obesity is an American epidemic, if not a worldwide pandemic. One out of five children is obese, and this will have a devastating effect on the world population. In the best-case scenario, an obese kid will live five years less than a nonobese person. However, with a host of other complications, many have a shorter life expectancy. Quality of life will likewise drop dramatically.[16] It is imperative that kids are taught about the perils of living an obesity-favoring lifestyle. Parents should be taught about this when all's said and done, because they are the ones who will have the most effect on their children's behavior over the years.

Why should childhood obesity concern anyone? If someone doesn't have an obese child, should it really be their problem? The facts are there for anyone to know, so childhood obesity is *everyone's* problem. For understandable reasons, children don't get to choose whether to become obese. They don't always have the judgment or willpower necessary to know when too much sugar is really "too much." Parents are instilling undesirable eating habits through bad example, and may be in denial about how an overweight child looks. Children are then learning to overindulge, and to this end, society is not teaching them to exercise properly. This is a social tragedy as much as it is anything else.

Think about how great a child's life can be. Unfortunately, obese children may not get to experience it all the way because of their situation. They have trouble playing as they get teased at school. They have a wide range of medical problems, and life becomes not only miserable, but far too short for them. This is so difficult on a child that eventually the wear and tear of everyday life becomes too much to handle, and the body succumbs.

Being obese can also affect the way a child views life. Obese children feel that life is harder for them and find it difficult to lose weight due to these negative feelings. Obesity can lead to difficulty performing everyday things such as going to the mall or climbing stairs. It can also lead to practical difficulties, including difficulty finding clothes that fit them or being unable to sit on standard bus seats or restaurant chairs. These issues can result in a level of self-esteem that is inhibiting enough to cause depression or anxiety disorders. Young obesity victims can get very moody when things get out of hand, and research confirms that these mood swings morph into more serious psychiatric problems such as borderline personality disorder and suicide.[17]

THINGS TO WORRY ABOUT BESIDES COLLEGE TUITION

Simply put, obese children are being deprived of many gifts in life. Their understanding of the world is a far cry from that of a healthy, fit person, and if it isn't enough to suggest that people need to educate the youth about childhood obesity, maybe the following statistics will. Obesity has already cost the American population more than $90 billion in medical bills, and 34 percent of the adult population is obese.[18] With the recent surge of childhood obesity, that number is sure to balloon someday. That's why America's medical costs for taking care of obese people will also increase. This is another reason why this is such a problem for Americans. Since children are prime representations of the world's future, childhood obesity will indirectly make the cost of medicine rise. Individuals who are not obese will have to pay for medical bills that are not their own. Therefore, the next question you have to ask is this: What is the government doing to solve this problem and what can the average citizen do to lessen the repercussions?

Worthy of the First Lady's Attention

Michelle Obama set a good example when she launched her campaign to eliminate childhood obesity.[19] All eyes were focused on her own children, whom she has subjected to certain lifestyle changes as advised by the family pediatrician. She cut serving sizes, switched to low-fat milk, provided fruits on the table, and banned weekday TV watching. Responses from the public were not all positive, and she was even accused of subjecting her own daughters to public scrutiny. Nevertheless, her message is that even small modifications in children's diets actually help. Adopting a healthier lifestyle will benefit children in the long run.[20]

Political icons from countries all over the world are getting involved in fighting childhood obesity. Mrs. Obama is trying to get the food budget for public schools increased from $1 billion to $2 billion. Because of the budgetary constraints placed on schools, educational institutions are forced to serve lower-grade, lower-quality, and less healthy food to students. By adjusting funds, schools can begin to purchase fruits, vegetables, and other quality ingredients. The First Lady considers the low budget to be the key factor in why children are being served obesity-causing foods in schools. She's also finding a way to increase children's physical activity levels while they are at school.

This is where budgetary constraints come into the picture again. For a public school to be fiscally sound, they often have to remove otherwise viable programs. Consequently, schools around the world may be cutting sports teams, physical education, and recesses, which result in children getting less exercise at school than normal. A child now has to take responsibility into his or her own hands and find a way to exercise when on their own time, but naturally, children don't want to do that. They would rather spend their time on social media networks, watching television, or playing video games. Here's another problem: Some states make it possible for children to avoid physical education classes. In 2010, Florida began letting children get a waiver to skip gym class and instead spend their time focusing on other things such as school work.

Mrs. Obama has noticed a problem in America that she wants to fix. She is involved inside out with the Let's Move initiative, intended to help with childhood obesity and increase school budgets to provide healthier meals for students. They provide more exercise opportunities for kids, but to fully approach childhood obesity, the work must be done within the family. Parents need to become more aware of the dangers.

The First Lady acknowledges that parents have busy lives and it is therefore tough to juggle all of the everyday tasks that come with raising a child. Some parents have to juggle multiple jobs, get their children to and from school, and take the children to extracurricular activities—all in addition to other daily stressors. Where exactly does shopping for fresh food and preparing healthy meals fit in? People may not have the energy to do all these things, so they take the easy the way out—fast food or microwave dinners. Mrs. Obama wants a law that makes food manufacturers put nutrition labels on the *front*, rather than the back of packages so consumers can easily identify what is and isn't healthy. She is hoping to collaborate with city mayors so communities can come up with a distinct, unique approach for answering the problems obese children are facing.

Political players like Mrs. Obama are putting a lot of energy into fighting childhood obesity. However, the most realistic approach to childhood obesity needs to come from within the family. People need to be more aware of the dangers, and parents have to be the ones who make the mindful decisions for obese children.

PARENTING BY THE DECADES

There are several steps you can take as a parent to approach childhood obesity. For at-home prevention strategies, try to be as direct as possible. Invest in (1) making sure what your child consumes is in fact healthy, (2) making sure healthy foods are available to the child around the clock, and (3) spending quality time with your child outdoors.

Exercise Is the Answer

Get your child to exercise daily. This can simply be done by playing and spending time with your children. Children have tons of energy and wild imaginations, so it's really easy for them to find something entertaining to do outdoors. This may include swimming, playing sports, wrestling, or whatever physical demands the child finds entertaining. Another way to keep him or her active is to limit TV, computer time, and video games. This will force them to spend quality time playing out in the open.

Repairing Your Child's Diet with Better Meals

As was discussed in chapter 3, diet is a huge factor in both adult and childhood obesity. Controlling diet in a young person can be easier than you think. It begins by reducing the amount of fast food that your child consumes. A single serving of fast food can have as many calories as two normal meals for a child. Everyone fancies the convenience of fast food, but the calories aggregate very quickly. Nutrition labels are found on the back and bottom of fast food containers. It is important you review these so your children can realize how unhealthy fast food is. Understanding the number of calories can also help you make better meals to counter any fast food later in the week.

Besides avoiding fast food while on the move, things can be done to improve diet at home. Spend more time shopping and looking at food labels and buying healthier foods for the family. Everyone has their own tastes and people want foods to satisfy these longings. Parents need to be aware that some of these meals, such as frozen microwave dinners, may be unhealthy. There are foods out there to satisfy your tastes that are far healthier. You need to come up with more creative solutions to solving these problems besides giving your children the same items over and over. Parents with little time on their hands during the week could pick a day when they do have free time and cook healthy meals for the week to freeze and serve later. Choosing healthy dishes that freeze well or keep for a few days in the fridge can be simple as there are many resources for recipes, such as cookbooks, online cooking resources, and other outlets.

Breakfast is an important meal, so remind your children to never skip this meal. Skipping breakfast is harmful, mainly because sleep itself requires energy. When you wake up in the morning, your cells need a fresh new supply of nutrients so they won't get overstressed during the first half of the day. Serving a child even a small breakfast every day will have a huge impact on his or her life. Research shows that children who eat breakfast regularly have a much lower BMI because breakfast jump-starts the metabolism for the day. Protein sources such as eggs speed up metabolism shortly after eating.[21] Children who eat breakfast have more energy in the morning and throughout the day; they are more inclined to play as they get a rush of energy and hence, they don't want to be cooped up all day long. Serving breakfast is a very simple task which takes up very little time. Children can be served low-sugar cereals, eggs, fruit, yogurt, whole-grain toast, English muffins, and so forth—all meals which take no longer than five minutes to prepare.

Try to balance the meals you make for your children. They will require a lot of nutrients, and following the food pyramid is a good way to make sure children are given what they need. A balanced meal will mean the child is eating healthy and will help prevent obesity. As you may have read in the earlier chapters, proteins speed up metabolism. Another benefit of adding proteins is that they slow down digestion and make children feel "fuller" for longer. Stay clear of starch-heavy foods since meals with too many of them usually have a lot of calories. This is why you should provide meals with only one or two servings of carbohydrates. A balanced meal will give your child proper nutrients and the right amount of energy to burn off the fat that their body is actively trying to store.

The Next Top Chef

Try to make cooking a fun and fruitful activity for your children. That's how you can teach them about healthy eating while helping them to re-member a list of healthy foods. It's all about paving the road for creativity and healthier alternatives to all those prepared and frozen favorites. It makes the child likely to eat what is in front of them because they took the initiative to prepare it themselves. Ask for his or her input when you decide what to make for dinner.

Calories

Take a good look at liquid calories. These calories are the easiest method for your kids to put on weight. Milk, soda, and juices high in sugar have a tremendous number of calories and can greatly affect your child's weight. Liquid calories are digested much quicker than nonliquid calories, so a child won't fill up on fruit juice or soda and will therefore have room to take in more calories. These empty calories are one of the biggest reasons for childhood obesity. Empty calories are calories without any nutritional value. If a child normally has a 1,000 to 2,000 calorie diet, which includes two cups of fruit juice or soda per day, he or she could gain thirty pounds over the course of a year. Don't let your child fill up on these empty calories. Encourage him or her to drink lots of water.

Have your children save calories, and lose weight if necessary, by giving them low-fat dairy products. Children need the calcium but don't necessarily need all the calories found in dairy products. Give them skim milk instead of whole milk. Use low-fat or reduced-fat cheese in their sandwiches and for snacks; serve them low-fat or non-fat yogurt. By swapping a cup of whole milk for skim milk, it can save a child seventy calories, which can later be used to indulge in favorite sweets and snacks, if you must.

The Fiber Essence

Here's another tip: Give your child lots of fiber. Insoluble fiber takes a long time to chew, thus allowing the stomach to more accurately reflect when it is full. Insoluble fiber adds density to food without adding bulk calories to a meal too. This is a good way to make children think they are full and thus reduce the caloric intake. Furthermore, fiber regulates the blood sugar level and decreases food cravings that children will have in-between meals, further reducing the overall amount of calories.

Juicy Foods

These foods are another way to "fill up" children without making them obese. Foods with plenty of liquid in them will make children feel as if they are full and will cause them to eat less throughout the day. Water will make them feel full but passes through the system very quickly, so it doesn't have the same effect as soupy foods. This is because food is a lot tougher to process internally than water. Water is absorbed through your large intestine (colon) so it gets distributed evenly before and after food passes. Pureed vegetable soup and watermelon are popular examples of juicy foods.

Snacks

Let's face it: children love to snack. They complain of hunger through-out the day and between meals. Give them vegetables for them to snack on in between meals. This serves a dual purpose because vegetables have few calories and lots of nutrients. In reality, your child is eating a healthy alternative to potato chips. When a kid complains about the veggies, he or she is probably eating out of boredom simply because he or she is a compulsive junk food eater. The point is to give him the op-tion of eating vegetables or waiting until dinner to eat anything. This is a good way to reduce caloric intake. A parent should always have child-friendly vegetables ready. Cherry tomatoes, bell peppers, cucumbers, and baby carrots would fit the bill here.

Ironically, a very important part of fighting childhood obesity is to continue to allow your child to eat unhealthy foods in small percentages. Around 90 percent of the time, the child should be eating healthy foods. This allows 10 percent of the time to be devoted to indulging but won't lead children into thinking that they are completely giving up their personal favorites such as ice cream, candy, and soda. The central goal here is to encourage healthy eating and to keep children from gaining unnecessary weight while enjoying their favorite foods enough to satisfy their basic levels of hunger. Human nature suggests that nobody is per-fect, and this concept is very important psychologically to get a child to eat a healthier diet.

THE RECAP

This chapter focused on the steps you can take both as an obesity suf-ferer or parent concerned with childhood obesity. Childhood obesity is a serious problem facing America today, but its far-reaching conse-quences are affecting the entire world. Therefore, one shouldn't idle around and let such a thing happen. One needs to educate the younger population on the dangers and seriousness of obesity.

Don't be satisfied if your son or daughter eats more than necessary or does not prioritize the quality of food at all times. This will keep your children away from the dangers of extreme obesity, which gradu-ally affects their health and physical mobility. Encouraging your children to engage in outdoor activities such as hiking, biking, swimming, and camping can increase their physical activity without compromising their innate need for fun and enjoyment. Have them participate in afterschool activities such as basketball, often a great form of exercise and physical activity. A child will develop a healthy, fit body and learn the value of teamwork, perseverance, and hard work. Note that children who are obese in early childhood are more likely to become obese as they grow up to be adults. Health risks pose a major threat as they reach their twenties or thirties.[22]

Childhood obesity is similar to a never-ending cycle where, once a child becomes obese, they may never return to a normal, healthy weight and lifestyle. Society has to let children know before they get stuck behind the eight ball. Children need to know what will happen to them, and people must understand what happens to children should they get obese. People need to know how to control childhood obesity so kids can live the happy and productive lives that they deserve.

8

OBESITY AND MENTAL HEALTH

Obesity might seem like a choice—a lifestyle option that many have simply elected to live. Many believe that obesity is about a result of overeating due to greed and lack of discipline, but this is often not the case. Studies show that obesity can be a side effect of a mental health problem,[1] which can occasionally be the main source of all the fat from the start. Let's look further into several types of mental issues that can cause obesity and vice versa.

Mental health can be defined as the level of emotional or cognitive well-being.[2] People often misconceive mental health issues as being mad or "nuts." In point, a mental health issue may be as simple as feeling depressed or unhappy, as well as more serious conditions such as obsessive compulsive disorder. There are several obesity-causing psychological disorders worthy of discussion here.

OBESITY-CAUSING PSYCHOLOGICAL DISORDERS

Anxiety Disorders

These are commonly known as any condition that can induce large amounts of situational stress, such as agoraphobia, acute stress disorder, and posttraumatic stress disorder. Obesity in the long run can be caused by anxiety, and is often a result of ways of coping with the stress. Foods high in sugar, fat, and calories alter the body's response to chronic stress. If you always go through high amounts of stress in your life, eating fatty food may make things worse. This is a vicious cycle, because the more fats you eat, the worse you feel and the more obese you become. In these cases, your anxiety disorder needs to be treated before the obesity gets out of control. Once you believe there is less or no more stress or anxiety in your life, only then will you be able to stop overeating in order to control it.[3]

Obsessive Compulsive Disorder

Obsessive compulsive disorder (OCD) is a mental health disorder that creates illogical thoughts and obsessions.[4] These thoughts, manufactured in the mind, make you compulsive and go through repetitive, irrational behavior. Is it merely a control issue? Many people develop OCD as a way to take control of their lives. OCD could serve as a coping mechanism for many obesity victims.[5] Obese people may not necessarily have a higher incidence of OCD, but medical research has noted substantial weight gain in mental health patients during OCD treatment.[6] Because of the compulsive thoughts and behavior, many OCD sufferers overeat and become obese. People with OCD also become wary of certain foods and often stick to one or two things that they can eat. If you are an obese OCD patient and are really wary of germs, then it's not uncommon for you to only eat canned or extra-sterilized foods.[7]

Unfortunately, food from aluminum cans and other metal containers is not the most nutritious of meals, and in such cases, OCD sufferers refuse fruit or vegetables because of possible pesticides or soil remnants. Pesticides can masquerade as hormones. These are known as hormone disrupters. When hormones are out of balance, the body can respond by adding fat, according to a study.[8] One pesticide linked to an increase in fat tissue in mice is tributyltin (TBT). This particular chemical is found in a variety of pesticides and is known to have an impact on a variety of species from insects to humans. For OCD to be treated, the person will need counseling and possibly medication to keep his or her compulsive behavior under control.

Depression

Depression, whether the person is obese or not, takes place for many different reasons. It may be due to a change in personal circumstances, such as a recent break-up. Whatever the reason, depression can affect anyone and its magnitude can vary greatly from person to person. On one day you could be feeling a bit low, but on the next, you feel almost suicidal.[9]

Many people who are depressed resort to "comfort" food. These foods can be fatty or high-sugar content items that reduce the stress and depression levels for a certain amount of time.[10] Unfortunately, these foods fail to reduce the levels for prolonged amounts of time, and therefore, the sufferer will eat these foods more frequently.

People often confuse depression with self-pity, and therefore don't feel as if help is necessary. Depression is actually a mental health disorder and should be treated by a health care professional with the use of counseling or medication. Clinical depression is not the kind of mental health disorder that just disappears quickly on its own, so obesity symptoms can often last much longer than those of depression. To summarize, a clinical investigation concluded that losing weight is bound to decrease symptoms of depression, irrespective of whether a person is obese.[11]

Learning Difficulties in Young Obesity Victims

Obese children can be susceptible to learning difficulties because they are at a very impressionable stage of their lives.[12] Many disorders such as autistic spectrum disorder (ASD) and attention-deficit hyperactivity disorder (ADHD) display pathological warning signs of obesity early on in life.[13] Solid clinical research suggests a high incidence of ADHD in obesity victims.[14] However, a study has also found that there is no difference in prevalence of ASD in obese versus nonobese children.[15]

For children affected by these disorders, it may be a confusing time and may create a lot of stress and anxiety for an obese child. The sequence causes children to overeat as part of a coping mechanism. Giving your kids extra food to deal with their problems can also be a way of showing your love for your children, but this is probably a wrong idea. Autistic children don't understand emotions completely, and as a result, parents feel as if they can show their love by spoiling their kids, however inadvertent their intentions. This can often result in feeding children junk food several times a week.

Remember that children with mental health disorders and learning difficulties have a tough time adjusting to their condition[16] and are in and out of clinics as they get diagnosed and treated. However, if the obesity isn't serious, it's easier to let the child eat whatever he or she prefers. This is especially true if the child is well treated and is comfortable with the situation. Making your child go on a diet when he or she is in a difficult time of life will only worsen any mental health disorder along with the obesity.

Stress

Stress is something that no one can permanently avoid. You might not find that stress is all too relevant to mental health, but any emotion could be connected to mental health, and as such, stress is one of the most common mental health disorders. Stress can occur during everyday events, at home, and at work, but as you may recollect, people take comfort in fatty foods because these foods lower the levels of stress. This can lead to behavior that results in obesity if used as a permanent relief from overwhelming work. To avoid getting obese while stressed out, take a look at all possible causes of your stress and try to deal with it directly if possible.[17]

Too much stress is not only a matter of your waistline, but is harmful to your heart and brain too. The idea here is to overtly block the stress rather than devour food to mask any mental health problem. If you cannot see yourself without stress in your life, then try to find something else that will allow you to let off steam without putting on the extra pounds. Exercise is very good for reducing stress as it releases endorphins, your natural pain-relief hormones. This has the same effect as junk food but is much healthier for you as you fight off the obesity.[18]

THE ODD COUPLE: MENTAL HEALTH AND FOOD

Mental health disorders are often a major factor for your obesity. However, the obesity can be an underlying problem originally triggered by a psychological problem. Many become obese in adulthood because they weren't introduced to the dangers of overeating while young. Keep in mind that overeating has a direct physiological correlation to obesity.[19] By not teaching your child how to eat properly, sensibly, and healthily he or she is unlikely to eat healthily during adulthood. Junior chef schools have always been around, but in the modern era, children need to learn the importance of nutritious food and how to eat healthy in ways that don't require cooking. If people are taught at a young age to cook simple and nutritious meals, then they would have no need to resort to junk food and they would know when to stop eating.

The Mentalities of Eating Disorders

Eating disorders are partly responsible for causing obesity and have psychological basis. While the term "eating disorder" is publicly associated with thin girls who never eat, this is in fact a misconception. Eating disorders can include overeating, binging, food purging, and other complications. Bulimia, in particular, can cause obesity when one repeatedly binges on high-fat and sugary foods. Each episode of binging can throw off a digestive system that barely ever gets any food at all, so your body clings to as much of the fat and sugar as possible. You put the weight on before it comes off, even with anorexia since your body reacts to starvation and bulks up its reserves in response.[20]

Selective Eating Disorder   Selective eating disorder (SED) is when a person is very picky about which foods he or she consumes; this type of behavior is also referred to as perseverative feeding disorder. It can affect a person at any age.[21] As a sign of restrictive preference, the person with SED will prefer one brand of food to another. Others have unnecessary concerns and will only eat food that's a certain color or softness. This can be a very harmful diet and may cause obesity.

Nevertheless, many people with SED are not held back by weight gain because it is sometimes more important to control the *type* of food that goes in than the quantity of it. The eating disorder likely to cause obesity (more than SED), is compulsive overeating, more commonly known as binge eating. Often linked with OCD, compulsive overeating is a behavioral problem that's more of a self-control problem than a weight issue.

Binge Eating Disorder   Approximately 2 percent of all adults in the United States suffer from binging problems, which can occur at any age but is common to teenagers and young adults. People with binge eating disorders are far more likely to have depression than an otherwise mentally sound obesity victim. Because binge eating is so easily hidden, many people find that their families and friends don't know about their condition. Therefore, treatment is often inadvertently delayed. Compulsive overeating needs to be treated by a mental health professional or counselor because there is usually a major underlying problem that needs to be addressed before the obesity is targeted.

Some eating abnormalities can go unnoticed for years while the person slowly gets obese. This is a characteristic of night eating syndrome, when a person goes on an eating spree very late at night, even while asleep. Night eating syndrome is attributable to the same brain activity as sleepwalking. There is often a longstanding problem that sometimes goes untreated due to the fact that the victims obviously don't realize that they are overeating. People who suffer from night eating syndrome usually go for high-fat and high-sugar foods or junk foods.[22]

Binge eaters will try to fill their binges with high-fat and high-sugar foods because it raises serotonin levels. Serotonin levels are reduced in many people with eating disorders, and this is believed to be the reason they choose fatty and sugary foods. A lot of antidepressant drugs are termed selective serotonin reuptake inhibitors (SSRIs) because they block serotonin. The common denominator here is that all people suffer from minor depression and anxiety at some point in their lives. In fact, depression and anxiety is a common feeling throughout the world population.[23]

Emotions   In dealing with your obesity, your doctor might tell you to avoid an emotional attachment to food since you may simply be eating whenever you feel sad.[24] Comfort eating is evidenced when someone is constantly depressed and turns to overeating. This is a clinical problem. The matter arises when the psychiatrist has to decide what exactly is causing your overeating. It needs to be dealt with using the above methods, and only then can subjects focus on getting better. Consider this: Many people who overeat don't even realize that they have a problem. People think that comfort eating is just a natural thing and that everybody does it. In truth, these people need counseling to talk about why they think that eating will make them happier.[25] Some will eat out of boredom and therefore require a little guidance to disclose ways in which they can keep themselves occupied. That's how you avoid eating all day and night.

Obesity and issues with mental health are closely associated. People who are obese often feel depressed and dislike the size of their bodies. Because of these feelings and thoughts, obesity victims look to food for comfort. These foods are usually high in fat. It is a cycle which is difficult to break. Extra food in one's mouth could be the easiest way to explain a disease such as obesity, since obesity can make people fatter when they don't have the simple willpower or mental strength to avoid overeating.

Body Dysmorphic Disorder   Many obese people suffer from body dysmorphic disorder, when they see themselves differently than the way they really are. Some obese people with this disorder will look in the mirror and see a thin person and therefore eat out of control, while others envision a morbidly obese person and feel depressed and begin to eat more. Every so often, people who are stuck in a cycle of depression and consume large amounts of food won't ask for help if they are content with their current diet. It's usually when a family member, friend, or health professional intercedes and reveals what's really happening that the victim will actually do something about it. Once the obese person decides to break the physical cycle, it's time to approach the problem at a psychological angle. Body dysmorphic disorder is a major mental health issue since the affected individual needs to have enough motivation to stop themselves from binge eating.[26]

FINDING MINDFULNESS

When you realize that you or your loved one needs more than just a diet club when it comes to obesity and you feel that there may be an underlying mental health issue, it's best to see a mental health professional right away. Sometimes you will be referred to an expert by your physician or weight-loss specialist. The expert will be able to get you going the right way and give you the much needed help. Several different types of mental health experts can help you get rid of any mental problems that are linked to your obesity.

Psychiatric and Mental Health Nurses

These health professionals are not simply nurses, but people who have spent years in college studying mental health. They work in a wide range of health care settings such as hospitals, community health centers, and outpatient medical clinics. These nurses are able to identify what is wrong with you and examine different cases of substance abuse and psychiatric disorders on a routine basis. They can draw up a treatment plan and help you to take charge of your clinical care. Psychiatric nurses get a degree in general nursing and then go on to specialize in mental health. A nurse must attend six years of schooling to qualify as a nurse practitioner.

Social Workers

Social workers are involved with caring for the obese mental health patient at home and the office rather than the hospital.[27] These professionals are dispatched to your residence to fully assess your situation and determine the outcome. Many social workers do home visits for a more comfortable setting or if you are unable to make it out of your home. This is necessary when the person has little or no self-confidence. It can also come from severe obesity and occasionally, it's due to a mental disorder such as OCD.[28] Social workers get in touch with the relevant mental health practitioners and advise them of the situation. They will then get together and decide what is best for you and decide the route of action. Some people will be admitted to a mental health hospital, while others will be able to receive treatment at home.

Home can be a much safer option because it makes the person feel more relaxed, but it makes it easier for him or her to cheat on a specific diet or routine. Social workers have to be educated with a master's or doctorate degree that's standardized for their specific field of discipline. A nurse works on the clinical health of a person, but the social worker emphasizes overall wellness from a social and personal standpoint. A social worker may suggest the services of a home health aide while a nurse can directly assist with matters of personal hygiene.

Counseling Psychologist

Counseling is a great way to vent about your problems. Counseling psychologists are trained to ask questions in a way that makes you reveal more about yourself than is already known. Through counseling, many obese people find that they have a lot more issues than they knew they had. The idea here is that by talking about them, you're actually addressing the issue in a positive manner. Therefore, it won't affect the subject's life any longer. Obesity victims may find that their problems stem from a childhood issue such as bullying. Part of your brain blocks out bad memories, so in trying to remember bad memories, you can often realize what's making you overeat in the first place. Counseling also works very well if you're willing to give it a go. Some obesity victims don't believe in talking about things and would rather "bottle it up." By talking about it, you can start to understand what is at stake, and with the help of a counselor, you can figure out how to change.

Your Psychiatrist

A psychiatrist is at the top of the food chain when it comes to treating any obesity-causing mental issues. They go through extensive training and have to spend roughly thirteen years in training. Psychiatrists focus on diagnosing people with mental health issues and handling such problems with medicine, cognitive behavioral therapy, or psychotherapy.[29] While a psychologist cannot prescribe any medications, a psychiatrist can. A psychiatrist will typically specialize in certain areas, including:

- Child psychiatry
- Adult psychiatry
- Forensic psychiatry
- Learning disabilities
- Emergency psychiatry
- Behavioral medicine
- Addiction psychiatry
- Neuropsychiatry
- Psychosomatic medicine
- Pain medicine

It is common for an obesity victim to visit more than one of the mental health professionals above. There are lots of different assistants, health care advisors, and others that will help with mental health issues and obesity. Some say that they have to treat the mental issue before targeting the obesity, a useful game plan if the mental issue is causing the obesity in the first place. Many health care providers believe that with a bit of self-confidence and a lot of education, their clients will naturally slim down after they begin treatment. Treatments can take years and years before the problem goes away. This is why it is a good idea to stay in contact with your psychiatrist. If any warning signs ever return, you can let them know.

Choose What's Right for You

A few obesity victims get treated at home more easily than others, while others require inpatient therapy, resident care, or hospitalization. There's no hard rule to how a specific mental health issue is treated at home, since this will depend on the person and the varying degree of the issue. Mental health professionals spend many years training and gaining qualifications in their specified field. That's why they know what they are doing and can decide if and when obesity victims with mental health issues are to be treated at home. Some mental health issues don't even need the attention of a specializing mental health professional and can be dealt with by your local physician.

Receiving the right treatment is essential, but there are more ways to approaching your obesity and psychological issues aside from seeing a mental health professional. By requesting the help of an expert however, you may notice that your treatment works much faster than approaching your obesity-related mental health issues on your own.

THE WONDER OF DIET CLUBS

To remain within the "comprehensive" shade of this book, one must include diet clubs in the discussion about mental health as it pertains to obesity. Joining diet clubs and focus groups are a good idea when you think you don't have the willpower to lose weight in the comfort of your own home. This may not cure your mental health issue right away, but it will help you lose weight. You gain a little more self-esteem as a result. Diet clubs could be a group of people in a local hall who chat with each other about healthy lifestyles, or a corporate club where fees are charged and a diet has been specifically formulated for each member. Remember that both of these methods have benefits and drawbacks.[30]

Diet clubs can track your progress. The clubs will generally give a helping hand if you need a bit of steering in the right direction. These diet clubs sometimes try to understand why you are always feeling hungry and what you eat throughout the day. You should be honest with them and not hide any information that will keep you from losing weight. Joining a diet club will give you the opportunity to make new friends and gain new life experiences. Obese individuals, especially those with mental health issues, often find it difficult to make friends who share something in common with them. Talking to anyone in general can be tough when you lack self-esteem.

At a diet club, you get introduced to people who all share the same interest with you, which is weight loss. No matter how badly you have done through the week, you generally get a round of applause for trying anyway. It's a good idea to tell your group leader that you have a mental health issue as it may need to be monitored. Other options include support groups that offer group counseling to its members.

Corporations

The corporate approach to dieting is very strict and may propose a diet that is guaranteed to work physiologically, but a smaller, local club may favor strategies for adding healthy foods to your lifestyle. Corporate diet clubs are expensive and your success can depend on what they offer. Corporate diet clubs that offer counseling, special client packages, food, or weekly weigh-ins, can cost a pretty penny. Others will ask for a few dollars a week to simply weigh you. With all diet programs, it is good to have someone keeping an eye on your weight throughout your workout phase.[31]

WHEN MEDICATION IS NOT THE GREATEST

Behavioral Therapy

As an obesity patient, it never hurts to try behavioral therapy. This can be in the form of nonmedicinal treatment by a psychiatrist. Behavioral therapy is similar to psychological intervention for overweight and obese people. Several studies have proven that the method works well and leads to positive results for many obesity patients.[32] Behavioral therapy works best when combined with exercise and healthy diet. This rids your obesity by focusing on the source. If your psychiatrist has diagnosed you with a disorder such as overeating, multiple personality disorder, or obsessive compulsive disorder, the therapist will give special focus to that particular illness.[33]

You could get referred to a therapist by your psychiatrist or physician and undergo therapy for a few years or more. Depending on how reversible the situation is, some obesity victims are scheduled with a therapist for up to five times a week. Behavioral therapists attempt to change the way you think and alter your whole mental pattern so that you can break free from a harmful routine. If you are afraid of heights for instance, your behavioral therapist will talk through your problem and take you out to places such as a building and slowly take you one floor higher each time you go out. He or she will constantly assure you that your fear is simply based on irrational thought, and that your imagination is responsible for instilling false ideas. Your therapist will continue to do this until your problems are gone.

This approach can be used to tackle a wide spectrum of mental health issues but has to be done by a trained professional. Otherwise, it may damage the person even more. All therapists have gone through extensive training and are often specialized in a specific field. This means that they treat people with the same mental health issue every day and know what is and isn't successful.

Get involved with group therapies that are known to assist obese people whose mental issues are not quite so severe. This is where a group of people who suffer from the same psychological problems will all join together and talk about their personal experiences. The idea here is for the therapist to convince the group to share thoughts with others, and by doing so, gives everyone some hope and understanding. It can be very scary for a person to see themselves mentally as the *only* one with an obesity problem, so when they are met by the group, they get a boost in self-esteem and plenty of confidence.

Whichever form of therapy is used, it's important not to miss any appointments. Therapists usually draw out a detailed treatment plan which may be set up in stages. Each stage might build onto the previous one. To this end, people who don't follow professional treatment plans will find it difficult to get better and could even relapse back to the way they were before treatment ever began. Behavioral therapy for obesity victims who suffer from mental health issues is very effective and can make a real difference. Trusting the professional is crucial to making all this work, and a bond that strengthens the treatment is usually formed between both the patient and the therapist.

Dietitians

You may be asked to see a dietitian for your obesity once your mental health issues are successfully treated by your psychiatrist. Dietitians are used to analyze what you eat and how you can go about putting healthier foods on your personal menu. They often have a challenge with obesity sufferers who feel the need to hide what they eat from them, for example, stating that they eat two bags of chips a day when they really eat five.

This of course does not help the dietitian, and he or she can usually tell a lie from the truth when a plan is not working. Dietitians are normally certified in their field and will bring a wealth of experience to the table. They work in both hospital settings and in the community, which is a plus for those who can't leave the house for specific reasons. A dietitian will write up a food plan for you to follow and will suggest taking fatty foods and sugary foods out of your diet. This is an ideal chance to discuss with them what sort of foods you like and whether you prefer vegetables or fruit. Being in a happy mood while eating helps with the digestive process because it triggers the release of the right enzymes and stress hormones.[34]

A dietitian can teach you how to include vegetables and fruit in great-tasting meals, as well as how to cook using the proper techniques and healthiest recipes. Dietitian's don't work exclusively with obese people, but also advise nonobese individuals on what they should and should not eat. For example, research has found that consuming vitamin C helps alleviate symptoms of knee osteoarthritis.[35] A dietician would then encourage osteoarthritis sufferers to eat citrus fruits that contain high amounts of vitamin C. This also works for mental health issues as it is known that certain foods can trigger different states of mind. People who have concerns about illnesses such as night eating syndrome can be helped by a dietitian because the latter can tell the victim when it's best to eat, what to eat before bed, and things to keep in the fridge to stop them from putting on so much weight. However, dieticians should know your economic and familial status before he or she creates any special diet plan for you.[36]

Dietitians are often used for therapy after a mental health issue has been treated. Taking on a lot of things at once make things really tough, especially if your mental health issue is ruling your life. This is why your first trip is often to the psychiatrist, followed by a behavioral therapist, and then finally, a dietitian. By getting better on the inside (improving mentally), you could focus on building your life back up again and boosting personal confidence by losing weight. Eating healthily and sticking to the dietitian's plan will help you lose weight, but incorporating exercise into your life will heal your mental health problems even faster.

Visit your dietitian weekly, or if possible, join a weight-loss boot camp. These camps are mostly for the morbidly obese who find it difficult to adhere to any exercise or diet plan. Boot camps will put you on a very strict diet and could involve several hours of exercise a day. It may seem a harsher option, but people have lost upwards of sixteen pounds by attending these camps.[37]

DRUGS, COUNSELING, AND THE COST OF OBESITY-RELATED PSYCHOLOGY

Your physician or psychologist may feel that your need to lose weight is just as important as your need to have your mental health issue treated. This is where medication enters the picture. Obesity victims will occasionally have other issues that have an added effect, such as high blood pressure, diabetes, and heart disease. These all need attention, and using medications for treatment is generally the road to take so you can focus on your mental health issues. Drugs will be given to help lower blood pressure, while insulin may be given for diabetes (if it is not diet controlled), and a blood thinner if you have severe heart trouble or wound-healing issues. Likewise, there are also a lot of medications offered to help you lose weight. Medication is often given only after you fail to lose weight by joining a diet club or because your BMI is greater than or equal to 30.

More on Drugs

Drugs are prescribed when you need all of your mental energy for focusing on getting better and don't have time to lose weight by routine exercise. Pills are usually taken three times a day after meals. The pills help you lose weight without putting in much effort on your part. Prescription weight loss drugs are much safer than the ones you find in stores or on the Internet and help you to lose weight if you have a psychological basis for your obesity, such as an eating disorder. Keep in mind that these are chemical drugs that have undergone many clinical trials and have been proven to work on your brain. When you eat food, fat is either digested or stored in the body. Stored fat, the type that isn't immediately used for energy, is what makes people obese. The more fat you consume, the more it gets stored and the larger you become. Weight-loss medication works by blocking some of the fat that never goes through digestion and gets rid of it through waste. By complementing these drugs with healthy diet and exercise, your weight loss will go much faster.

Weight-loss pills obtained online are usually designed to speed up your metabolism to burn the calories at greater speeds. This is not a healthy way to lose weight and these pills can become dangerously addictive. They can also fluctuate your energy levels, which is a bad sign for any obese person who suffers from a mental health disorder. By taking the medication prescribed to you, it means that you can focus on getting better mentally. When your psychiatrist or physician believes you are well enough to cope with the weight loss yourself, you will be discharged or referred to a long-term prevention program.

Counseling

Counseling is an amazing opportunity to talk about your obesity issues and your mental health issues. You may find a group in your area that deals with mental health issues and obesity—all rolled into one. Counseling is often very helpful for any mental health issue, not only obesity. It's a good way for discussing your problems and sharing it with everyone. Obesity victims sometimes get caught up "in their own mind" and can't see a way out of their problems, but counselors offer a fresh view of things and suggest different methods to cope with any mental health issues you may be experiencing as an obesity patient. They make you feel better mentally and physically and instill a great sense of hope deep inside of you. Once you realize that you *can* do something about your situation, you can then discuss how to go about treating it yourself. Your counselor will talk about the different options, how your days are normally spent, and how obesity has affected you.

Group counseling is often helpful for people since it can reveal hints and tips on how to cope with mental difficulties. Group counseling allows people to try to help *each other,* not just the individual. In some cases, you have to watch out for competitiveness between members, which can be a good *and* bad result of bringing up personal issues among your peers. By attempting to improve your obesity-related mental health problem in less time, group counseling may mean you're getting better more quickly than normal. Or, it could uncover new mental health issues you thought you never had. In contrast, things may turn out for the best as those who are reluctant to discuss issues will now talk for hours, trying to "vent" and get positive attention from others. The counselor is usually aware of this and will recognize it when it surfaces.

Face-to-face counseling is also very good if you have a really sensitive issue at hand. This type of counseling also works well when you have very low self-esteem or are shy about talking in public. By having a face-to-face session, you can talk about anything and get more quality time. You can talk about sensitive topics with your counselor. There should always be an element of trust between your counselor and yourself as this helps you to release your thoughts. You can also combine both group and individual therapy. Keep in mind that a therapist will ask questions and devise a treatment plan for you to stick to, whereas a counselor is there to listen to you and prompt you to find your own way through the issue by listening to your answers and encouraging you to see the end result.

There is a wide selection of group therapies that you can attend. Some are there for treating mental health problems, some specialize and provide therapy for a specific problem such as OCD, and others focus on obesity and the psychological toll which the disease takes on you. Group and one-on-one counseling are also designed to help you lose weight. The idea is to help you know *why* you are eating— whether it is emotional, habitual, or a mental health disorder—and address it so that the next time you are upset, you don't go running toward the refrigerator.

Costs of Obesity-Related Psychological Problems

Consider the amount of strain that obesity is putting on the health care system. Mental health issues are difficult enough to treat without the addition of a dietitian, eating disorder specialist, group therapy, and gastric band surgery. All of this costs a lot of money, and, even if countries with free health care services are unable to cope with demands, they still have a duty to treat everyone equally. They have to treat the mental health disorder in addition to treating obesity.

THE PROOF OF THE PUDDING IS IN LOVE OR HATRED OF FOOD

If one would talk at such a great length about obesity as it relates to mental health issues, the very *real* food obsession that some people have should be included. When an eating disorder is mentioned, most people think of anorexia. This is incorrect because anything that involves both eating and obsessions can be unofficially considered an eating disorder. While anorexics refuse to eat anything so they can feel in control of their bodies, people with other eating disorders will only eat a certain type of cookie, or only canned foods. These actions may not make any sense to many, but to some, it creates, or at least attempts to create, a perfect world.

A person who cannot eat foods of a certain color, for instance, probably had a prior incident with something of that color before and now has an irrational fear. It's almost similar to the fear people have of harmless spiders. Though mostly an irrational response, people still "freeze" when they see a scary-looking spider running across the floor.[38]

The relationship between food and your mental state is much more than what people give credit for. Some eating disorder victims spend their lives trying to battle obesity while others can't eat enough to keep the weight on. The next time you see an obese person at the ice cream stand and think they shouldn't be there, why not think a bit further? They may not be eating because they like sugary foods, but rather because they literally cannot stop themselves from eating because of a psychological disorder.

Is Gastric Banding Really a Quick Fix?

While this procedure has been discussed in-depth in chapter 4, it is important to know that gastric banding is one of the most unconventional ways of dealing with obesity, especially if the latter is rooted psychologically. These bands are placed over the stomach to make it smaller and make you feel "stuffed" a lot quicker. They get inserted under general anesthesia and require surgery. While in theory the band *does work*, it isn't very suitable for people who have a mental health issue such as an eating disorder. Obesity victims who are severely depressed and need to lose weight to gain some self-esteem and help them with the depression are likely to succeed with a gastric band, while an overeater will probably just damage it by eating too much.[39]

These bands are not permanent fixes, so if you have a relapse and begin to eat heavily again, then you will put the pounds back on. A gastric band will succeed when you are getting help and responding well to mental health treatment. If an obese person is unstable and feels that he or she can binge out at will, then isn't gastric banding only a waste of time? Here's the key: don't look at gastric bands as an "easy way out" simply because you no longer have to diet or exercise to relieve your obesity. Anyone who wishes to put themselves through surgery without a real need should seek medical counseling first. That said, your doctor may decide to send you to a therapist *and* a dietitian before resorting to a band procedure.

THE LAST CALL

Remember that mental health issues and obesity can be approached concurrently. Mental abnormalities such as depression and anxiety can leave you in a hole that will only lead to more weight gain and depression. The first step is to acknowledge that you or a loved one really has a problem. There are warning signs, such as substantial weight gain, odd conduct, and mood swings worthy of concern. Once a problem has been identified, you should seek the help of a general physician or social worker, who will refer you to the appropriate staff and get you the help you require. Depending on the outcome, you will be referred to a psychiatrist, therapist, or counselor to chat about and address your situation. While counselors can help get rid of your addictions, you cannot rely solely on them for your obesity problems, especially since recent research argues that obesity is in fact a result of the body's neurobehavioral processes, and not from personal choices.[40] These processes involve determining your neurological status by checking your behavior. People who conjointly suffer from mental health issues and obesity may see all three of these professionals, which is nothing to worry about since it could just mean that your problems are being approached using all available options.

Note that when an extreme mental disorder is linked to obesity, psychiatric hospitalization may even be required.[41] This again is not as scary as it may seem, since you'll be receiving nonstop care and constant attention to make you better. The key to any physical or mental obstacle is that you keep on top of it, and once treated, don't let it come back. You will eventually get to know the warning signals so keep an eye out and don't go into denial. Find treatment quickly so that you are able to return to normal within a reasonable amount of time.

In the end, you need to understand that obesity-related mental problems are becoming increasingly common. You'll be surprised by who these problems affect without them even knowing. Try to remain a good friend or family member and look out for any warning signs[42] so that your loved ones can receive psychological treatment as soon as possible.

9

BLAME AND GUILT

There are health risks from obesity that make it nearly impossible for people to lose weight.[1] Furthering this problem are of course the food manufacturers. Many food companies try to get people to eat their food so that they can make money, possibly without giving much attention to the well-being of the consumers. They often don't care about the nutritional content of their food, nor is there enough of a focus on people who suffer from the damage caused by unhealthy foods. Major food corporations use many different tactics to get people to purchase and consume their items. They already know about their unhealthy products, but one way to cheaply produce and maximize profit is to use low-grade, unhealthy ingredients. Food manufacturers are tricking the consumer into thinking that their products aren't that bad for them, and one of the tricks is to sell "low-fat" foods.

HAS SOCIETY BEEN BRAINWASHED?

How It All Works

Food manufacturers advertise calorie-rich food by advertising it as "low in fat." The man in a famous submarine sandwich maker's commercials, who apparently lost weight by exercising and switching to the company's trademark sandwich diet, is a prime example of this. The ads don't really focus on the exercise part of this man's diet. Instead, they show the consumer some mouthwatering pictures of their subs and claim that these subs have only around seven grams of fat. This sounds great, but in reality, the sandwich has quite a large amount of calories in it. A typical foot-long sandwich has over 600 calories[2] when adding up all the additional items that don't come standard with it. These items can include soda, chips, and fries. The bread itself contributes 400 calories.[3] Consequently, keep in mind that the man exercised quite extensively. Focus on the importance of working out consistently just like he did.

In addition to using preservatives that make you gain weight[4] and whatever they can find to make their product inexpensive and appealing, food companies try to convince the public that they are on their side and care for their health by occasionally airing commercials that caution against overconsumption of a product. They spend money to promote school sports and physical education programs simply to preserve a superficial sense that they are doing what they can to help fight obesity. When they come under fire, however, they get defensive. It's as if they "help" society just to gain public trust and deflect attention away from the real dangers of their products.[5]

Assumptions Are Not Necessarily Based on Reality

People assume that most of their daily caloric intake comes from the fat in food. This seems to be reasonable, considering that fat is very high in calories. As stated before, fat is the way that the body stores calories, so food fats are almost like dense clusters of calories. An interesting fact about eating fatty foods came to light many years ago. According to a studies that began in the 1960s, the US population received 45 percent of their calories from fat[6] and during that era, 13 percent of Americans were considered obese.[7] Americans now receive 33 percent of their calories from fat,[8] while 34 percent of the population is considered obese.[9] Let's avoid downplaying the reality of obesity and fat since there's a growing concern about the two.

Abstinence from Fat Fuels the Brainwashing Cycle

Fats provide nine calories per gram, so they can be solely responsible for causing obesity.[10] However, your body needs them, and they should account for roughly one-third of the average person's caloric intake. There are four types of naturally occurring fats, and only one of them is consistently processed artificially by food companies in the United States.

Monounsaturated Fats These fats are not harmful to your body. Instead, they should be chosen over all the other types of fats because they are known to lower the risk of cardiovascular disease. There are many health benefits behind monounsaturated fats such as quelling insulin resistance. These fats reduce low-density lipoprotein (LDL) cholesterol, which leads to heart disease. Eating food that contains oleic and monounsaturated fatty acids are great for preventing cardiac disease while reducing cholesterol levels in your blood. Natural foods, which are rich in monounsaturated fats include olive oil, whole grain wheat, nuts, whole milk products, avocados, oatmeal, cereal, peanut butter, canola oil, and seeds. Monounsaturated fats contain nine calories per gram and should be eaten with moderation to avoid getting overweight. They are good for you in small or moderate quantities.[11]

Polyunsaturated Fats These fats are slightly less beneficial than monounsaturated fats but are still useful for the body. Omega-3 fatty acids are found in polyunsaturated fats. These are important because they have anti-inflammatory properties. The body cannot produce omega-3 fatty acids. That's why they are known as essential fatty acids. Furthermore, omega-3 acids are found in very few foods.[12]

Trans Fats These fats are also known as hydrogenated fats. As covered in chapter 6, food manufacturers use trans fat in many of their products. They use this type of fat so the food stays fresh longer. In other words, trans fat is a preservative. It is made through a process called hydrogenation, when vegetable oil is warmed with heated hydrogen. Trans fats are not the same as saturated fats. From a scientific standpoint, the term *trans* refers to the arrangement of atoms in a molecule of fat, opposite to the term *cis*. In contrast to saturated fats, trans fats are artificially processed and created to prolong shelf life in store-bought products by combining hydrogen atoms to vegetable oil. Trans fats are found in many baked goods, chips, crackers, and cakes. It can also be found in many fried foods. Trans fats are known to increase your bad cholesterol levels while lowering your good ones. Because trans fats are solid, they have a dangerous chance at clogging arteries. These fats lead to considerable weight gain, and that is why it's very important to check the nutrition label for them. Check the label thoroughly to know whether the item has trans fat in it.[13]

Saturated Fats   The fourth type of fat is saturated fat. This type of fat is commonly added by meat-producing companies. It is unnecessary for the body to consume saturated fat because the body can produce the required amount if enough of the good fats are already there. Too much saturated fat intake increases the chance of coronary heart disease. Consumption of saturated fats, which have almost but not the same negative effects as trans fats, increases the chances of getting heart disease.[14]

THE MARKETING FACTOR

False Nutrition

Another way that food manufacturers contribute to obesity is through nutrition labels. There are many tricks that food manufacturers use to make their food look healthier. Food companies use nutrition labels based on a single serving. A package usually contains a lot more than just one serving. A single serving is usually far less than anyone would eat in one sitting. For instance, Gatorade has 50 calories[15] per serving, but there are 2.5 servings per bottle. There are really 125 calories for every 20-ounce bottle, so many people might normally drink a full bottle's worth of calories in one sitting without really knowing.

See You after the Elections

Food companies have lobbied congressmen to get laws concerning nutrition labels passed in their favor. Businesses no longer have to include certain substances in nutrition labels if it is below a certain amount. People can be tricked into eating food that they think is far healthier for them when it is not. Trans fat is a perfect example of this. If an item has less than one half gram of trans fat per serving, it is considered to be free from any trans fat, and food manufacturers don't have to include it on the nutrition label. People will end up consuming trans fat in spite of clinical recommendations to avoid it. The consumer thinks he or she is getting a very healthy meal, but is instead eating far more than the recommended amount of food.

Food manufacturers are trying to be successful and make a profit. Realistically, they want to protect their interests at all costs. Through advertising and donations to schools and charitable institutions, the companies are able to deflect some attention from the unhealthiness of their products. That said, government is the only organization with the power to instill guidelines by which the food manufacturers must abide. In an effort to get congressmen on their side, food businesses spend money and endorse politicians' campaigns. Politicians help get bills in the corporations' favor passed. Since most lawmakers don't have the near-endless fiscal resource that the food industry has, companies are the ones holding tremendous power. In one fiscal quarter of 2010 alone, a soda industry giant spent $1.2 million on lobbying against more strenuous nutrition laws.[16] It would be very easy for government to place tough restrictions on nutritional requirements and outlawing certain substances, but they don't because the food manufacturers indirectly have lawmakers in their pockets. Another proposal that a congressman put forward was to "traffic light" food products. It would be easier for the consumer to tell what's healthy and what isn't by the color of the nutrition label. For instance, if a package contains a green label, it is healthy; yellow, it is moderately healthy; and red, it is unhealthy. Once again, food manufacturers flexed their monetary might and were able to successfully lobby enough support to stop that bill from getting passed.[17]

Food manufacturers use the government almost without any limits to their benefit. The manufacturers know that as people start to know the things about their food, the population will want some of these harmful substances banned. In a way, it is legal for food manufacturers to lie about the ingredients in their products. The manufacturers worm their way through the loopholes to make a product that is very appealing to the public, but it is really far different than what's on the label.

Here's another example of how politics are partly responsible. For food to be classified as low fat, it must contain less than three grams of fat per serving. This seems reasonable, but the Food and Drug

Administration (FDA) does not have a rule that specifies what a serving size must be.[18] That is at the food manufacturers' discretion. It allows for businesses to imply that any given food is low fat. Food corporations could make a high-fat item but make the serving size so small that there is less than three grams of fat per serving, and then advertising right on the label that it's low in fat. This is a really easy way for food companies to trick consumers into eating what they think is healthy, low-fat food. In reality, consumers are getting something not much different from its "high-fat" counterpart.

Another law that food manufacturers must abide by, which appears to be a good idea, is that they must list ingredients on the food label in order of decreasing quantity. Food companies have found a loophole in this law also. A prime example of this is jam. For jam to be purely made of fruit, the name of the fruit must be on the top of the list of ingredients, meaning it has the highest quantity in the jam, right? No. "Pure fruit" jams can have as little as 30 percent[19] fruit, and the rest be made of syrup from cheap fruit juices. Roughly 70 percent of the jam is made from sugary syrups.[20] Food manufacturers will label their products as "20 percent fruit," but the sugary syrup that the product is based on will be made from various amounts of apple juice, grape juice, and pine-apple extract. The manufacturer can claim the jam is pure fruit because, technically, the ingredient in the highest quantity is fruit.

INTERNAL AFFAIRS

What Goes On in Factories?

As trans fats turn increasingly unpopular, food companies are craving for a substitute. With baked goods, the texture and taste comes from hydro-genated oil, which is how to get trans fats. That is why food manufactur-ers in the past were using a process called interesterification. Through this process, food manufacturers are able to create something that has the same effect as hydrogenated oils, but since many people don't rec-ognize it, they don't know it hurts. Food companies use hydrogenated and interesterified oils to give people the softness and texture they love in baked and fried goods. Since hydrogenated oils are chemical precur-sors to trans fats, they are slowly becoming banned as obesity victims are starting to realize their potential danger. By including interesterified oils, food manufacturers are labeling their products as trans fat free, but still give the consumer the same taste. This all sounds great, but in reality, interesterified oils have similar side effects as hydrogenated oils.

Here are two major "side effects" that interesterified oils are guilty of: The first is that interesterified oils lower HDL cholesterol and boost your harmful "bad" cholesterol in the body. That in turn increases your chances of getting heart disease. Interesterified oils also provide more calories than regular fats do. Food manufacturers are contributing to obesity by using a different process that doesn't have to be disclosed on the nutrition label, but is still genuinely harmful for the body.[21]

Troublemaking Stickers

Food corporations mislabel their product to entice obesity sufferers to consume more of it. People who are trying to make an effort to eat healthy may not be getting the healthy food they think they are because the label could be misinterpreted. Recently, the FDA has been trying to crack down on this kind of misrepresentation because it is contributing to obesity at an alarming speed. You can't make a healthy choice if you don't know the actual nutritional information associated with the product. Sometimes, food manufacturers charge more for a low-fat alternative but mislabel its actual fat content, saying it is low fat but really having the same fat content as the "high-fat" product.[22]

Corporations omit a lot of information about their food processing techniques from their labels. Most store-bought salmon is unhealthier than one is led to believe. People assume that salmon is very healthy because it contains omega-3 fatty acids, protein, and many other nutrients. Salmon caught directly from natural waters is good for you because it contains nutrients. Food manufacturers take advantage of this belief because most salmon purchased in stores is farmed, not caught in the wild. The salmon are hatched in a plastic tray, raised in crowded, unsanitary cages underwater, artificially fattened, and treated with antibiotics and pesticides. As if that weren't enough, the salmon are fed a substance that artificially dyes their meat pink.[23] This pigment contains canthaxanthin, which used to be used for tanning lotions, but was outlawed for human use because it causes serious eye problems and eventually makes you go blind in high dosages. At greater amounts, canthaxanthin causes aplastic anemia, which is a potentially fatal blood disorder. Food manufacturers make food that looks natural and appealing by using artful stickers, but in reality are lying about the healthiness of the product by omitting important facts.[24]

TOXIC COMMITMENTS

The Chemical Verdict

Fifty years ago, people ate many of the same foods as they do now, so why were people far less obese back then? Part of this can be contributed to the fact that chemicals are being added by food industries today. Chemicals used as additives are very damaging to the human body and are also contributing to obesity. Fatteners are called obesogens[25] and many recent studies have showed that these chemicals are causing obesity. Obesogens disrupt the functions of your hormonal system. These hormones control appetite, digestion, and burning of energy. Obesogens are very detrimental to your health, and they are known to cause heart disease, diabetes, high cholesterol, and obesity. Obesogens find their way into your foods in the form of pesticides. Farm-raised fish and commercially grown fruits have these obesogens.[26]

Paper or Plastic?

Plastic compounds are another source of obesogens. Many containers are made with plastic, from microwavable trays to bottles, and each one of these are contributing to the obesity problems of the world today. Antibiotic farm feed contains obesogens, and they are given to chicken and farm-raised fish because the animals are raised in tight, unnatural conditions. Obesogens are also found in hormones that are periodically added to food.

Hormones

Food hormones are another way in which companies contribute to obesity. Again, food manufacturers are chasing monetary profit. The way to make it in the meat industry for instance, is to fatten the animals and make them as heavy as possible. It's a common practice for food manufacturers to add growth hormones to animals such as pigs, cows, turkeys, and chickens. Studies have shown that growth hormone can be absorbed through what you eat.[27] Therefore, the hormones that manufacturers are feeding to animals, which are being consumed all the time, are being transferred to the body. The problem with this is that people don't grow taller after reaching physical maturity. The only way for your body to grow is outward. It's very straightforward. People are in part becoming more obese because they are eating food that is doused with growth hormones, merely because manufacturers want their products to look better for consumers.

THE BUSINESS OF OBESITY: FOR BETTER OR FOR WORSE

Marketing Gurus

The economics of obesity will be covered in the following chapter, but for now, let's investigate how Corporate America itself is making people fat. Food manufacturers go to great lengths to contribute to obesity, and advertising campaigns are one of the oldest tricks in the book. Companies need to sell their product, and the more product they sell, the more money they make. One way they do that is by advertising their food as being very low in fat. As discussed earlier, their ads are more likely to be untrue. In reality, you would still eat as poorly as you would if you ate the other high-fat product. When people consume less fat, they feel better about themselves and what they are eating. Therefore, they are prone to eat unhealthily with more meals on the horizon.

Furthermore, companies direct their advertising schemes toward both adults and children. They hold contests and give kids rewards when they collect enough cans or boxes of a product. Simply put, it is very difficult to get any tangible reward from this. Food manufacturers also advertise with beautiful women, famous athletes, and others who are idolized in society, just to get certain products across to both adults and children. Celebrities use very little of the product, but the commercials convince people on the contrary. Many people use products just to be like the celebrity that is apparently using it, but without understanding that these cultural icons only exist virtually in the consumers' personal lives.

Food businesses prefer to target their advertisements at children, since children are the most susceptible to the power of suggestion. Corporations like to prey on the innocence of children and like to take advantage of any persuasive power that children hold over their parents. Food manufacturers know what children like to eat. Therefore, they advertise to children with cartoons and show food that is loaded with sugar. Children may not know the dangers of eating sugary, unhealthy foods. They know they like the food, so they beg their parents to give them what they want. Parents are willing to comply for a multitude of reasons. Children and parents don't know that once someone becomes severely obese, it becomes nearly impossible for him or her to return to a healthy weight without the right approach. Food corporations are contributing to obesity by convincing kids to eat their unhealthy product, after which the children are getting stuck inside the cycle of obesity that was mentioned earlier.[28]

Judging Food by Its Cover

Food manufacturers also know that their product won't appeal to everyone, especially when someone can make a similar item at home. The food companies do ridiculous things to make their product look very appetizing in their commercials. They make steam come out of a reheated item because they know everybody loves a hot meal. They will spray the product to make it look moist and do a lot of other things to it.

Think about when you go through your nearest drive-thru. How great do all of their products appear before you actually receive the meal? Usually, it looks dull and bland once you hold it in your hands. Food manufacturers do the same thing in their commercials. They want people to feel the urge to buy their product, either now or later. To leave a lasting impression, the corporations make their food look irresistible. It is a ploy to get people to consume their product, irrespective of whether or not it's healthy. Using the power of cosmetics to make their food look irresistible, they are contributing to obesity by making people want their food no matter the harm.

Food companies want to keep customers in the dark about how they are contributing to the massive obesity problem. They don't want you to know how unhealthy the commercially prepared food is for them. They prefer not to let you know the facts of the matter or the laws about presenting information on the nutrition label. They keep you from knowing the unsanitary conditions where livestock is raised, and how they artificially dye products to get them to look tastier.

Fast food restaurants are some of the worst offenders here. Consumers choose their food not only because it's going to taste good, but because it's appealing to the eye. Food businesses create an amazing picture of every meal on the menu—so amazing in fact—that the consumer can almost taste, smell, and imagine devouring it. This is the companies' objective since the real product is typically a far cry from that which is shown on TV.[29]

Don't Go with the Rest of the Crowd

Society itself is the fast food manufacturer's advantage. As society gets more modern, it turns into a fast-paced machine. People don't have time to take their foot off of the gas pedal. There is always something involved beyond the taste. They stay up later and spend more time on what they consider to be more important. Though responsible for causing obesity, fast food has the advantage of being constant and convenient. Restaurants usually close at reasonable hours so if someone is busy until after 10 pm, they have to eat something at home or opt for fast food. Individuals want shorter lunches so they can be on the clock more and make more money, so they subconsciously choose the convenience of fast food. Not only is fast food easy and quick, it seems like there is a franchise on every corner. You don't have to drive far to find a fast food meal. Neither is it going to be too expensive.

As if things are not already going in the wrong direction, the ingredients that food companies use are very low quality when it comes to recommended nutrient levels. Everything is either cooked in fat or deep fried. Everyone wants to get a soda, which is filled with sugar and calories. Worst of all, serving sizes at these places keep getting larger. Everywhere you go, it's, "Would you like to super size that?" or, "Would you like a jumbo meal," or whatever the nickname they use for extra-large orders. Food manufacturers prefer that because they profit when people put in such orders. These mega-size meals have over 1,000 calories, half the daily allotment for an average-size human being. Trans fats are very common in fast food. Although some fast food companies are cutting down on trans fats, there are still high levels of trans fats in all items found on the menu, especially fried items. Many food companies are reverting to the equally dangerous *interesterified* oils. The reduction in trans fats could just mean that fast food chains are not making their meals any healthier. Instead, the companies are making the food appear and sound healthier.

THE BEVERAGE SAGA BEGINS

The Soda Guilt

Serving large and extra-large sodas is the norm for fast food companies. If a 12 ounce can of soda has approximately 140 calories,[30] then large fountain sodas (32 ounces) each have at least 400, which would account for somewhere between 20 and 25 percent of an average person's caloric intake. At the midpoint of the twentieth century, Americans were consuming four times as much milk as soda. Now, Americans drink four times as much soda as milk. Soda is a major contribution to obesity in America. One of the problems is that the body responds differently to soda than it does to food.[31]

When you eat, your body releases a combination of hormones which signal that the stomach is getting full. When your blood sugar is lowered and your stomach empty, your body releases a hormone called ghrelin, which signals the brain that it's time to eat again. When you consume soda, you have to deal with a massive dose of calories *and* a huge increase in sugar. Your sugar level rises rapidly once you drink soda. Your body goes into panic mode and overcompensates to correct the dilemma by releasing insulin which breaks down the sugar. By overcompensating, the insulin breaks down too much sugar, and the blood sugar level drops. The body releases ghrelin and other hormones, making the person want to eat again. Food companies design their products to affect ghrelin levels, among other appetite-regulating hormones. Consequently, you end up with a fluctuating diet once you routinely start drinking soda.[32]

Added Fructose

Scientists believe that another big problem with soda and many other sweet foods is the use of high-fructose corn syrup. The syrup is a very popular substitute to sugar because it's cheaper and extends the shelf life of beverages. With the increase in consumption of fruit juice and soda, food and drink manufacturers are using it often and people are consuming more of it. Peer-reviewed research indicates that high-fructose corn syrup contributes to obesity.[33] When people consume the same amount of calories but consume different types of sugar (e.g., sucrose versus fructose) the person that consumes the high-fructose corn syrup tends to be more obese. Add this to the fact that more liquids that are sweetened with high-fructose corn syrup are being ingested, which leads to greater numbers of obese people. Children are especially in danger of this.

More on Sugary Drinks

Because children crave sweet and sugary products, they consume large amounts of juice and soda. Unlike food manufacturers, many parents are unaware of the inherent dangers of sweetened juice and soda and make the two readily available for their children. If you were to decrease your intake of juice or soda by two cups a day, you would decrease your daily caloric intake by over 200 calories, and therefore, lose over thirty-two pounds in the course of a year. It is difficult to monitor children all the time. Children spend time in school where there are soda machines. They spend time over at their friends' homes where they might have access to soda and juice. Children also spend time at home where they have access to similar items. They could walk to the local market and buy it themselves if they so choose. Aside from the instant, constant access, it is a known fact that food manufacturers market to children who are susceptible to certain marketing tactics. That's why it is not easy to free the youngsters from the habit of drinking soda and juice.

There's a lot more to the story here: carbohydrates and glutens. While a study has found that there is no correlation between addiction to carbs (sugar) and eating disorders,[34] carbohydrates in general are known to cause weight gain. Keep in mind that many sugary drinks continue to make up Americans' diets. Carbohydrates can be found in products such as cakes, ice cream, and potato chips, just to name a few. However, carbohydrate imitators are substances such as alcohol and sugar substitutes. Food companies add carbohydrate imitators to their products all the time. When someone consumes too many of these imitators, the body starts to crave foods with carbohydrates. Excessive carbohydrate consumption yields a similar reaction to high-fructose corn syrup. The body releases too much insulin and the blood sugar level plummets, causing you to feel hungry and eat more food. Some carbohydrates break down quickly, while others take a lot longer to break down.

Whether you drink "fast" or "slow" carbohydrates, your ongoing weight gain does not accelerate any faster than it already is. "Fast" carbs pertain to easily digestible sugars, and "slow" would mean the opposite. It would seem that you could consume only the "fast" carbohydrates and be fine, but people who consume more "fast" carbohydrates tend to accumulate fat a lot more easily. The weight gain may be the same, but the type of fat is different and the results are not too great.

Glutens are proteins that are found in wheat, rye, barley, and oat products. They are also found in some breads, alcohol, and cereal, just to name a few. Glutens cause the body to release chemicals called exorphins. These molecules have addictive properties (since they are derived from opioids) and, in turn, signal to the brain to crave more gluten products. It's as if you are unintentionally eating something that makes you hungrier.[35]

When food industries produce sugary drinks with low quality ingredients, they know that their product won't satisfy your appetite upfront. They add fillers such as sugar, starches, and carbs to make sure you're satisfied, even though it's probably just healthier to keep the meal the way it is.

The problem is that people naturally don't like meals that leave them hungry because they would otherwise lack any need to eat. Americans want hearty portions. School cafeterias serve as prime examples of this. Schools are on such a tight budget that they are forced to use poor quality ingredients to make sure each child has a full stomach and (supposedly) gets all the day's necessary calories. They fill the children up with corn syrup and carbohydrates, both of which are scientifically proven to have links to obesity.[36]

Caffeine and the Unbounded Quest for Energy

It's not just the increase in calories, sugar, and salt that is the problem with caffeinated drinks. Caffeine is very bad for a child's development, and food corporations know that. Caffeine can be very problematic for children who have more than a small dosage. The drug can lead to a myriad of medical problems such as osteoporosis and hypertension. It can make children restless and inattentive in school. Caffeine is addictive, and when people consume too much of it, they need their daily fix just to get started in the morning. Children are in danger because the energy drinks and sodas they consume contain more caffeine than the average grownup needs. This intake of caffeine in a smaller body leads to far greater dependency. It is very hard to kick the habit, and once children are sucked in, they will continue to find sources to get their caffeine. This means that they will consume more soda and energy drinks and will continue their typical caloric intake and eventually increase it.

Children are starting to consume mass quantities of energy drinks that are presently very popular in society. It's an easy way to get energy in something that tastes reasonably good. In fact, a leading energy drink company has inventive marketing strategies to get the public to enjoy their beverage. The company has amusing commercials that usually depicts someone escaping from an awkward situation simply by taking a sip of their product. They also sponsor air races, humorous contests, and extreme sports, which kids love because of all the action. Though a study noted improved memory, cognitive, and physical performance from consuming this company's flagship energy drink, other research suggests that energy drinks in general may be responsible for the growing obesity problem altogether.[37]

Since energy drinks are much sweeter than coffee, children are turning to them rather than consuming coffee. Most adults agree that children should stay away from coffee since the caffeine is too much for a child to handle and will stunt the child's growth and development. However, some parents are content with a child drinking soda or energy drinks that contain similar amounts of caffeine. Energy drinks and sodas are worse than coffee because they contain many more calories and sugary additives, including the notorious high-fructose corn syrup noted earlier. You may think you are giving a treat to a child, but are really providing your child a disservice.

The Salt Notion

Beverage consumption is also responsible for world obesity because of the salt intake. Medical research has shown that salt levels have a very strong correlation with obesity.[38] According to a lengthy study, salt intake increased by 50 percent between the 1980s and mid-1990s.[39] The problem with a salt increase in your diet is that is makes people very thirsty. Hydrating drinks that athletes consume, for instance, are supposed to quench one's thirst. However, consumers are usually just as thirsty after drinking one because of the salt in the drink. By increasing daily salt intake, people get thirstier. This increases the amount of beverage consumed daily. People consume more calories because of the increased amount of drinks consumed daily. This is one way in which salt is contributing to the obesity epidemic.[40]

PRESERVE LIFE, NOT OBESITY

Preservatives, which food manufacturers use with ease, are one of the largest contributing factors to the obesity problem. Food manufacturers like to employ preservatives in almost anything they produce because it makes their product taste better and have a longer shelf life. These companies don't lose as much income to products that go bad while waiting on the store shelves. Items such as frozen foods, cake mixes, and canned goods all contain some sort of preservative. Each preservative needs to get approved by the FDA before it can be used publicly. There are plenty of approved preservatives used today in everything from fruits to ice cream.

Monosodium Glutamate

Better known as MSG, this preservative is added to a variety of foods as a flavor enhancer, usually in fast food places. The FDA has concluded that MSG is safe, but many scientists agree that it is unhealthy. MSG has many side effects including increased dreaming and drowsiness. Its most devastating effect however, is obesity. Scientists carried out an extensive study in rural China where most people grow, raise, and prepare their own food.[41] Participants were broken down into three groups based on their MSG intake. Among the three groups, the scientists found that the group that consumed the most MSG was three times more likely to be obese than the next group. There are three factors that can explain this phenomenon, and all three play a part. First, MSG makes food taste better. People eat more foods with MSG simply because they crave the taste. Second, MSG as a preservative causes the body to release more insulin into the blood stream. This causes your body to break down too much sugar and lowers the blood sugar level. Your body is tricked into thinking that it needs to eat more just to gain enough energy to get through the day.

MSG not only attempts to make food taste better, but has addictive properties similar to narcotics. This is the third reason. When people consume food with MSG, they get a euphoric feeling, causing them to overeat. They use foods with high amounts of MSG to artificially sweeten everything. They know that both children and adults love sweet flavors. They also know which additives, such as trans fats, make the texture of food really appetizing. Even though they know that trans-fat is unhealthy, they still use it because it gets them the results they desire.

MSG has highly addictive properties. MSG works similar to when narcotics react inside of you. It causes the body to release increased amounts of adrenaline, dopamine, and serotonin. Look through your cabinet and see how often MSG will be on the nutrition label. It is in everything from canned soup to potato chips. Ask restaurants for ingredient lists and you will notice MSG is hidden in almost every item on the menu. Food manufacturers admit that they use it because it causes people to eat more of their products.

APPEARANCE AGAINST REALITY

Food companies will do whatever it takes to make sure their interests are protected. They will also do whatever it takes to make sure they generate massive revenue so they deliver to you whatever they choose.

They give you something that tastes great—something irresistible. The more consumers eat, the more money that food companies will make. They use subtle tricks to make sure that the same products continue to stock the shelves. They make sure that people are still satisfied with it, and that people still feel the need to eat these products.

Does the food industry want the American populace to turn obese so that people will consume more and slowly gain larger appetites? If anything, food corporations use doctored pictures to make the product look tempting, as if you can taste it by literally licking your television screen. The corporations try to use low-fat food to assuage people's guilt, and thus obesity victims overeat because they think they are losing weight by consuming just one healthy meal. Food businesses use promotions and have famous people endorse their products to make you believe everyone could be famous in a very short time. They do that knowing quite well that once someone becomes obese, it's tough to ditch the pounds. They know that obese people are good for their business so they get people addicted to the products. They use ingredients that make people crave what they have, such as carbs, which are addictive, and people tend to overeat because of the amount of insulin that carbohydrates make your body release.

Food corporations are constantly doing extensive research behind the scenes to separate unhealthy foods from healthy ones, but why do they still choose to use obesity-causing ingredients? The answer is this: it's what they claim consumers prefer. The manufacturers use inferior ingredients because it is cheaper, but they add in "fillers" to spruce up the taste. It is as if people are forced to favor something that they are not naturally designed to like.

Food businesses want consumers who don't ask questions and just accept and be happy with whatever is placed in front of them. The companies simply want to "fatten" the planet. They continue to increase portion size with lower prices and trick you into thinking a container has only one serving, though each package usually has multiple. People eat a lot more than they should and consume more of food companies' products but sadly, these companies are the ones gaining from all of this. All things considered, you have to remember that your health may not be on food companies' minds, but should definitely be on yours.

10

THE ECONOMICS OF OBESITY

Economies are typically made up of financial activities taking place within a nation's own borders. The economic condition of a country, no matter its geographic location, has a certain level of influence on generalized global markets and specific domestic markets. Economics can be separated into two categories: the microeconomic (small-scale) and macroeconomic (large-scale) levels.

At the microeconomic level, the basic factors are supply and demand. To begin determining the economic impact of obesity in the world, you look at supply and demand that's linked to food production. This involves the economic food-market trends. The following is a quick review of what happens when there are changes in food supply and demand.

SUPPLY AND DEMAND: MICROECONOMICS OF OBESITY

Two things take place because of changes in the supply and demand of money: inflation and deflation. When there is a rising price for foods and services, inflation often occurs. Because of a decrease in currency value, the purchasing power of a country will take a dive and interest rates will subsequently rise in times of inflation.

Inflation

There are mainly two types of inflation affecting the food industry:

1. Demand-pull inflation: This type of inflation happens when people want to buy more food than the economy can actually produce. This usually happens in a strengthening economy, and because the demand is so much greater than the amount of food being produced, food prices go up.[1]
2. Cost-push inflation: This type of inflation happens when the prices of raw materials used to produce finished goods increases. This is the main cause of cost-push inflation. The food companies or suppliers need to increase their selling price to compensate for their own buying costs. This causes food retailers, such as grocery chains, to pay more for getting the goods. They also have to increase selling prices to make up the difference from the end user, which in this case is you, the consumer.[2]

It's difficult to imagine how obesity could negatively affect an economy. To obtain the statistics of inflation, the prices of thousands of consumer items, such as groceries, are evaluated each month. These goods are symbolically called the "market basket" to represent the economy of a country. The costs of these items are compared from time to time. This comparison will result in a price index, which takes into account the price of a certain item in a given period.

In the United States, two price indexes are used to measure the country's inflation:[3]

- Consumer Price Index (CPI): This index measures the change of price from the purchaser's point of view. When it comes to food suppliers, the index measures price changes in foods typically found in local grocers and international retailers.
- Producer Price Index (PPI): This index measures the change of price from the seller's standpoint. It measures price change in selling prices of goods and services produced by domestic producers.

Deflation

Simply put, deflation is the opposite of inflation. Deflation ensues when prices of goods and services decline continuously. Such a slope will actually cause a higher supply of food but with a slower market demand. As a result, demand comes to a standstill in wake of the higher purchasing power customers hold. Food prices have to drop to match the limited demand. Usually, CPI is the preferred index to use when calculating the inflation rate.

DECISION MAKERS: MACROECONOMICS OF OBESITY

At macroeconomic levels in general, the two types of economic factors a government normally addresses are monetary and fiscal policies. The principle idea of monetary policy is that price levels are determined by the amount of money available. That means the foundation of monetary policy is, in a way, the money supply. The real goal is to maintain the economy's growth at a steady pace without huge fluctuations and price instability.

The principal driver of all monetary policy decisions in America is the Federal Reserve Board. The Federal Reserve Board oversees the US money reserve when the federal government chooses to either expand or tighten our monetary supply. All the above situations, along with the actions of the government, affect the economy. Lower interest rates indicate an easier access to financial credits. Food businesses will usually try to expand under these circumstances. Such an expansion will get the country's economy going. Similarly, lower tax rates will lead to more food consumption as society has a lot more money to spend.[4]

Economic Indicators for Obesity

There are several economic factors contributing to monetary policies. Analysts normally use these economic factors to determine the economic situation of any specific time frame:

- Leading indicators: These economic indicators predict changes in the economy. However, these indicators are relatively inaccurate when compared to others. Leading indicators include industrial food production rates and averages of weekly unemployment insurance claims.

- Lagging indicators: These indicators measure changes in the economy, especially when it begins to follow a particular trend. Lagging indicators are good for analyzing the future performance of a country's economy. Lagging indicators include interest rates, unemployment rates, corporate profit, and labor cost per unit of output.[5]
- Coincident indicators: This is an economic factor that changes directly with the health of the economy. Coincident indicators therefore give the best depiction of the current economy. Coincident indicators include non-agricultural employment and personal income.[6]

The above indicators have a great influence on both the domestic and global food market.

Economic Status and Personal Health

So far, this chapter has discussed the fundamental knowledge of economics in order to refresh what factors affect a certain market. In general, each individual impacts the world's economy in a small but definite way, and in turn, the economic market affects everyone's lives. Experts have investigated a causal effect of obesity and the economy, and, through medical studies, have documented a positive correlation between good health and desirable economic status.[7] There's quite a debate out there about the connection between economic status and personal health.

Obesity research suggests a cause-and-effect scenario that can travel in many directions. For example, high-income consumers tend to invest more in their own health. When income increases, they pay for effective nutrition, healthier diets, better health care, and improved hygiene. A healthier person is more likely to be alert and energetic and will probably be more productive and have a higher standard of living.

To a greater extent, attention has been given to the increase in personal health care costs because of problems which obesity is responsible for. This topic is likely to become more popular in the future because the impact of health care costs for obesity on the large economic scale will become more obvious. Valuing your own health should be a main concern, and this involves allocating your resources and finding the right balance between your health and personal finances.

The reality of obesity is that it is a major life-threatening situation with the same serious risk factors as diabetes, high blood pressure, and related problems. Therefore, the disease should be given the same medical *and* financial attention as other diseases. The National Center for Health Statistics presents data for the United States suggesting that about 30 percent of adults older than twenty are obese.[8] That accounts for more than 60 million people in America. Consider how this affects a US economy that, at the time of this writing, has to provide for more than 311 million people.[9]

THE YOUNGSTERS' STORIES

In addition to adult obesity trends, there is also the shocking increase in the rate of obesity among children. A 2008 update reports that 10 percent of the world's kids are either obese or overweight.[10] Although research about the negative economic effects of obesity has remained a challenge in the United States, the obesity problem *has* been noticed and labeled as a life-threatening situation. A lot of attention has been given to the increase in personal health care costs linked to diseases such as childhood obesity, but this topic is likely to become more popular in the future. The impact of health care costs of childhood obesity at the macroeconomic level has a lot to do with the worldwide obesity problem. However, valuing your own health should also be a priority, and this means finding the right balance between your personal finances and health.

YOUR BANK IS CALLING YOU

Type 2 diabetes, high blood pressure, and heart disease are becoming more frequent due to obesity. Just decades ago, these illnesses were common only among adults. Using public health records, experts have found that medical expenses used for treating health problems caused by obesity and being overweight makes up about 10 percent of total US expenditures. That is over $100 billion,[11] half of which is paid for by Medicaid and Medicare.

The Economics of Obesity and the Cost of Living

Obesity shortens your lifespan and could negatively affect your career. Since governments are normally there to serve their nation, it is important for the former to reduce the economic burden created by obesity. Obesity has led to many long-term problems that have drastically risen. Both federal and state governments are likely to go bankrupt because of the costs of obesity and its subsequent illnesses.[12]

In fact, an experiment shows that obese people spend much more on health care than healthy people.[13] In the obese group that was studied, more finances would go toward treating weight gain in as little as three years. However, chronic illnesses such as diabetes, asthma, and heart disease are also taken into account here, so in this situation, you cannot really put all the blame on obesity. Even depression can take place when there are other economic, medical, and personal stressors in someone's life. Medicare made a statement that health care costs and treatments for obesity will be paid for using taxpayer money. This suggests that public funds will soon be depleted if things continue the way they are.

Diseases linked directly to obesity can be prevented if proper care is taken, but everyone needs to help. To slow down obesity, government, parents, schools, and related organizations should all get involved. To prevent obesity early, the education system must get involved. Children should learn about good eating habits, as well as the benefits of exercising. Nowadays, children eat junk food until they're stuffed instead of eating a proper meal. Most of the time, these children come from families with no concept of a healthy diet or families that do not monitor and promote better eating habits. Proper education about diet and nutrition should be included in every school's curriculum in order for children to have a good fundamental knowledge of what they eat. Since children are a massive share of the world's population, you can avoid the toll which obesity takes on the global economy if you educate them about healthier eating habits.

People who are deprived of wealth usually have a difficult time affording basic necessities and have to decide between spending on food or using hard earned money to pay the rent. While you might think that these folks are malnourished and are severely underweight, you must remember that many of them live right here in North America—not some other continent. To make matters worse, cheaper groceries and foods don't really provide proper nutrition, as most of the affordable options are overprocessed by commercial procedures. They are mostly high in fat and sodium, but low in vitamins and minerals. This is the main reason there's a direct correlation between economic poverty and obesity.

Nowadays, families with average incomes are struggling to balance great food with the right level of nutrition. Unhealthy foods can often cost less than healthier alternatives. Even membership prices for local health clubs have shot up over the years. If exercise facilities don't cater to the lower and middle class, most of us won't even be able to afford a simple workout, especially if there are no local parks or safe outdoor areas for exercise. On a larger scale, this could be contributing to obesity. Incentives should be offered to encourage people to stay healthy. If the government can provide things such as parks and city pools, perhaps it could also design low-cost local fitness initiatives through parks and recreation departments.

REDUCING THE ECONOMIC COSTS ISN'T FUTILE

Training and education must be used to avoid both obesity itself and rising health care costs. As obesity increases, many organizations should educate their employees about how to live a healthy lifestyle. Some companies have on-site gyms or offer discounted fitness-club memberships for their employees. Corporations can also give away healthy snacks instead of junk food to their employees to release work-related tension. This is in fact a win-win situation for everyone because employees in poor health might not do as well as those who are already fit.[14] This problem can lead to increased health insurance spending, a risk for the organization *and* society itself. In the end, training employees to get fit and stay healthy is a good way to fight obesity and ultimately strengthen the economy.

A nutrition expert at the World Bank, believes the growing trend of obesity could cut off the gross domestic product (GDP) of a country.[15] Malnutrition takes away 2 to 3 percent of the GDP in the hardest-hit regions. For example, in 2000, obesity cost California $22 billion.[16] This figure included indirect costs and was said to have a massive impact on the economy since obesity can reduce life expectancy, too. A British study predicts that men would live five years less by 2050 if obesity continues to grow at its current rate.[17]

To come up with economic costs of obesity, a few researchers published their findings in a peer-reviewed journal.[18] Many consider their research to be the first reliable study about the economic cost of obesity using simple calculation methods. The investigators took into consideration obesity-related illnesses such as high blood pressure, coronary heart disease (CHD), Type 2 diabetes, gallbladder disease, breast cancer, osteoarthritis, and endometrial cancers. They divided total costs of each of these illnesses into direct medical costs for prevention, diagnosis, treatment services, home care, and the like. Indirect healthcare costs included costs resulting from a reduction of physical and financial productivity.

Table 10.1 provides an additional breakdown of disease costs.

The total expense of obesity and overweightness to the US economy in 1995 was $99.2 billion, of which about $50 billion went to direct costs and about $45 billion went to indirect costs.[19] Because the diseases listed in the first column of table 10.1 are strongly linked to obesity, you could conclude that obesity has a major influence on the US economy. The

Table 10.1. Costs of Obesity-Related Diseases to the Economy

Illness	Direct cost in billions (approximate)	Indirect cost in billions (approximate)
Type 2 diabetes	30	31
Coronary heart disease	7	N/A
Osteoarthritis	4	12
High blood pressure	3	N/A
Colon cancer	1	2
Postmenopausal breast cancer	0.85	1.5
Endometrial cancer	0.29	0.5

Source: A. Wolf and G. Colditz, "Current Estimates of the Economic Cost of Obesity in the United States," *Obesity Research* 6 (1998): 97–106.

researchers came up with an important estimate by using 1994 National Health Interview Survey (NHIS) data. They pointed out that about 40 million workdays were lost nationally each year due to obesity-related causes. About 240 million restricted-activity days, 90 million bedridden days, and some 60 million physician visits were devoted to obesity. These figures, when converted to percentages of the US population, are: (1) around 35 percent for restricted activity days, (2) around 30 percent for bed days, (3) about 50 percent for lost workdays, and (4) about 85 percent for physician visits.[20]

More on Medical Costs

Of the total estimated health care costs in 1995, about $50 billion of direct medical costs are believed to originate from obesity. In addition, Columbia University experts suggest that around 4 percent, or approximately $40 billion, of total yearly US health care costs were obesity-related.[21] They stated that direct medical costs may have gone down due to the higher death rates of obese people. The loss of physical productivity among society may also add to the costs of obesity.

Body mass index (BMI) also matters when it comes to the economics of obesity. An analysis of more than 17,000 members of a major pharmaceutical company found that a BMI of 30 or greater resulted in: (1) higher inpatient and outpatient costs for the patient and provider, (2) increased medication costs, (3) more laboratory services, and (4) frequent physician visits. The total cost for obesity was $220 million.[22]

In 1998, peer-reviewed research exposed the economic burden obesity brings on US businesses.[23] The study examined the steep health insurance costs, sick leaves, higher life insurance premiums, and common disability insurance policies. The total yearly cost of obesity to American businesses is said to be about $12 billion, with the largest share of this being a stunning $7.7 billion in higher health insurance premiums, followed by almost $2.5 billion in paid sick leave, and around $2 billion in life-insurance premiums. Lastly, approximately $1 billion was spent on disability insurance.

Aside from the growing economic burden of obesity in adults, there was also an increase in youth obesity which directly affects the US economy. Based on information from the National Hospital Discharge survey from 1979 to 1999, doctors calculated the economic burden of obesity in youths in their preteens to age seventeen.[24] There were also other conditions in which obesity was labeled a secondary diagnosis. Primary diagnoses include diabetes, obesity, gallbladder disease, and sleep apnea. The percentage of obesity-related diagnoses went up. Illnesses such as diabetes nearly doubled during the twenty-year testing period, and gallbladder issues and obesity tripled. Sleep apnea increased by five times. Hospital costs went from $35 million in 1979 to 1981 to $127 million in 1997 to 1999. These figures give a rough estimate of what rehabilitation and mental health centers have to face if they consider getting obese people some real help. It's a strong example of why society needs to provide more funding for helping obese people, even if this simply means making a few minor economic changes.[25]

The huge rise in obesity cases has alarmed the global health care system, which relies heavily on the economy. Injuries among nurses, physical therapists, and other home health aides continue to unfold as they care for the morbidly obese. These injuries typically include tissue tears, sprains, and falls.[26] In addition, more expenses are made for special beds, lifts, scales, electric wheelchairs, and other hospital facilities to cater to overweight people. When facilities are not suitable enough to serve obese people, symptoms can go undiagnosed.[27] As a result, there may be a lack of preventative measures and overall care. The high figures of morbidly obese people have caused certain sectors of the health care system to be unable to provide adequate services. Also, obesity may lead to higher premiums for life insurance policies that are subject to economic disadvantages.

WHO'S EATING ALL OF YOUR TAXES?

According to a major news report, the George Washington University Weight Management Program advises how obese people suffer from related complications.[28] Consequently, the added disability quickly results in added cost. Medicare and Medicaid don't directly compensate for the medical treatment of obesity, but they do pay for resulting diseases. Therefore, the economic load of these two programs still continues to spike. According to the university's weight management program, private health companies may actually refuse to pay for obesity treatment. Even if the client's obesity somehow disappears, these companies still have to pay for other chronic illnesses obesity causes. People can have serious financial burdens if their health care plan *does not* cover them for conditions unrelated to obesity.

The Social Security Administration plays a major role in government spending. In 2000, about 135,000 people collectively received $77 million per month for disabilities related to obesity.[29] Similarly, obesity costs can be indirectly linked to the taxation system since treatment of the disease can be claimed on your tax returns.

LONG-TERM ECONOMICS AND LONG-TERM DISEASE

The current economic recession in the United States is really a worldwide dilemma. It has caused serious financial crises everywhere. Obesity rates in America are an epidemic that may cause serious economic destruction like any large scale financial crisis does. Regardless of whether scientists find a cure for obesity, remember that in 2004, 70 percent of all healthcare costs in the Unites States were due to chronic illness.[30] As covered in chapter 3, many chronic illnesses are caused by obesity.

A Few Studies to Add to the Discussion

Preventative actions, diagnostics, and treatment protocols related to obesity are considered healthcare expenses affecting the global economy. However, these costs and expenses can be examined from a microeconomic (a smaller, domestic) point of view. An expert study assessed the spending of obese and nonobese people.[31] The researcher in this study found that obese people spend about $400 more per year on personal health than nonobese people. Obesity is more closely related to the occurrence of chronic illnesses, lower quality of life, and expensive medical bills than are smoking and alcohol.

In one study, a scientist conducted research where he compared effects of obesity (due to alcoholism, poverty, and heavy smoking) on chronic disease and health care expenses.[32] The findings suggested obesity was the most serious health problem for chronic illness and health care spending. The author of these findings completed his research using a national household telephone survey that Healthcare for Communities conducted. They obtained data from approximately 10,000 respondents. Participants with a BMI of 30 or greater (obese category), reported an increase of close to 70 percent in chronic conditions that included diabetes, heart disease, high blood pressure, asthma, or cancer when compared with normal-weight individuals with similar social standings.

Reports demonstrate that poverty also heightens the effect of obesity, allowing for about a 60 percent increase in chronic conditions.[33] Obese people stated spending around 35 percent more on health care and around 75 percent more on prescription drugs than normal-weight participants. Normal-weight smokers and heavy drinkers reported 25 percent and 12 percent more chronic conditions, respectively. The smokers spent more than 20 percent on health care services and nearly 30 percent more on prescription drugs. The authors of the reports remarked that this was shocking, and that in 2003, health care expenses in the United States were at about $117 billion.

Another study showed that obese female workers in Chicago with other health issues spent more than $170,000 on medical expenses while their nonobese counterparts only spent roughly $100,000 in undiscounted costs.[34] Meanwhile, obese males paid about $125,000 in medical expenses while normal-weight males spent slightly over $75,000.

Economics of Obesity and Kidney Disease

Chronic diseases that occur concurrently with obesity cannot be predicted. For example, chronic renal disease (also called CRD or kidney disease) is asymptomatic. This means the disease doesn't always present with noticeable symptoms until things really get out of hand. The rate of having such a disease continues to climb alongside the increasing rate of obesity. When you have chronic conditions such as high cholesterol (hypercholesterolemia), Type 2 diabetes, high blood pressure, and obesity for a long period of time, kidney disease often comes hand-in-hand. Many people with chronic illnesses may not take proper recommendations due to a lack of money or time. After a lifetime of failed treatment on chronic illnesses such as diabetes and high blood pressure, kidney problems can ensue. If obesity were curable, the costs of long-term disease such as kidney failure would be avoided.

Tufts Medical Center released an analysis of federal health data in November 2007, which states that roughly 26 million people, accounting for about 13 percent of American adults, suffer from chronic kidney disease.[35] A decade earlier, this number was about 20 million, or 10 percent of the US adult population. Cost for chronic dialysis or kidney transplantation is painstakingly high. The strain on the health care system is huge, and the situation is only getting worse as weeks and years go by, not to mention that the current state of the economy is causing dialysis centers to struggle to meet national demands.

Most people don't know kidney disease caused by obesity comes with a wide range of symptoms. There are two criteria that pertain to how the kidneys can effectively process the body's waste and the presence of protein in your urine (referring to proteinuria). These additional symptoms pose an indirect threat to the drastic affect that obesity already has on our global economy. In 2005, more than 485,000 people were suffering either from a dialysis or a transplant, spending a total of about $30 billion. Medicare spends more than a quarter of its annual expenditures on kidney disease, renal failure being an example. Medicare also offers more than $30 billion in coverage for people younger than sixty-five years of age who need dialysis or kidney transplants. If obesity can be controlled, costs associated with hypertension and diabetes can be eliminated. This would save the health care system at least $20 million.[36]

HEALTH INSURANCE AND BMI: NOT A COINCIDENCE

A study incorporated a microeconomic model that compared health insurance and obesity using two separate methods.[37] In the first method, people paid their insurance premium based on their body weights. The second required everyone to pay the same exact health insurance premiums. The researchers didn't find any obesity spillover costs under the first method, but they did find them using the second, in which the personal welfare for nonobese participants had been significantly reduced. This experiment implies that normal-weight people are, to a certain extent, financially pressured by obesity victims when everyone, regardless of their weight, is offered equal insurance premiums.

Researchers working at Stanford University concluded that obese individuals actually receive a lower salary.[38] Obesity-induced health care expenses are supposedly high enough to generate discrimination when it comes to obese employees' salary ranges. However, this finding only pertained to women, and the salary discrimination was greater than the extra health expenses resulting from obesity. Another report supports this finding.[39] Of the $80 billion of US medical care expenses in 1998, nearly half had gone to obesity-related causes through private insurance (40 percent) and payments from the consumer (about 15 percent). The report concluded that a single taxpayer gives up about $180 every year just to finance obesity-related medical costs for Medicare and Medicaid consumers.

Now, let's dig deeper into the study described earlier, which looks at Medicare data in more than 9,000 males and about 7,500 females.[40] You look at the relationship between the BMI of young and middle-aged obesity victims to medical expenses during later years of life. The researchers found that males with higher BMI tend to have lower education, are older, and have higher blood pressure and cholesterol levels. For males, there is a correlation between BMI and inpatient and outpatient medical expenses. However, one must keep in mind that obesity is less prevalent in females than it is in males. From an economic standpoint, females have less inpatient and outpatient medical charges. Similar statistics are true for women with diabetes and heart disease. Severely obese males incurred expenses totaling more than $6,000 higher and females around $5,500 higher than those with normal weight.

A 1998 study tested future health care costs among more than a thousand members of Kaiser Permanente Northwest.[41] In an initial survey in 1990, members were thirty-five to sixty-four years old, reported having a BMI of 20 or greater, were nonsmokers, and lacked any history of cancer, heart disease, or AIDS. The health care costs were tallied over a nine-year stretch until 1998. For comparison, the researchers used three BMI ranges—20 to 24.9, 25 to 29.9, and 30+. They found that throughout the course of nine years, total health care costs increased dramatically with BMI. The total costs for those with BMIs of 20 to 24.9 were at least $15,000 whereas BMIs of 25 to 29.9 cost around $18,000 and BMIs of 30 or more cost approximately $21,000. Higher cumulative costs were documented for pharmacy costs, outpatient services, and inpatient care.

CAN YOU LIVE FOREVER WITHOUT RULES?

Years of Life Lost

A Johns Hopkins University professor used the concept of "years of life lost" (YLL) to link obesity to death rates.[42] The results of the expected YLL because of increased weight were that twenty-year-old white males with BMIs higher than 45 lost about thirteen years as compared to white males with a BMI of 24 at the same age. If an approximately twenty-year-old male is expected to live for seventy-five years, his life may be reduced by thirteen years if he is obese. For twenty-year-old white females with a BMI greater than 45, the YLL is eight. However, this supposed effect was considerably smaller among black people. The YLL effect is much smaller and only happens when BMI is more than 32.

These statistics differ from that of another medical study, which concluded that YLL due to obesity increased with age but decreased once you are seventy-seven to seventy-nine years old.[43] Financial experts would agree that life-expectancy trends shift the economy in different ways. Owing to poorer health conditions, the likelihood of death can increase with obesity. The investigator in this study used data from the American Cancer Society's Cancer Prevention Study to shed light on this theory. More than 60,000 males and about 260,000 female volunteers were part of the experiment, which went from 1960 to 1972. Researchers found evidence that being overweight really heightens the risk of death regardless of any health problems such as heart disease, diabetes, or high blood pressure. The comparative risk was slightly greater for males and seemed to decline as they get older.

On the subject of YLL, a shorter life expectancy also means a reduction in combined working years for a given obese population and could therefore signal a decrease in the general economic contributions of obesity victims. The tendency of people to get fat has become a long-term problem which stands at an alarming level. Both state and federal governments stand to be bankrupted by the increasing medical costs related to obesity and other chronic diseases obesity causes.

If the management and treatment of obesity is paid for by taxpayers, public funds could be drained out in the name of lifelong obesity treatment. The economic cost of obesity goes beyond individual cost because many of the health care procedures in America are paid using taxpayer dollars. It is like saying that while medical costs are covered under a health insurance policy, this "personal" insurance is actually funded by others. This is one of the responsibilities that the general public has to carry rather than have only the obesity sufferers pay all related costs.[44]

Obesity at Work

A prospective report discussed how young obese women had lower education levels, lower income, and were less likely to marry.[45] Additional research stresses that young obese adults don't generally fall into the same socioeconomic categories as their nonobese peers. According to research, the socioeconomic costs of obese employees for businesses, such as loss of salary and productivity, may even be slightly greater than the above medical costs.[46] Money making potential of obese people may be limited by discrimination, but it's still impossible to measure when exactly discrimination enters the picture here since many of these cases go unreported.

Now let's analyze socioeconomic trends using numbers. Between 1991 and 2000, the number of obesity victims in the United States grew by 60 percent. From 1980 to 2003, the number of overweight teenagers tripled from 5 to 15 percent. By 2003, 65 percent of adults and even children two to five years old were found to be overweight.

The above figures not only represent the potential cost of obesity-related illnesses, but also the general economic impacts of obesity. The socioeconomic influence of obesity includes the indirect costs of worker productivity losses such as absenteeism and lack of employee turnover. A weight-gaining work environment can result in loss of earnings, and even more serious, premature death. In fact, health professionals interpret these possibilities as collateral costs of *any* disease, not just obesity.

The rate of obesity in America doubled in only thirty years, and at least 30 percent of US adults are now categorized as obese. A labor economist from the Conference Board Management Excellence Program warns that Americans must realize obesity isn't just a simple health matter in today's economy.[47] Health problems concerning obesity cost businesses billions of dollars every year in workers' absenteeism or sick leaves and other medical expenditures. For their own good, employers have to pay attention to their staff's weight control.

There are several conclusions in the economist's report:[48]

- More than 40 percent of US companies have started obesity-reduction programs. More than 20 percent agree that they planned to do the same in 2008.
- Return on investment (ROI) estimates for wellness programs range from $0 to $5 per $1 invested. With the ROI in mind, the programs may offer provider companies a bottom line to recruit or retain suitable staff. Some companies prefer to present giveaways to employees who lose body mass by paying them in cash or providing some other form of compensation.
- Employers have to weigh the risk of getting involved with employees' obesity problems against the risks of not taking care of the issues at hand. There is evidence that weight gain lowers salaries, so employers should be informed of any potential legal matters before mentioning their staff members' weights.
- There is still much debate about employers' costs versus benefits for employees' surgery expenses. Though obese employees are obviously eligible for weight-loss surgery (about 9 percent of the US workforce), employers may not be able to pay in full before these employees leave for other jobs.

It is imperative that employers know how to design their wellness program the right way and be able to communicate it to their staff. It may be a good idea to let workers participate in logistical and socioeconomic planning of such programs rather than implement the program from the top down. In the meantime, personal information should be protected.

STOP OBESITY, NOT THE ECONOMY

The First Step Is Always Prevention

A better way to get rid of some health care costs is to make investments in prevention, rather than simply searching for cheaper drugs or negotiating for lower cost care. These routine tactics won't necessarily resolve the problem in the long term. Prevention is known to be the most economical step in fighting off the world's obesity problems, and the advantages of practicing it are vast. By using proper prevention strategies, people will avoid paying for expensive hospitalization, pharmaceutical products, and surgery. With prevention, you won't lose so much of the normal work productivity and will thus reduce medical leaves. In the end, keep in mind that everyone tends to take care of themselves at their own discretion by choosing a lifestyle with the level of fitness they desire and figuring out how to control their health and diet.

Though the concept of prevention sounds great, prevention is extremely uncommon in today's health care. This may be due to the fact that taking preventative steps is unprofitable to certain parties involved in health care systems. For example, pharmaceutical organizations, hospitals, surgeons, doctors, and even small clinics are focusing on business expansion for meeting increasing demands. Ironically, implementation of health care strategies to improve public health will inevitably affect the growth of their business and profits. This could be why prevention hasn't been encouraged so much at schools or during visits to the doctor. Sounds scary, right?

Using prevention to suppress the economic drawbacks of obesity is a good idea, but it has to be done through education and subliminal advertising. In addition to improving body image, people should be informed on how to better their health and quality of life. Exercise, discussed in the next chapter, is a really inexpensive form of prevention. The bottom line is that prevention is also necessary for letting health care systems focus on widespread issues such as obesity.

What Needs to Be Done

Obesity is a growing financial issue as it sits on top of the ballooning national debt from the second Bush administration. Disturbing obesity rates and the demand for obesity care could cause a worldwide economic disaster. In addition to having domestic economic issues, the United States continues to pump out disease-causing items such as soft drinks and cigarettes. Fast food businesses are sprouting everywhere very rapidly. This leads to global obesity problems, and the World Health Organization has recently suggested that governments tell their citizens to consume less food, period.

Dietary guidelines have passed at the World Health Organization despite strong opposition from food companies in America. Nonetheless, industrialized nations keep supporting corporations such as hospitals, pharmaceutical suppliers, junk food manufacturers, and health care suppliers in ways that harm the consumer. They also neglect to educate their consumers on the dangers of obesity. A global financial and medical crisis may be impending because of out-of-control medical costs.

Major businesses such as airlines and food companies have their own concerns about the economic impacts of obesity. Airlines always have problems with rising fuel costs, and they keep getting pressured to increase seat width. Restaurants are facing accusations of causing obesity. In 2005, members of Congress proposed legislation to prevent obesity lawsuits against the food industry but did not succeed.

Governments have to take the necessary steps to educate people and influence public belief in order to eliminate the worldwide economic effects of obesity. Everyone should be notified about unhealthy foods and demand positive reforms for the food and restaurant industry. The United States experienced tremendous change in dieting habits during the 1950s and 1960s, when fast food was still making its way into pop culture. The world's economy is bad enough right now, so remember that you can share the cost of meals and still get a lot more food nowadays. Having simple meals at home rather than your local restaurant can save you money.

The world's largest retail corporation is already taking action on this matter.[49] The company plans to set up a nutritional consultant on its website so customers can get ideas about health and diet. Similarly, local government agencies are starting educational campaigns. Even the Health Department for the largest city in America is putting up posters in the subway, intent on educating people about calories and other diet-related information.[50] Health insurance companies have a financial interest in fighting obesity. It is a well-known fact that being obese increases the risk for many diseases. However, many insurance companies do not offer reimbursement for treating obesity. Ironically, they will cover treatment for the diseases it causes. Obesity treatment, or weight-loss regimens to be more precise, can be very expensive and by not covering it, health insurance companies risk the health of those they insure.

Health insurance companies can help decrease obesity rates by considering and paying for obesity treatment just as they would any other disease. However, it may take time and effort to convince them to do this. In order for changes to be made, health insurance companies must acknowledge, in a more transparent fashion, that obesity is the cause of other problems such as diabetes, high blood pressure, and heart disease. They should then adjust their billing policy and structure it so it covers direct, obesity-related medical costs as a separate entity in addition to covering the expenses for treating the underlying diseases. Such a policy would work when an individual's weight and fat content are monitored over an extended period of time. If state and federal governments around the world were able to get more involved in all of this, one would be able to see a great deal of economic improvement. These types of initiatives have to be consistent yet exciting to keep everyone interested. The media should also become proactive about obesity, as this is a very good way to relay the right information to the masses. In the end, remember that reducing the economic impacts of obesity is only possible if and when people get serious about it.

III

KEEP IT UP!

THE ART OF EXERCISE

Physical activity is considered a necessary part of the daily routine at school, work, and just about anywhere else you can imagine. Obesity victims don't normally incorporate exercise into their daily routine unless they are on a diet or a rigorous fitness plan. Most cultures incorporate exercise in the form of social sports, such as the typical Sunday afternoon football or tennis match.

Some consider fitness as a form of physical activity that includes a rigorous daily exercise regime, while others consider it as being slim and trim or having the stamina to finish a whole marathon. "Fitness" signifies a fit body and healthy mind amid the worldwide expanse of obesity. As you have read in previous chapters, obesity is rapidly becoming the center stage of the health care industry. Today, obesity is a disease that brings lots of medical complications that can become a life threat. You can overcome these complications by staying active and exercising with a lot of self-discipline.

DETERMINING WHETHER YOUR PHYSICAL ACTIVITY IS ENOUGH

There is the notion that obesity is only related to your weight. People check to see if they are obese by simply looking at the numbers on a scale. However, the scale doesn't exactly calculate body mass and height, important signals for someone who is overweight. This could lead to a serious miscalculation. That's why you should calculate precise body mass, height, and age to really know whether you are obese. If you have excessive body fat, then you would be tagged as someone suffering from obesity. Generally speaking, when you weigh more than the average weight of someone else of the same height and age, then you are considered overweight.

Excessive body fat leads to overweightness and is the major contributing factor for obesity. To overcome obesity, you need to lose weight, and one of the simplest means to lose weight is to routinely exercise. Weight loss relates directly to burning more calories than you eat. For true and effective results, it is necessary to know the basics of weight loss, which type of exercise needs to be done, and how it should be carried out. The most important aspect of exercise is consistency. Let's go over some other tools needed for exercising specifically for the purpose of weight loss.

EXERCISE REDUCES WHAT MATTERS MOST

Leptin and Exercise

According to a study that was funded by the National Institutes of Health and conducted by obesity researchers at the University of Michigan, exercise not only gets you fit and in shape, but helps reduce appetite when certain hormones are in the right amounts.[1] The study was presented at the Endocrine Society's 90th Annual Meeting in San Francisco and focused on the relation between exercise, obesity, and leptin, the hormone linked to appetite reduction. Observers conducted the test on a group of postmenopausal women. These women are generally prone to increased central adiposity (belly fatness) because of the hormonal changes that they go through. The scientists put the study participants on treadmills in the mornings and afternoons and recorded specific data. The volunteers performed either a high intensity workout or a traditional, low-intensity cardio exercise. Throughout the day, all the participants were instructed to rank their level of hunger on a scale of one to ten. Blood samples were taken to measure the level of leptin in their circulation.

Other research has suggested that compared to a woman of "normal" weight, there is a lower level of leptin in the blood sample of obese women who recently lost weight.[2] This supports the functions of leptin mentioned earlier, that for normal-weight people, an increase in the level of leptin leads to a lack of appetite. However, the individuals participating in the research did not report experiencing any appetite suppression after going through exercise, despite having high leptin levels. This research therefore shows that once you are obese, leptin has minimum effect on your appetite control. While the quantity of leptin produced may be greater, obese individuals' resistance to leptin makes this hormone almost indifferent to appetite. This kind of pattern bears an awfully close resemblance to Type 2 diabetes symptoms in obese men and women.

As the experiment continued, researchers found that both types of workout (high- and low-intensity cardio) reduced the levels of leptin in normal-weight women. Technically, that means there should be an overall increase in appetite, but despite the level of leptin dipping during exercise, these women didn't feel hungry at all. It appears the high-intensity workout resulted in appetite suppression in lean women. This could suggest that overweightness and obesity interferes more with your appetite control system than with hunger, and that exercise may not reduce hunger in obese people after all.

The scholars were trying to establish a direct link between leptin, exercise, appetite, and obesity, but only succeeded in doing so partially. For example, the study mentioned before didn't include any male participants and thus failed to account for gender and additional hormonal factors.[3] Appetite control and obesity is definitely a complex issue, and as you try to find out more about this relationship, things get increasingly complex and confusing. The one result you can draw from this research is that as an obesity victim, you cannot depend exclusively on suppressing appetite if you want to get rid of your obesity.

LET'S GET GOING

Your daily activities may just be your key to weight loss. See table 11.1 for a better understanding of how you can fight obesity by doing simplified daily routines.

Table 11.1. Physical Activities and Calories Burned

Physical activity	Calories burned per ½ hour (approximate)
Getting groceries	120
Moving furniture	190
Vacuuming	120
House cleaning	100
Going for stroll	100
Biking	250
Gardening (outdoors, in summer heat)	150

Table 11.1 demonstrates that many forms of activity result in burning calories. Most people can begin gradual, moderate exercise such as gardening, on their own. Gardening is one activity many people enjoy that requires time and effort, but results in calorie burning and the satisfaction of seeing a garden grow.

About Gardening

There are different forms of exercise and movement when it comes to gardening:

- Raking and edging the lawn
- Moving piles of mulch around
- Digging holes
- Pulling out weeds
- Planting seeds

Gardening will exhaust all the crucial muscle groups in the body, and studies even show that an hour of gardening can help a 180-pound obesity sufferer to burn around 200 calories. (A person who is 180 pounds can be obese if the fat levels are above the normal range for his or her height.) Various research studies revealed some astonishing findings: gardening, and any other activity that involves a significant amount of physical activity, could reduce insulin resistance, but elevations in insulin resistance could lead to metabolic conditions such as diabetes, which in turn can vastly contribute to heart disease.[4]

If everyone had a garden, wouldn't the global obesity problem theoretically disappear? Gardens in both rural and urban settings should not only be used to improve public health and provide fresh produce, but also to provide a good means for exercise. To improve your gardening, remember to use gadgets such as electric weed trimmers, which make the process go a lot smoother.

Sitting and Reading

This may sound strange at first, but sitting and reading can in fact demand more calories than sitting quietly on the porch or sleeping. If you can attribute your obesity to sitting and doing practically nothing for hours at a time, then sitting down and reading would be a good starting point. Brain activity increases when you consciously interpret what you see or read, and you need a certain amount of energy to do this. Increased brain activity burns a lot of carbohydrates and thus, total calorie levels remain untouched. This is in stark contrast to other metabolic processes that burn tremendous amounts of overall body fat as fuel, such as extended runs on a treadmill. Reading is estimated to burn about one to two calories per minute, which is really very low as compared to intense fat-burning exercises.

Light Housework

Light housework can burn up to two to three calories per minute. Light housework isn't usually thought of as a super-fast way to lose weight, but it can help in speeding up your own metabolism. Doing household activities such as washing, cleaning, and sweeping requires lots of energy outflow, as a result of more fat burning. The end result is a decent amount of weight loss. Light household work can boost your metabolism, and once you start losing weight, your opinions about household work may also change in a positive way.

Speed Walking

Walking is considered to be one of the best exercises for weight loss. Walking daily for the long term can help to burn around 55 percent of all your body fat. However, the amount of fat burned depends heavily on the intensity of your walk. Walking aggressively, or for a long stretch of time, burns through a bigger amount of calories. You can choose the type of exercise based on the amount of calories you prefer to burn off. Walking can be the exercise of choice for *anyone* who wants to lose some weight.

Aerobic Exercise and Light Jogging

Another option for weight loss is aerobics, an exercise that's a little more intense than it may initially seem. It falls under the same category as any workout which is designed to enhance your heart rate. It improves your oxygen intake, thus benefiting your entire body. A night of aerobics could morph into a week of walking, running, and swimming. Aerobic exercise can burn a large amount of energy in a single go, but for obesity patients with breathing issues, this could turn out to be a little too intense. This is also true when you are trying to keep up with others who are already fit but just trying to stay in shape. What is the downside of intense aerobics? You could experience heavy breathing that will turn fats to carbohydrates and slow fat burning to as low as 30 percent. That's why you should start off your exercise regimen with gentle walking. Move up to brisk walking after a few weeks. Once you get in shape, switch to aerobics exercise for more noticeable results.

Aerobic exercise helps you absorb oxygen while you do workouts. This helps to increase muscular stamina rather than overall muscle strength. Aerobics is a major form of exercise because it burns maximum calories during activity. This directly reduces your obesity. The nature of the aerobics makes it really easy to perform, depending on your level of intensity. These days, small children can swim, ride a bike, and do other aerobic exercises with a lot of enthusiasm. Aerobics, even for a child, is a very realistic way to get in shape. There are certain exercises which are complex and beyond the scope of children's capabilities, so it might take a little time to convince them to get involved. A study found that children can get rid of sleep problems such as snoring by participating in aerobic exercise for twenty to forty minutes a day.[5]

Aerobic exercise can help you:

- Boost your bone's mineral density levels
- Lower your body fat more than that achieved from resistance training
- Elevate your submaximal and maximal endurance time
- Slightly raise your HDL levels
- Avoid drastic changes in lean body mass
- Lower your overall heart rate
- Increase insulin's responsiveness to glucose challenge tests
- Lower your basal insulin levels
- Increase insulin sensitivity[6]
- Lower your LDL minutely
- Boost your VO_2 max (aerobic capacity or max oxygen consumption)
- Boost your basal metabolism[7]

Why is aerobics considered the exercise of choice for a lot of people? The answer is this: It has the ability to increase the duration for physical activity leading to longer hours of workout, so you can remain active for a lot longer and burn more calories while at it. The longer you do aerobics, the more calories you burn.

Water Aerobics

Water aerobics is usually a later addition to aerobics. Though some may have varying opinions for water aerobics, it can prove to be a lot of fun and excitement for children and adults. There is no age restriction for this type of exercise, as long as you can swim. It all depends on your individual needs and capabilities. Water aerobics involve movement of just about every muscle and joint of the body. It's also fun because you don't have to worry about getting overheated as you do when working out in a gym. When you float in the water, you are putting less strain on your joints and allowing your muscles to work more freely. Obesity victims who are unable to do weight-bearing exercise can opt for water aerobics.

There are a few things you have to keep in mind when it comes to water aerobics. The routines should be formulated with the help of your doctor, especially if you have diabetes. The water temperature should be checked so you have the right conditions for calorie burning. Try to warm up prior to the exercise and take a shower afterwards to avoid any chlorine-related issues. Drink a lot of water because you could get severely dehydrated if you swim too much without drinking anything. It is always advisable to have an instructor while doing water aerobics. Follow all rules and regulations that are there for your own safety. Floating devices not only save your life, but can be used to focus your exercise routine.

Water aerobics boost your physical strength. Walking, jogging, or running in the pool helps develop cardiorespiratory fitness, as does treading water. Various games associated with this type of exercise provide for a wide range of movements and therefore also improve your flexibility. As the training progresses, you can go to deep water exercises depending on the workout routine and your instructor's advice. A maximum of twenty to forty minutes of treading per session should be enough for the day. You could burn around 340 calories while "jogging" in chest-deep water for thirty minutes, compared to the 240 calories you burn when jogging on land. A well-qualified water aerobics instructor will know how to teach water aerobics and acknowledge any special health concerns you have at the time.[8]

Running for Exercise

Running a mile in seven minutes could burn more than fifteen calories a minute.[9] After watching long-distance runners during marathons, one could infer that *running* is by far the best exercise for losing weight. Most long-distance runners are slim and carry around a small amount fat. Marathons are suitable for them because of their training. Their muscles have adapted to this level of intense running year after year. These athletes use up more oxygen than people who don't run too often. This accelerates fat-burning mechanisms even at higher levels of physical activity typically observed in long-distance running. Distance running may not be the right exercise for you when you first get into the gist of things because you could lose about 80 percent of essential carbohydrates and only 20 percent of fat. Losing higher percentages of carbohydrates may speed up your appetite rather than to suppress it.[10]

Sprinting

This form of exercise aims to burn many calories within a short period of time. Medical research proves that sprinting is a realistic form of exercise for losing weight when you are obese.[11] Sprinting will have different, faster effects on weight loss than mild speed walking or jogging. However, sprinting necessitates a lot of rest between the training sessions and can ironically burn fewer calories overall. Due to rapid muscle exhaustion, sprinting is usually performed for very short intervals.[12]

Aerobics account for the other side of the story here since it can be performed regularly. The physical exhaustion associated with aerobics is spread out evenly over time. That's why aerobics can burn more calories compared to sprinting. An obese person can get favorable results by exercising lighter but longer. Regular exercise does help one lose weight, but the idea is to exercise sufficiently longer and strenuously so the body ends up burning more calories than it generates.

Weight Training

Intense exercise affects your metabolism rate even though they involve an "on-off" type of calorie burning with repetitive breaks. Building lean muscle by using weights can help your metabolism and allows a little fat burning even when you take a break. If your fitness level is OK and the doctor clears you for it, then weight training exercise may be the way to go.

THE WORKOUT MANIFEST: FOUR REASONS TO EXERCISE

Regular exercise is a must for healthy operation of your body systems and parts. Mild activity helps maintain the size, tone, and shape of muscles, whereas laborious exercise strengthens them significantly. Exercise makes the joints more flexible and improves your scope of movement. Five minutes of squats and pushups can help build up your muscle mass. The stronger your muscles get, the higher your metabolism will be because you can burn more calories in any given day. A fitness consultant[13] and author of a high-impact book about diet believes that an elevated heart rate lets you burn more calories after a cardio workout. The more intense the workout, the longer it would take for your metabolism to return to its original state. A moderate-intensity aerobic exercise done for forty-five to sixty minutes at least five times a week would give you the best results.[14] The following is a list of four great reasons for working out.

Strengthened Immune System

When people exercise, they have a 40 to 50 percent reduction in sick leaves from work. This should tell you that exercising boosts the immune system quite a bit. When you exercise, your heart starts pounding faster and the blood pressure increases in normal response, driving disease-fighting immune cells into the blood. These cells have markers to detect troublemakers such as flu viruses and bacteria and fight them off the body.

Happiness, Stress, and Energy

Research at the University of New Orleans shows that exercise can make you happier.[15] Scientists asked forty-two participants how they felt before and after a fifty-minute aerobics session. The result? Most of the participants felt relieved after exercising. A simple workout can lessen stress and anxiety. At Indiana University, a professor used psychological and hormonal evaluations to measure the anxiety levels in people who work out.[16] Fifteen participants were asked to report how they felt before and after a twenty-minute workout session. They reported feelings of considerably less anxiety during an hour and two after the exercise session. Exercise was found to (1) increase the brain's serotonin, the hormone responsible for giving you positive moods, and (2) increase body temperature, thereby causing relaxation.

Another significant research study found that a brisk ten-minute walk can provide you with more energy than consuming a single candy bar.[17] This is because exercise boosts a hormone that increases energy. Physical workouts strengthen the lung's capacity to pump more oxygen, which eventually adds strength to muscle and increases both respiratory (breathing) stamina and endurance. That is why you feel more energetic a few hours after a very tiring workout.

Lower Cholesterol

A study has found that the intense workouts such as running reduces the level of cholesterol, which reduces the risk of heart disease.[18] High-density lipoproteins, associated with your good cholesterol, helps clear the body of low-density lipoproteins (LDL), the notorious cholesterol-causing protein. Although peer-reviewed research experiments suggest that HDL levels are not always improved by exercise,[19] HDL is very important for the body. Exercise really adds to the positive effects of HDL. There is another fat particle in the blood called triglyceride, which is associated with heart disease. The lower the level of triglycerides in your circulatory system, the lower the risk of heart disease. Exercise converts triglycerides back into a fatty acid form so they can be easier to burn during energy expenditure. You burn calories when you work out, which leads to a loss of weight.

A Stronger Mind

Exercise can strengthen your mind and enhance your reasoning capabilities. Research conducted on approximately sixty volunteers gave some very impressive results.[20] Participants were tested after they did some aerobics and finished watching a video. They said their minds were a lot sharper once this was completed and they scored much higher on creativity tests after exercising.

EXPLORING YOUR OPTIONS

As you may know, exercise comes in different forms such as walking, jogging, aerobics, tai chi, tennis, gardening, and swimming. The point here is to choose the best option for you. The more you enjoy a particular form of exercise, the more likely you are to take it up for as long as you can. You may have heard the saying: "Variety is the spice of life," which means life is far more appreciable when you try different things.

However, being inconsistent with exercise can throw your metabolism off balance.

Exercise Balls

Many people use exercise balls to work out. Also referred to as orthopaedic balls, these spheres are highly efficient exercise tools. They come in handy and are convenient enough so people can do workouts almost anywhere, such as the office, home, or while watching television. These are just some preliminary ideas to get started, but as far as exercise balls go, you need to talk about where the rubber really meets the road.

Because of the balls' ergonomic properties, they provide support and straighten your spine. This paves the way for good structural balance and lets you sit with a posture that's correct and healthy. You can sit on these exercise balls in the office comfortably. Exercise balls are part of a new wave of antiobesity campaigns everywhere. These brightly colored, oversized plastic balls can be used to do many different exercises that help you improve your:

- Balance
- Strength
- Movement
- Flexibility
- Coordination
- Posture

Exercise balls also help boost your core muscles such as that of the back, abdomen, and sides. Working out with an exercise ball for hours on, you sit continuously in the same position. This is unhealthy for your back and will make simple tasks such as writing at a desk or sitting at the kitchen table very uncomfortable. An orthopaedic ball forces you to change position in order to balance your body the right way, thus providing motion while keeping your bones and joints in good shape.[21]

This brings people to the million dollar question: Why should anyone use orthopaedic balls as a major tool for exercising? The answer is very simple: When you're trying to balance your body on the ball, you stretch your muscles and joints without feeling any serious physical tension. The ball can be more useful when it's used as a long-term exercise machine. Using these balls in the course of exercise boosts your metabolism and blood flow. Proper flow of blood and water in your body keeps your internal organs clean.[22]

Exercise balls are also less costly compared to other exercise equipment such as treadmills or weight-bearing devices. Even an oversized but sturdy beach ball can serve the purpose, and since exercise balls are like toys, you can have more fun while exercising and can burn calories, gain muscles, lose weight, and finally stay fit. There are lot more benefits of exercise balls in addition to those mentioned above, but in light of the economics of obesity that were covered in chapter 10, these balls are simply cheaper and more affordable than gym memberships. They can be kept anywhere in the house where you can have the luxury of using them whenever you want.

PILATES AND RESISTANCE TRAINING IN COMPARISON TO AEROBICS

Pilates

The origin of pilates dates back to the twentieth century, but you have to admit, Pilates is very trendy these days. It was developed by a German man named Joseph Pilates and focuses on supporting the body's core muscles as you move through a large range of motion. This form of exercise makes your muscles more powerful and flexible. It also improves your posture. Pilates is done using mats, but there are some Pilates exercises requiring other large equipment involving pulleys. Pilates is very popular among celebrities and professional dancers. It also helps keep you slim.[23]

Resistance Bands

In reality, using rubber bands to exercise is a lot more common than one may think. Children play with rubber bands all the time. They stretch the bands with their index finger and fling it all the way across the room to the other person just for fun. The same concept is applied to resistance bands but in your case your entire body's muscles get a decent workout. During resistance band training, you use your own body weight to gain resistance instead of external weights such as dumbbells.

To use a resistance band, slip the band around your arm or foot and extend or lift the limb against the band's resistance. It can also be attached to the door or fixed strongly to a bar for doing exercises. Resistance bands are a cheap and portable exercise tool. They come in different sizes and varying degrees of resistance. Shorter bands strengthen your hips, ankles, wrists, and hands. The longer ones are used mostly for working out your upper and lower extremities. Distinctive colors identify the level of resistance offered by the bands. Yellow bands are identified as least-resistance bands. Others are green, red, blue, or black.[24]

Muscle strength can be improved by introducing muscles to a stimulus which is greater in resistance than they are normally designed to encounter. Even so, "tweens" and teens benefit a lot more from the resistance training than younger children do. Men have to go through bigger changes from resistance training than do women. This is all owing to the release of hormones after puberty and new bone development. Resistance training not only increases bone density but also helps to reduce body fat.[25]

This type of training is divided into three categories (see table 11.2).[26]

In truth, any of the exercises described in table 11.2 will counter your obesity in some way. To lose as much weight as possible, you have to burn more calories than you absorb. Resistance training and aerobic training should be in the best interest of everyone, unless circumstances do not allow for it. Both of these workouts have their benefits, but remember that such advantages may still differ for each individual.

Table 11.2. Types of Resistance Training and Their Descriptions

Isometric	Resistance is held at an angle for a period of time.
Isotonic	Performed by using free weights and machines. You have a set of weights and move them around through the range of motion.
Isokinetic	Perform concentric (muscle shortening) and eccentric (muscle lengthening) movement through ranges of motion at set speeds.

Resistance training and aerobics are comparable to two siblings cycling between fighting and caring for one another. Resistance training builds muscles, which in turn helps burn up more calories than aerobics does. While aerobics burn more calories, resistance training leaves room for more potential energy for burning calories in the future. Strength itself has so many different meanings that it's mind boggling, but resistance training increases muscular strength, which after all is the ability of your muscles to produce force against any resistance.

HOME TACTICS

Cardio

In-home cardio exercises are considered to be the best regimens for maintaining proper health and body fitness, but the idea of a gym workout is sometimes difficult to grasp due the costs and time needed to travel to the facility itself. However, exercising doesn't always require a trip to your local gym; it can be done in the privacy of your home if you have enough willpower and perseverance for consistent workout. Once you get in the flow of things and you can exercise at least every other day for about an hour, you can get fit right from home.

Step Aerobics

Step aerobics are one of the best cardio exercises presently available to fitness fanatics. Intense step exercises completed for approximately half an hour will help you get rid of around 400 calories. Though it is mostly performed by women, this can be a good option for men too. This is an excellent exercise that will help anyone, irrespective of their gender, overcome obesity.[27]

Jump Roping

A jump rope can be a very useful addition to any home gym. It takes up only a small amount of space and can be stored very easily. It also helps improve body parts such as limb coordination, speeds up eye movements, and boosts your overall endurance and stamina.

Stationary Cycling

This form of exercise allows you to burn about 500 calories in a single go. This is not a new type of exercise. It's been around for decades. In contrast with traditional bikes, stationary cycles require a lot less surface area to operate and let you exercise in a private atmosphere.[28]

POPEYE'S CREED: EXERCISE AND CHILDREN

The percentage of obese children in the world has increased drastically in the last thirty years. The cause is a lack of exercise, less involvement in extracurricular activities, and sitting and watching television or playing video games for long periods of time.[29] As a parent, you should try to develop an exercise plan for your child in a way that fits your schedule as well; simply going for walks or taking a trip to the park can ensure your child gets exercise every day. Impose a time limit for watching television or playing video games and let them spend copious amounts of time outside when weather permits. Children should be encouraged to do physical activities such as walking to school with a caretaker rather than taking a bus and using stairs instead of elevators. The list could go on forever, but everyone knows that children learn a lot from watching adults.[30]

The Norm

A child with proper upbringing would normally participate in physical activities without ever knowing. Children subconsciously run and play as part of normal everyday routines. It's when they stop and replace this with something much more sedentary, that diseases such as obesity may occur.[31] Moreover, children enjoy playing indoor and outdoor games. These games provide lots of movement, and thus, give children flexibility and stamina. Parents and teachers can help encourage healthy living through the promotion of exercise and responsible eating habits. Limiting junk food and sedentary time will go a long way to helping encourage children to incorporate healthy habits into a lifelong lifestyle.

Exercise Gets Things Going for Kids

Remember that fitness comprises three different elements: stamina, strength, and flexibility. The effects of all three are witnessed when children go through a growth spurt after years of chasing each other, crossing monkey bars, and bending over to tie shoe laces. Make sure your son or daughter participates in various activities that have all the elements of fitness.

Exercise is one among the many approaches to combating childhood obesity and is in the running to become the most important treatment option. While children need to be careful with what they eat, exercise should also become a normal thing in their life so they can have a healthy adulthood. Physical endurance and stamina builds up when your child practices aerobic activities. Aerobic activities increase heart rate and speed up breathing. If done regularly, aerobic activities enable a child's body to provide oxygen to all the cells and helps to strengthen the muscles of the heart. Running, skating, walking, cycling, playing basketball, soccer, swimming, and tennis are considered oxygen-gaining activities that, if carried out regularly, can benefit the body immensely. In addition to being very useful, these activities provide fun and excitement for the otherwise bored child.

Weight Lifting   This is not the only tool for gaining strength, and children who want to do this should always perform it under adult supervision. Medical literature dictates that too much weight training at a young age is not recommended.[32] Children can gain muscle mass while climbing or wrestling, so why not do that instead? They can do sit-ups, crunches, and push ups to tone muscles as they get older and can master the proper form.

Stretching   When you stretch your arms and legs, its helps improve flexibility and toughens your bones. It's one of those things children do automatically from an early age. Smaller children start stretching when they reach for things or when they do somersaults as a toddler. Static stretching is done by stretching and holding the stretch for about thirty seconds. Dynamic stretching makes your children's movements swifter and increases physical momentum. It isn't necessary to have all your children do the same stretching routines or spend the same amount of time on exercising.

Yoga   Yoga is another form of exercise that promotes flexibility and a healthy attention to the body. Many facilities now offer youth yoga programs. How does yoga decrease obesity? Yoga is the union of both mind and body. Regular practice of yoga helps achieve balance between the two. At the very least, the yoga asanas (poses and postures) and the breathing techniques increase physical activity and the supply of oxygen to the body. This increased physical activity and the extra blood oxygen burn up the excess fat in the body. However, yoga goes beyond that; it calms down the mind thereby reducing mental stress. This way yoga fights the obesity caused by the emotional factors. The yoga breathing techniques strengthen the lungs and alleviate the illnesses in the body that are caused by improper breathing patterns. Yoga practice is the natural way of losing weight. When practiced properly, yoga not only fights obesity but also helps cure other health-related problems. Best of all, proper practice of yoga does not cause any adverse side effect on the body.[33]

Why Should You Encourage Children to Exercise

As you can see, exercise is not only beneficial for adults but also has many benefits for obese children. Children who perform physical activities are less prone to developing obesity and Type 2 diabetes. Exercise leads to strong muscles and bones even though it makes children leaner. Exercise helps to control blood pressure and cholesterol levels. This of course paves the way for children to be healthier by the time they reach adulthood. Exercise makes children sleep better at night and helps cope with stress during the day.

The increasing threat of childhood obesity is visible in the United States as well as around the world, in developed *and* developing countries. Obese children who never exercise are at a greater risk of severe medical complexities. Chronic conditions pertaining mostly to adults, such as osteoarthritis, diabetes mellitus, and cardiovascular disease can cause severe health complications when you age, but avoiding exercise will lead to poor quality of life and increased personal burden even as a child. That's why it is vital to consider exercise and other physical activity as a weapon against childhood obesity. A child's family and community impact the accessibility of physical activity.

Schools should stress the importance of exercising for a healthy and active lifestyle. There are lot of causes for childhood obesity, so a single blame won't cut it, but everyone must come together and vouch for the incorporation of exercise into society, including new activities in schools. In any case, society has a duty to increase children's quality of life from both physical *and* psychological venues.[34]

THE PERSONAL TOUCH

Personal Fitness Trainers

If you suffer from obesity, some of the advantages of getting personal training, as compared to a gym membership are:

- Gyms don't allow you to negotiate schedule and price. They usually set non-negotiable membership prices for you.
- If you go through a personal trainer, you could negotiate the price, length, and frequency of workout sessions.
- Personal privacy could be a big reason to ditch your local gym and get a trainer. You can get trained with personal attention without having a concern about any distractions.

Personal fitness trainers are sometimes trained in various approaches to obesity, so he or she could come to your home, workplace, or set up an appointment at their studio to help you lose weight fast. If you're really serious about losing weight, personal training is an excellent option. While it involves cost and time, it could still prove very beneficial. Now let's review a few of the personal training options available to you as an obesity patient.

Therapeutic Exercises

This is when personal trainers help ease movements or make you lose weight in specific areas. It also indirectly improves musculoskeletal function and maintains a condition of well-being all throughout the body. Therapeutic exercises can improve:

- Respiratory capacity, the amount of air your lungs can hold
- Blood flow
- Balance
- Performance levels during exercise
- Stamina
- Nerve coordination
- Muscle viability

Therapeutic exercises help reduce hypercontractivity of muscles and removes unnecessary tension from tendons and fascia. They are easy to perform and may be recommended by your trainer to be any of the following: playing tag, bike riding, playing football, or basketball. These exercises can be imitated by the child easily. Therapeutic exercises aim at achieving and maintaining good health in two different ways: stamina training and flexibility training. Here are some basic parameters you need to know about each.

Stamina (Endurance) Training

Endurance training is recommended by most personal trainers to be done around three to five days a week. Each interval should go on for approximately ten minutes and could be longer if the exercise is low intensity. Endurance training can be performed by experienced individuals for much longer duration, but it should still be done in intervals.[35]

Flexibility Training

This concept is commonly overlooked by many but it is a very important way to lose weight since it provides full range of motion during any training. The greater the range of motion involved during exercise, the greater the loss of energy and fat. Flexibility training can involve a special type of program called proprioceptive neuromuscular facilitation (PNF), which is done by alternating the muscles between contraction and relaxation. This form of personal training requires licensed therapists and caters to many people with paralysis. It is commonly used by chiropractic physicians and athletic trainers.[365]

THE UNAVOIDABLE MATCHUP: EXERCISE, DIETING, AND WILLPOWER

The Physiology Behind Exercise and Diet

Research conducted at Wake Forest University Baptist Medical Center attempts to understand what really reduces the size of abdominal fat cells.[37] These cells are generally located between muscle layers and skin in your abdominal region. Abdominal fat cells (adipocytes) play a major role in developing diabetes and heart disease. The study went on for about twenty weeks and gave researchers important facts about burning calories. The scientists confirmed that burning calories is only one of the remedies which are suitable for reducing abdominal fat and that altering lifestyles is equally required.

It is a well-established fact that exercise can help in reducing fat cell size. Since more women suffer from obesity than men do, studies usually involve female participants. In the study at Wake Forest University, the objective for the participants was to lose 2,800 calories per week.[38] The participants were divided into three groups. Each group had a different set of instructions for losing weight. The first group needed to burn off their calories by dieting on meal plans designed by dieticians. The second group was instructed to walk at the speed of one to two miles per hour on a treadmill three times a week for around fifty minutes. Participants in the third group were required to walk at three-and-half to four miles per hour. They did this thrice a week for around thirty minutes for each run.

Body size, weight, total fat, and abdominal fat cell size were measured before the experiment. The first group was only using dietary measures to lose weight, but the second and the third group was performing exercise. After the experiment, researchers found that all the study volunteers from the three groups were able to lower their body weight, fat body mass, waist circumference, and hip girths. The second and the third groups were able to reduce around 18 percent more abdominal fat cells than the first. Both the second and third group were able to fight off 400 calories a week merely by walking.

The Willpower Incline

It can be assumed that everyone on Earth, be it a man or a woman, longs to have a great physique and attractive body, but this can only be achieved by having the willpower to exercise properly. Some obesity victims may not have such longing for a great physique, but at least everyone among them understands the importance of daily exercising in order to maintain good health. This is more so relevant in today's world when many people have sedentary jobs that involve very little physical activity.[39] Health is wealth, and this is true because a simple exercise schedule can keep out hundreds of possible ailments which may cost you hefty medical bills.

Despite this common sense, most people simply do not exercise. Believe it or not, it doesn't take much to start exercising and staying fit. All that's required is finding the right willpower. Lacking spirit is the number one reason most people don't exercise despite understanding its importance. So how can you overcome this problem? You must realize that this problem is very internal to you and your solution for the same lies within yourself. The mental barrier can be overcome if you sincerely think about the problems associated with obesity. You need to ask yourself what you want from your body. Ask yourself honestly without the typical, "I don't care." The truth is, you do care about how you look and so does everyone else. You would definitely prefer to look similar to the person who has a great physique, who is adored by every beholder, and whose body exhudes confidence and glamour. One of the most effective ways to keep motivated is to look at "past pictures" of fitness daily. In the end, envy may drive you to the gym.

Now that you have convinced yourself to exercise, the next excuse is usually, "I don't have time." This doesn't hold much truth. You can manage at least ten to twenty minutes for exercising every day. The problem is that you prioritize everything else over exercising. This might even include watching TV or chatting on the Internet. When you do so, just ask yourself if you really lack the time or are simply being lazy.

At last you have scheduled some time and also convinced yourself to start exercising, but then you fall into the trap of saying, "Oh! I don't have gym membership. I don't have sports shoes. I don't have a trainer," and so on. To reverse these excuses, simply start exercising with whatever you have at hand. You can buy things from equipment retailers or make other arrangements later when you have progressed into a steady state of mind and body. If you have nothing to commence with, then you can at least start off with a basic exercise routine which includes push-ups, crunches, spot-jogging, and stretching. These exercises don't require any special accessories since they can be done at home.[40]

SUMMARY

Besides physical disability or disease, there's really nothing to stop you from exercising. Exercise requires perseverance and strong spirit to initiate. If you are able to maintain these two, the rest will surely fall into place and hopefully, exercising will become a habit. Lastly, keep in mind that while research proves that exercising makes you live longer,[41] it may not be the only solution to all of your obesity problems. Sometimes obesity sufferers have difficulty finding motivation for different reasons. As you all know, a multistep plan is never complete without long-term maintenance. Conquering obesity symptoms and pains can make one feel much better, but being able to keep the weight to a minimum will make you a true winner. Chapter 12 will explain why the most formidable challenge you can encounter as an obesity sufferer is learning to maintain and stick with motivational strategies.

12

FINDING MOTIVATION

THE NEED

By now you should be familiar with the most common reason for obesity: overeating. When the consumption of food is much higher than the rate of calorie usage, anyone can easily become obese. As you have read in previous chapters, other causes of obesity include serious eating disorders, genetics, and family history of the disease. In such cases, the mental aspect for an obesity victim becomes difficult as feelings of helplessness begin because he or she cannot control weight by just managing their diet or exercising. Moreover, there are other causes such as diseases like hypothyroidism, which may cause obesity indirectly due to the slow rate of metabolism. That's why people should be aware of whether their illnesses lead to obesity before trying to motivate themselves.

Prior to motivating yourself to lose weight, it's always a good idea to get educated about the inner workings of the human body. You should try to understand where the calories come from and how to get rid of them. There is an explanation on why people lose weight and gain it back—people have adipose tissue where excess fat is stored. When additional calories are consumed, fat cells will grow larger and accumulate for storage. When you lose weight, the additional fat cells don't disappear together with the weight. This may explain why some people gain weight a lot quicker than others do, but this issue cannot be addressed in the absence of personal motivation.

Besides heredity, some medications or drugs may lead to obesity. Taking too many painkillers, mainly corticosteroids,[1] such as those given for arthritis, as well as sedatives, will cause your overall body fat levels to spike. If it's necessary to consume such drugs, you must be careful with the amount of consumption and keep track of any negative effect after use. As you can see, there are several factors for obesity, and some may exist beyond your control. All the above symptoms can be overcome at least partially by using motivational techniques.

WHAT MAKES OVERCOMING OBESITY SO DIFFICULT

The Roadblocks

The growing number of obese people in the United States has led the way for another issue to enter society through a hidden door—the lack of sympathy and understanding. While obesity rates in the United States are mounting, things would be better if the general public understood obesity sufferers. This would undeniably help them find more motivation. A study found that society is far less tolerant with the obese population than nonobese groups.[2] Obese participants of the experiment felt more discriminated against today than they did a decade ago. Sadly enough, 620 doctors were questioned as part of this experiment and more than half of them felt that obese clients are awkward, ugly, unattractive, and noncompliant. One-third of them described obese people as lazy, weak-willed, and sloppy. Professionals who specialize in offering obesity treatments are surprisingly among those showing negative attitudes toward obesity. This makes it all the more difficult for obesity sufferers and their loved ones to find motivation.

Discrimination and stigmatization can happen to obese people in every aspect of daily life. Even within the family, an obese child may not receive academic encouragement. Parents will often provide less financial support to their obese children when it's time for the child to go to private school or college. In the workplace, obese people are being discriminated against in nearly all aspects of employment, including employment processes, salary negotiation, and work-related benefits.[3]

Medical research has also determined that overweightness draws out more discrimination than other appearance-related issues such as age, race, and gender.[4] According to a book on clinical obesity, more than 25 percent of individuals who were 50 percent above their ideal weights reported that their benefits were cut by employers.[5] These benefits include health insurance. Many studies show that some employers prefer hiring unqualified, thinner candidates over an obese person who has better credentials.[6] Similarly, a study conducted in 1988 revealed that people would choose to marry an embezzler, a shoplifter, a drug addict, a blind person, or a handicapped person rather than exchange vows with a victim of obesity.[7]

Obese groups have been blamed partially for causing the outrageous fuel prices seen today, weight gain among friends, and global warming, according to a report.[8] Such bias and blame is unfortunately spreading at almost every corner of the world and will ultimately damage and hinder obese people as they struggle to tackle obesity on the mental front. The report goes on to say that there are legal protections for gender, race, or age-based discrimination, but none really exist to protect obese people from being discriminated against. As always, the blame for creating the problem should be directed to the source, not toward the obesity victims who are trying to find motivation.

Motivating by Denouncing Discrimination

The attitudes of anti-overweightness by various levels of society can be studied in many ways. Written surveys, covered in the upcoming paragraphs, serve as good examples here, and a countless number of them have been handed out to physicians, nurses, and medical students. The negative attitude portrayed on the surveys implies that obese people are lazy, awkward, and lacking in self-control. It also suggests that obesity is caused by serious flaws in character and people fail to lose weight because they ignore clinical recommendations.

A medical study used the Implicit Associations Test (IAT) to really get to the bottom of this issue.[9] The IAT uses powerful techniques to measure implicit attitudes on obesity bias among health care professionals, including those specializing in obesity treatment. This test showed implicit discrimination against obese people, including those who are apparently devoted to treating obesity. These professionals are not consciously aware of their bias, and ironically, they all specialized in obesity.

In another experiment, more than 1,000 physicians took a survey assessing their interventions, attitudes, and referral practices for obese people.[10] Though these physicians are aware of their own role in helping obese people, they try not to intervene as much as they should and are unlikely to encourage obese people to go through rigorous weight-loss programs. They are only willing to discuss weight management with overweight (but not clinically obese) people.

Original research reveals why some physicians are ambivalent about treating obesity patients: They claim to be short on time, have a lack of medical training, or experience some insurance reimbursement issues.[11] Attitudes of physicians affect their client when it comes to seeking treatment. Negative attitudes may cause obesity victims to avoid getting health care treatment altogether, in addition to other outcomes of demotivation. Here are some facts from a study done among physicians on willingness to provide pelvic exams to obese women: 17 percent were reluctant to do the exams on severely obese clients, and 83 percent didn't want to provide the exam if they were unsure of weight status.[12] This shows that many obese people may not receive the necessary preventive health care treatments. Other studies show that more than 12 percent of obese women delayed or canceled their physician appointments.[13] Women with higher BMI have a much higher rate of delaying or canceling appointments due to the embarrassment faced when being weighed. Again, this adds to why motivation is difficult to come by.

It's quite clear that bias against the obese continues to increase.[14] Obese populations are unfortunately internalizing societal antiobese and pro-thin biases. It is as if they agree with society's inner negativity that an imperfect body represents an imperfect mind. People should try to manage stigmatization by confirming negative stereotypes, providing socially acceptable explanations for being obese, avoiding hateful situations, and promoting weight loss through medical or surgical treatments when necessary.

The Surgical Cover-Up

A researcher writes that before undergoing bariatric (weight-loss) surgery, more than fifty obese patients in her experiment complained about experiencing biasness for their obesity in both professional, social, and family life.[15] After losing more than 100 pounds after surgery, they reported almost no bias in their lives. This further exemplifies that discrimination against the obese does exist in reality. It's strange enough that with so many obese people in the world, there could be so much discrimination against them. Can this be explained by how obese people rate themselves and perceive their own body image? If you stare into a mirror and say, "Yes, I look horrible," it really won't help your cause all that much. This kind of self-assessment may or may not serve as sarcastic encouragement, but it won't help you to find motivation as an obesity sufferer either.[16]

Going Shopping

Scientists conducted a study to evaluate how and why obese shoppers are likely to experience discrimination.[17] By noting the sales clerks' interactions, including eye contact with shoppers, investigators found that obese customers wearing casual clothes go through interpersonal discrimination more frequently than obese shoppers in professional attire. Both the casually dressed and professionally dressed customers were treated normally if they weren't obese. In the second phase of study, the mystery shoppers carried either a diet soda or ice cream. The results showed that obese shoppers who ate the ice cream or drank the soda experienced a greater amount of interpersonal discrimination than nonobese shoppers. These two phases of the experiment may serve as proof that obesity is perceived as social trouble and victims are stereotyped as being lazy and weak-willed. When sales clerks encountered obese buyers, they would mostly ignore or sidestep these particular groups of customers.

The third phase of study was a generalized shopping survey. The survey asked about the shoppers' experiences with the sales associates, how much they had planned to spend versus the amount *actually* spent, and their body type. Unsurprisingly, those who experienced bias spent less time and money than intended and chose not to return to the store in the future. Besides picking out discriminatory practices, the study also served as a stark reminder for business owners to take note of their employees' behaviors for ethical and financial purposes.

Research at Rice University on people's attitudes toward obesity victims was done in individual and interpersonal settings.[18] This is different from the traditional way of conducting similar studies in large-scale environments such as social gatherings. Therefore, the findings are more consistent with modern conceptualizations of prejudice. The research doesn't really suggest that overweight people should control their obesity just to avoid getting stigmatized. Nor does it imply that obese people bear entirely the responsibility for reducing discrimination though they should learn to protect themselves from negativity at all times. The research noted a certain level of damage from discrimination. As discussed earlier, obesity victims may be able to adopt some methods to avoid certain forms of discrimination and find motivation. Businesses that stigmatize obese people should become proactive and take actions to reduce discrimination by their employees. Only then can obesity patients realistically find motivation.

Under long-term discrimination and harassment in public places and even at home from members of family such as parents, brothers, sisters, children, and spouses, obese people suffer from depression, stress, and low self-esteem. The worst of it can be suicidal thoughts and behaviors.[19] Also, motivation can be difficult to come by if obese subjects handle their anxiety by overeating unhealthy food and avoiding physical activities. A report emphasizes that obese people need to show others that they can be successful and ambitious for reaching their goals.[20] The report also notes that obese subjects should try to stay hopeful and happy with their lives, even with obese body types.

GOING FOR THE GOLD

As obesity rates have doubled worldwide in the last thirty years,[21] people should look for ways to eliminate the current rates of obesity besides getting motivated enough to have a higher quality of life. Nearly all regions of the world are experiencing an increase in obesity rates regardless of age, sex, race, ethnicity, social status, and so forth. Obesity not only results in physical consequences, but also has psychological and social consequences in all age groups of the population.

Finding Motivation in Any Environment

The situation in the United States is laid out in different levels. These levels include social, economic, environmental, and individual. Harboring an environment that promotes unhealthy dieting, lack of physical activities, and too much food consumption has been characterized as obesogenic. To penetrate healthy diet and practices into public of different levels, corrective public health approaches should be published in schools pamphlets, community groups, and work places. A simple and more affordable way to provide motivation here would be to support environmental change. Getting rid of obesogenic settings would be very difficult, but not impossible, to achieve on a global scale.

Besides straying from harmful environments, individuals who are having obesity problems should find motivation primarily through weight loss. A change of diet and lifestyle can be tough for most obesity sufferers who have adapted to their old living methods. Certain people are familiar with the right way to avoid obesity and other chronic diseases, yet they would prefer to have delicious but nonnutritious food. That's why efforts should be made to motivate you to consistently stay motivated on weight loss. It can be demotivating when regaining weight if it was an uphill battle for you to lose the weight in the first place.

Learning the Ropes

Here are a few rules to keep you motivated and ready for weight loss:

- Set a major goal and stay on track—break down your major goals into minor ones which you know you can keep. Initially, try to succeed in each of the minor goals so you're really prepared for the challenges associated with major objectives.
- Always try to finish what you start. Easily giving up on things can turn into an ill-advised habit, so you should avoid stopping halfway through progression. Get in the habit of completing something you

start out doing. Going back to the first rule, try to proceed with minor goals first, since they are generally easy to complete. This will create a future environment in which you're able to take on larger projects and finish them accordingly.

- Try to socialize with others of similar interest. People are generally affected by and learn from each other's actions. Close friends with positive attitudes tend to influence people around them in a good way. Socialize with people who have similar goals and are very focused on what they really want in life. Mutual interaction is important in overcoming obesity.
- "Learn how to learn." People have the ability to teach themselves. Sometimes, depending on others for knowledge may cause more procrastination and lack of progress.
- Use your natural talents to find motivation. Talent creates motivation that will eventually help you reach your weight-loss goals. For example, if you can play soccer really well, continuing to do so will make you fit as time goes by.
- Don't be afraid to take certain risks, as failure can be a great learning tool. While weight loss may be a risk you are willing to take, worrying about not losing any weight could make you gain even more of it. If you never try, how will you know the best way to get rid of your obesity?

To lose weight, you have to make a plan that is as realistic as possible. This plan should include a target weight that you wish to reach.

SELF-NOTE, MILESTONES, AND PRACTICALITY

Know Where You Stand

Ask yourself, "What is the minimum weight I want to lose, and how long do I intend to take?" Write down a list of steps you feel you can take on a piece of paper, and place it inside this book or in a diet magazine when you're not using it. Once you finish the list, get started as soon as possible. Remember that, slow, gradual weight loss is in many ways better than getting thinner rapidly. Losing weight very quickly leads to a higher chance that the weight will return very soon when you return to your past eating behaviors. Losing weight through exercise is similar to a long day's hard work that later rewards you. It would have been easier to simply get "a free pass" for losing weight, but such a pass doesn't really exist.

Milestones

If you end up getting enough motivation to lose a few pounds, it won't hurt to get a little leeway by rewarding yourself with a rare large meal. This is to compensate you for going an entire week with proper eating habits. However, food is not generally encouraged as a treat for reaching your personal weight-loss milestone. Remember that self-discipline is important to getting back on track during the weekdays while not overdoing anything on the weekends. Make it your job to keep active, since calories will burn much more evenly when you remain constantly in motion.

Choose walking over driving when you want to go somewhere close. Take a few more steps and more calories will be burned. If there are friends or family members who need to lose weight, then make plans with them for the weekend or other days off from work. You could have a basic weight-loss contest and check everyone's weight after approximately three months. If your friends or family members do not need to lose weight, you can let them know about the weight-loss plan and ask for their help in monitoring your progress. Having more active participants make the whole plan more interesting and challenging. After reaching a smaller goal, such as five pounds, get yourself something that reminds you of reaching a major milestone. For instance, next time you go shopping, buy yourself clothing that fits your smaller body size.

Practicality

A good weight-loss program should not be too rigid, for such a program will make the whole process only temporary. If your program is really strict and you stop abruptly, you will quickly gain back the weight. You may need a lot of motivation just to start all over again. That's one of the reasons why many obese people are unable to lose their weight for the long term. In fact, maintaining body weight is a lifelong affair. Obesity victims need to have a mind-set of developing a healthy lifestyle and think positively that all nutritious foods are great despite possibly lacking good taste. In the meantime, don't worry too much over what you let go—those junk foods or tantalizing items that you're used to eating. Objectives get unrealistic when you set standards too high. Again, this makes you revert to your old ways, and that's something one should always stay away from.

REASONS FOR MOTIVATION

While a professional study confirms that people lose weight to improve their appearance,[22] there are many other reasons for finding the extra motivation in your dealings with obesity.

Fighting Off Related Diseases

Motivation for obesity is essential for those who want to reduce the risk of high blood pressure, strokes, high cholesterol, and other chronic disease. Obesity is linked to many leading causes of death in the United States alone. Deaths from obesity are more specifically linked to cancer, stroke, and heart failure. Studies show that when you are overweight, it puts you at risk of serious illnesses including heart disease and diabetes.

Things Can Worsen

You can get demotivated when you are unable to determine the difference between appetite and hunger. Determining what your body really needs can help you set up a proper diet plan while helping you to discover how appetite differs from hunger. Many people eat even after their hunger has been satisfied, simply because appetite takes over. Realistically, appetite is a strong desire or craving for food. Most of the food that stimulates your appetite is saturated in calories and fats. When you consume too much food, it can make you gain weight and leave you in need of further motivation.

Better Nutrition

In every phase of life, good nutrition is important to your health. Nutrition is defined as a process that the body uses for certain provisions. Ideal nutrition promotes better health. Even when your body has the nutrients it needs, it has room to grow and develop. Without proper nutrients, your body lacks the ability to fight off dangerous diseases, such as heart failure.

When you set up a proper diet plan, your body gets the proper nutrition it needs to function properly. Healthy nutrients encourage energy flow by boosting your metabolism. You can feel and look your best when you eat healthy and maintain your weight. Healthy nutrients encourage mental alertness and smoother skin. More importantly, a healthy nutritional diet will help reduce the risk of certain cancers, heart disease, diabetes, stroke, and other chronic disease.

In order for your body to survive, it needs nutrients found in food supplies. Knowing the specific kinds of nutrients that cause or fight obesity helps you get motivated because it gives your weight-loss program a greater sense of purpose. Nutrients act as a number of life-sustaining functions. Nutrients are divided into six major categories, namely carbohydrates, water, minerals, vitamins, fats, and proteins. Carbohydrates essentially make up energy components of your daily diet, since they provide carbons, hydrogen, and oxygen. They serve as food and energy supply. Water is necessary to help you sustain life since the body is made up of 70 percent of it.[23] Minerals are inorganic (lacking carbon) materials found in nature, so they help you stay healthy. Vitamins are organic substances that are essentially there to boost your metabolism. You need them to help you fight off viruses and disease.

Your body requires a decent, but not excessive, amount of fatty foods to survive. Fats are nutritional components found in foodstuff. Fats provide nine major calories per gram of energy. Fats offer the nutrients the body needs to sustain the right amount of energy. Ironically, many fatty foods contain healthy vitamins such as vitamin A, D, E, and K. Finally, proteins are complex natural compounds. These compounds have a fibrous structure composed of amino acids. Proteins are essentially needed to help living cells ward off viruses. Since amino acids are important for cell growth, it is important that the body gets a balanced measure of proteins daily to sustain life.

Carbohydrates provide energy and nutrition very quickly. Being obese can interfere with the body's ability to digest them. Carbohydrates are found in foods such as bread, potatoes, and pasta. They are essential for keeping the body full of life, but when you consume too many, obesity can occur.

CHILDHOOD DISCOVERIES

What Makes It Tougher

Aside from adults who are obese, children who are used to eating too much face problems with getting motivated to lose weight. How this disease affects a child depends primarily on his or her parents and other relatives' general feelings toward overweightness. It also depends on how acceptable obesity is within the family's specific culture. If the overweight children's family perceives overweightness as a bad sign, they may keep pressuring the child about weight control. If you blame children for being obese, they can get emotionally distraught and might show very low self-esteem. If that is the case, there would be no way to find genuine motivation.[24]

From a Youngster's Standpoint

Sometimes, it really depends on how children perceive their disease themselves. Some children don't mind the extra weight and it may feel as if they are fitting in if the rest of the family is equally obese. Others may be very particular with their weight and get upset if they are a few pounds over. Girls are generally very concerned about weight. That is why the relationship between weight and self-esteem is more pronounced in young females than it is in males.[25]

Instilling Motivation in Obese Children

Children remain under the guidance of parents and it can be at times easier to motivate them and change their perception. First of all, parents should pay attention to their child's weight fluctuations and daily activities. Are these children getting used to watching television all day long, glued to video games, or "working" as a full-time Internet surfer? If they are one of the above, you should try to find some physical activity for them. Try to advise them on what foods to eat and take a family walk after dinner. Even if the walk only goes for about twenty minutes, everyone will benefit for the long term. Think of some chores such as sweeping, mowing the lawn, or gardening for the children to do when they are free.[26]

Don't let children fall asleep in front of the TV or computer. Figure out how many hours should be allowed for watching television or playing video games and remember that children should also spend a reasonable amount of time doing outdoor activities. Motivate them to invite their close friends to go for outdoor activities such as hiking and camping, help out with chores, or have them walk to and from school or the bus stop with someone instead of driving there.[27]

If you have good neighbors, talk with other parents who live nearby to let the children walk together and have a different parent accompany them each time. To motivate children to lose weight, parents themselves should have a routine to exercise and let the children see that exercising regularly is really all part of a daily routine. Children will likely adopt these habits for the rest of their lives. To make things a bit more interesting, teach your children how to play board games while they are really young. Have them fly a kite, ride a skateboard, or use a jump rope. If the children have a pet, give them some quality time to spend with it.[28]

Obese children need to be encouraged to do their best and ignore how others perceive them. Despite getting picked on by schoolmates, obese children have to remain optimistic about the future and make the best of everything at hand. The key is to avoid things that you know the kids won't have any control over. Slowly, the children will build up their own confidence and understand that they can still do something successfully, rather than letting others get to them just because they're overweight.[29]

NO SHORTCUTS: MOTIVATION FOR GROWNUPS

Living with adult obesity is a reality that may come at a great personal cost. For children, it depends greatly on how parents perceive, motivate, and help them deal with the disease. Adults must occasionally face personally induced consequences. However, some may be obese due to hereditary or some rare illness, which lead to hormonal imbalances that are obviously not their fault. If the obesity isn't due to your own actions, don't be afraid of telling the reason for your obesity to others. This may make them accept obese people into their lives more easily. Tell them you've put in a lot of effort to reduce your weight and, if they are health care professionals, ask them if there's a better or new treatment to help get rid of the extra fat.[30]

Sweetness of Self-Esteem

The term self-esteem is mentioned very often in motivational articles, but what exactly does it mean? If you live with a lot of self-esteem, you live with confidence and satisfaction. Of course, not everyone will have self-esteem all the time. Sometimes, you feel frustrated or upset and thus may present with low self-esteem. Obese people should remain in a solid state of self-esteem to avoid the urge to overeat.

Low self-esteem can unfortunately be attributed to a close relative, a particular object, or an event that took place a long time ago. Obese people, regardless of their weight or BMI, should know what can and cannot change about self-perceptions and the attitudes of the general public. In simpler terms, you should learn to accept the way he or she looks. Let's face it: you can feel much better when you're satisfied about your physical identity.

Obesity victims incidentally allow others to put a "lazy" label on them. No one's appearance can be changed overnight (except in the event of direct trauma to the body), but obese people could start out by making sure they have proper hygiene and "tidy up" to avoid looking clumsy. Wear clean clothing and avoid giving off any strong body odors. This will make people more willing to interact with you all the time. This is also advised for normal-weight people as well. It's really about having fundamental etiquette. First impressions are very important, and while you can't change your features 100 percent, you have to at least gather the self-esteem needed to find the motivation to get rid of your obesity.

Only a few manufacturers make oversized clothing designed specifically for the obese market. The low numbers may be responsible for creating the low self-esteem found in many obesity sufferers. Some overweight people, especially females, might only be familiar with a single retailer that sells plus size clothing in the neighborhood.[31] It all depends on the situation and one's self-esteem, along with the desire to actually attract attention from others. Is keeping a low profile in public the best way to go for you? Absolutely not, because it would defeat the whole reasoning behind why an obese individual should always dress right. The goal here is to deny others the opportunity to look at you in a negative way. Failure to present yourself the right way will only bring on more stigmatization that will lower your self-esteem. You have to understand how to deal with negativity before you find out the best way to motivate yourself. Toughening your self-esteem is a sensible starting point.

FOOD FOR THOUGHT?

Food Addictions Hinder Your Motivational Spirit

Research suggests that the reason for obesity, aside from heredity, is overeating.[32] Therefore, you should avoid eating too much in public and at home. Ironically, eating out can at times provide more motivation for losing weight than staying at home all day. When out dining at a restaurant, there are usually other people there looking at you. You get only the amount of food you can order. At home, however, you can dig into your fridge whenever you want, especially if you live alone.

Judging by body size, people have already stereotyped that most obesity victims are addicted to food. If you continue to act out public assumptions, it makes it harder for you to lose weight while obese. To obese people, both the lack of diet control and stigmatization from others are unsurprisingly demotivating factors. Stigmatization will lower an obesity victim's self-esteem, and reducing his or her food consumption may depress them even more if they do in fact have a food addiction.

The Dangers

Compulsive overeating is clinically considered an addiction.[33] Food addiction could lead to a self-destructive cycle where some people will eat more and get increasingly depressed, putting on extra pounds and completely ignoring their weight. Obese groups who fall into this cycle find it very difficult to change. The bottom line is this: you have to be aware of this unhealthy and destructive way of living at all times. You must gain a strong will to fight off your urges and remember that taste buds aren't the only thing you need to satisfy in life.[34]

If you cannot find a way to get rid of your food addictions in a short period of time, try to focus on long-term goals. Avoid having high-calorie foods. High-calorie foods can increase appetite and make you want more of whatever you just finished eating. It sounds easy, but the quest to get motivated for fighting food addiction is a long and bumpy road for obese people. It is easy for a normal-weight person to have diet control, but you have to realize that some obese people are really addicted to food. Such an addiction is very difficult to overcome because when someone cuts down on food, this will also lower the consumption of important sugars and essential fats. An abrupt reduction of sugar in meals can lead to depression by altering your serotonin levels.[35]

Self-Motivation and Food Addictions

Obese people with food addictions often don't get enough motivation. You need to have more than just a positive attitude and personal responsibility. As an obese parent, your children will follow your lifestyle and eating habits. However, as a responsible person within a community, you have to realize that being obese involves many internal and external problems that have been mentioned in the earlier chapters. Suffering from obesity yourself, you must avoid having your children go through the same disease.

Obese parents should understand and know how to self-motivate and lead their families to better physical, mental, and emotional health. Single parents with food addictions may think that the best compensation for their children who are not living with their mother and father is food. It's almost as if food has been used to replace the love of a parent who is never present in the lives of his or her children. Without motivation, these children may have obesity problems for the remainder of life.

MOTIVATIONAL EXPERIENCES

Growing Support

Martha Lyons (not her real name) grew up in in Carmel, Indiana, and was an overweight child.[36] She was picked on heavily at school and didn't have many friends. Her closest friend during school was a physically disabled girl in school. The class that Martha most feared was gym.

Her life was settled afterward but she was married and then divorced, and had to raise her two children by herself. She was alone for many years with the children, and only after the children grew older did they encourage her to have her own social life. Starting in 1998, Martha decided to meet someone who wouldn't focus too much on her weight. When she went to local organizations for obese women and discovered a group of overweight people having fun, happily meeting people as if body size didn't restrict them in any way. After the events, she read a lot of self-motivation books and listened to a few tapes. She decided to start a similar group in Indianapolis. Initially, this was an Internet group, and in 2002, the organization grew to more than 1,000 members consisting of people from all different weight ranges. She set up a very nice picnic and had gatherings every week that followed.

Martha discovered that many of the members didn't exactly have a social life until they joined the club. Most of the members regained their confidence for socializing with people, and several of them even found their soulmates among the members. Though she was running the club quite successfully, she had a problem with finding sponsors to help her organization survive in the long term. Most of her events were popular and while she considered herself to be a lucky person, she was very surprised to know that some businesses that were selling large-sized clothing weren't willing to promote her group. As one can see, Martha is a great example of self-motivation and improvement of social life in an obese individual. She not only helped herself, but motivated those who had problems similar to hers.

Motivation the Natural Way

Mark Rosenfeld (not his real name) slowly began to gain weight in 1986.[37] He had personal reasons for not controlling his diet. From what he recalled, he ate a lot of processed food, high-calorie items, and skipped normal meals, eating at the wrong time of day. His body size peaked in July 2000. He had tried several different kinds of weight-loss methods, losing about thirty pounds but quickly regaining the weight. One day, several people from a fitness company came to his workplace for the purpose of creating an ad. They were looking for someone who was interested in a serious weight-loss plan. Because Steve seemed as if he was just the guy, they approached him and asked him to try their weight-loss plan for a month. He was instructed not to tell anyone about the plan before it was underway.

After a month, Steve lost approximately twelve pounds and started to discuss his weight-loss plan on the airwaves. He continued to be on the weight-loss plan and successfully lost a total of 110 pounds. This is an ideal example of weight loss in the absence of pills. The program mainly instructed its participants on how to change their lifestyle and suggested what to eat. After losing just a few pounds, Steve already began to feel much more energy than he always had. He realized he had to carry so much fat on his body when walking around all those years that he felt exhausted all the time. Steve himself didn't notice any change in his emotions or behavior, but friends around him told him that he had gained more confidence. In fact, the weight-loss plan helped him to understand how the human body works, and more importantly, gave him a little motivation for a whole lot of change.

Some diet plans don't really mention how much food to take and how many calories you would gain after eating a specific type of food. Steve soon realized that having *too much* control on a diet could make you feel very unhappy. He would eat a burger in the morning and later in the day would only have fruits and vegetables to balance the diet. Steve was content with his weight loss and he could now wear the same size jeans he wore when he was in high school. Even so, he hoped to lose a little more weight.

READING BETWEEN THE LINES: DIRECT VERSUS INDIRECT TALKS

The Communication Mesh

With all the advanced technology nowadays, you can communicate with others through the Internet without going out or bending over backwards to get information. However, you can also get stressed if you don't possess the motivation to join a support group, or get a blog, forum, or any online platform. Obesity victims can receive positive advice or talk specifically with others with the same agenda and team up to make a change in their lives. Through communication and discussion, you could gain some knowledge on how to handle your life and stay motivated.

Sometimes, it's really not so easy to find someone to talk to for motivational purposes. Take the initiative to look for obese people who are in the same town or city as you are. If you share the same interests or hobbies, organize a couple of activities such as a simple walk in the park. Start up a small reading group, dancer's union, picnic, or travel club. Hobbies are especially helpful if you cannot get motivated enough to work out. The purpose of this is to redirect all your focus from overconsuming food to getting rid of your obesity completely.

THE FAREWELL

In conclusion to this comprehensive journey of realizing the true nature of obesity, remember that obesity is serious business no matter where in the world you live. When you're overweight, you increase your risk of heart failure, cancer, diabetes, and other life-threatening disease. Being overweight can also affect your quality of life, which is why it is important to consider finding motivation for your obesity. The disease in the United States alone plays a large role in causing common health risks, and motivation is required to avoid such risks. When you find motivation to get rid of obesity, you also find a way to reduce the risk of diabetes, high blood cholesterol, high blood pressure, cancer, atherosclerosis, hypertension, and other diseases. Set up a good diet plan now, incorporate exercise into your daily life, and put forth a realistic effort to eradicate obesity.

APPENDIX A:
OBESITY-RELATED WEBSITES

www.americanheart.org/presenter.jhtml?identifier=3053103

www.bodypositive.com

www.cdc.gov/nccdphp/dnpa/bmi/index.htm

www.health.gov/PAGuidelines

www.ific.org/nutrition/obesity/upload/obesitybackgrounder.pdf

www.mayoclinic.com/health/fitness/SM99999

www.mypyramidtracker.gov

www.obesity.org

www.obesityresource.com/

www.shapeup.org/

www.smallstep.gov

www.win.niddk.nih.gov/index.htm

www.ymca.net

www.ywca.org

APPENDIX B:
RESEARCH AND TRAINING

American College of Nutrition

300 S. Duncan Ave., Ste. 225
Clearwater, FL 33755
(727) 446-6086
Fax: (727) 446-6202
office@amcollnutr.org

**National Digestive Diseases
Information Clearinghouse (NIDDK)**

2 Information Way
Bethesda, MD 20892
(301) 654-3810
Fax: (301) 907-8906

**Canadian Institute of Food
Science and Technology**

3-1750 The Queensway, Suite 1311
Toronto, ON M9C 5H5
(905) 271-8338
Fax: (905) 271-8344
cifst@cifst.ca

**National Food Service Management
Institute**

The University of Mississippi
6 Jeanette Phillips Drive
P.O. Box 188
University, MS 38677
(800) 321-3054
Fax: (800) 321-3061
nfsmi@olemiss.edu

Institute of Food Science & Technology

5 Cambridge Court
210 Shepherds Bush Road
London W6 7NJ
+44(0) 20 7603 6316
Fax: +44(0) 20 7602 9936
info@ifst.org

Institute of Food Technologists
525 W. Van Buren, Ste. 1000
Chicago, IL 60607
(312) 782-8424
Fax: (312) 782.8348
info@ift.org

International Food Information Council Foundation
1100 Connecticut Avenue NW
Suite 430
Washington, DC 20036
info@foodinsight.org
www.foodinsight.org

North American Association for the Study of Obesity (NAASO)
8630 Fenton Street, Suite 412
Silver Spring, MD 20910
(301) 563-6526

National Kidney and Urologic Diseases Information Clearinghouse (NIDDK)
3 Information Way
Bethesda, MD 20892
(301) 654-4415
Fax: (301) 907-8906

National Mental Health Association
1201 Prince Street
Alexandria, VA 22314
(703) 684-7722
Fax: (703) 684-5968
www.nmha.org

National Weight Control Registry

Brown Medical School/The Miriam Hospital
Weight Control & Diabetes Research Center
196 Richmond Street
Providence, RI 02903
(800) 606-NWCR (6927)
tmnwcr@lifespan.org

Office of Health and Nutrition US Agency for International Development
Ronald Reagan Building
Washington, DC 20523
(202) 884-8722

Fax: (301) 587-2365

www.naaso.org

National Center on Sleep Disorders Research

National Heart, Lung, and Blood Institute

Two Rockledge Centre, Suite 7024

6701 Rockledge Drive, MSC 7920

Bethesda, MD 20892

(301) 435-0199

Fax: (301) 480-3451

National Diabetes Information Clearinghouse

1 Information Way

Bethesda, MD 20892

(800) 860–8747

Fax: (703) 738–4929

ndic@info.niddk.nih.gov

Fax: (202) 884-8977

linkages@aed.org

Society for Nutrition Education

9100 Purdue Road, Suite 200

Indianapolis, IN 46268

(800) 235-6690

Fax: (317) 280-8527

info@sne.org

Weight-Control Information Network

1 WIN Way

Bethesda, MD 20892

(877) 946–4627

Fax: (202) 828–1028

win@info.niddk.nih.gov

www.win.niddk.nih.gov

APPENDIX C:
OBESITY-RELATED ORGANIZATIONS

American Anorexia/Bulimia Association, Inc.

165 West 46th Street #1108

New York, NY 10036

(212) 575-6200

www.members.aol.com/amanbu/
index.html

American Dietetic Association

120 South Riverside Plaza, Suite 2000

Chicago, Illinois 60606

(800) 877-1600

American Sleep Disorders Association

1610 14th Street NW, Suite 300

Rochester, MN 55901

Healthy Weight Network

402 South 14th Street

Hettinger, ND 58639

(701) 567-2646

Fax: (701) 567-2602

www.healthyweight.net

National Association to Advance Fat Acceptance

P.O. Box 22510

Oakland, CA 94609

(916) 558–6880

www.naafa.org

National Eating Disorders Organization

6655 South Yale Avenue

Tulsa, OK 74136

(507) 287-6006
Fax: (507) 287-6008
www.asda.org

American Society for Metabolic Nervosa and and Bariatric Surgery
SW 75th Street, Suite 201
Gainesville, FL 32607
(352) 331-4900
Fax: (352) 331-4975
info@asmbs.org

American Society for Nutrition
9650 Rockville Pike
Bethesda, MD 20814
(301) 634-7050
Fax: (301) 634-7892

American Society for Parenteral and Enteral Nutrition (A.S.P.E.N.)
8630 Fenton Street, Suite 412
Silver Spring, MD 20910
(301) 587-6315
Fax: 301-587-2365
aspen@nutr.org

Council on Size and Weight Discrimination, Inc.
P.O. Box 305
Mount Marion, NY 12456
(845) 679–1209
www.cswd.org

(918) 481-4044
Fax: (918) 481-4076
www.laureate.com/aboutned.html

National Association of Anorexia Associated Disorders
P.O. Box 7
Highland Park, IL 60035
(847) 831-3438
Fax: (847) 433-4632

National Center for Health Statistics
Division of Health Examination Statistics
6525 Belcrest Road, Room 1000
Hyattsville, MD 20782

School Nutrition Association
120 Waterfront Street, Suite 300
National Harbor, MD 20745
(301) 686-3100
Fax: (301) 686-3115

The Obesity Society
8630 Fenton Street, Suite 814
Silver Spring, MD 20910
(301) 563-6526
Fax: (301) 563-6595
www.obesity.org

Eating Disorders Awareness and Prevention, Inc.

603 Stewart Street, Suite 803

Seattle, WA 98101

(206) 382-3587

www.members.aol.com/edapinc/home.html

APPENDIX D:
SELECTED STUDIES

Americans Consume Too Many Calories from Solid Fat, Alcohol, and Added Sugar
U.S. Department of Agriculture (USDA), Center for Nutrition Policy and Promotion
Nutrition Insight 33, June 2006.
www.cnpp.usda.gov/Publications/NutritionInsights/Insight33.pdf

BMI—Body Mass Index
Department of Health and Human Services (DHHS), Centers for Disease Control and Prevention (CDC), National Center for Chronic Disease Prevention and Health Promotion
www.cdc.gov/nccdphp/dnpa/bmi/index.htm

Defining Overweight and Obesity
DHHS, CDC, National Center for Chronic Disease Prevention and Health Promotion
www.cdc.gov/nccdphp/dnpa/obesity/defining.htm

Do You Know the Health Risks of Being Overweight?
www.win.niddk.nih.gov/publications/health_risks.htm

From Wallet to Waistline: The Hidden Costs of Super Sizing
National Alliance for Nutrition and Activity (NANA)
www.cspinet.org/w2w.pdf

Obesity among Older Americans
Georgetown University, Center on an Aging Society
Data Profile Number 10, July 2003.
www.hpi.georgetown.edu/agingsociety/pubhtml/obesity2/obesity2.html

Obesity and Disability: The Shape of Things to Come
RAND Health Research Highlights (RB-9043-1), 2007.
www.rand.org/pubs/research_briefs/RB9043-1/index1.html

Overweight and Obesity: Economic Consequences
DHHS, CDC, National Center for Chronic Disease Prevention and Health Promotion
www.cdc.gov/nccdphp/dnpa/obesity/economic_consequences.htm

Overweight and Obesity—Statistics
American Heart Association
www.americanheart.org/downloadable/heart/1197994908531FS16OVR08.pdf

Statistics Related to Overweight and Obesity
NIDDK, Weight-control Information Network
www.win.niddk.nih.gov/statistics/

The Contribution of Expanding Portion Sizes to the US Obesity Epidemic
Lisa R. Young, PhD, RD, and Marion Nestle, PhD, MPH *American Journal of Public Health* 92, no. 2(2002):246–50.
www.steinhardt.nyu.edu/nutrition.olde/PDFS/young-nestle.pdf

The Health Risks of Obesity: Worse Than Smoking, Drinking, or Poverty
RAND Research Brief (RB-4549), 2002.
www.rand.org/publications/RB/RB4549

The Price Is Right: Economics and the Rise in Obesity
Jayachandran N. Variyam
USDA Economic Research Service, *AmberWaves*, February 2005.
www.ers.usda.gov/amberwaves/february05/features/thepriceisright.htm

U.S. Obesity Trends 1985–2007
DHHS, CDC, National Center for Chronic Disease Prevention and Health Promotion
www.cdc.gov/nccdphp/dnpa/obesity/trend/maps/index.htm

Weighing In on Obesity
Food Review 25, no. 3 (Winter 2002).
www.ers.usda.gov/publications/foodreview/dec2002/

NOTES

PROLOGUE

1. "Obesity: Preventing and Managing the Global Epidemic," *World Health Organization Technical Report Series* 894 (2000).

2. World Health Organization, "Obesity and Overweight: Fact Sheet No. 311," www.who.int.

3. Bloomberg School of Public Health, "Medicare Changes View on Obesity: School Researchers Explain the Significance of New Policy," June 30, 2004, www.jhsph.edu; S. Heshka and D. Allison, "Is Obesity a Disease?" *International Journal of Obesity and Related Metabolic Disorders* 25, no. 10 (2001): 1401–4.

4. J. Hildebrand, "Too Fat to Fly: $60m Cost of Obesity to NSW Ambulance Service," *Daily Telegraph*, 2009, www.news.com.au.

5. World Health Organization, "Obesity," www.who.int.

6. J. Siedell et al., "What Aspects of Body Fat Are Particularly Hazardous and How Do We Measure Them?" *International Journal of Epidemiology* 35, no. 1 (2006): 83–92.

7. D. S. Kirschenbaum, "Misguided Diplomacy: Getting Past the 'Fear' of Telling a Child They Are Overweight or Obese," 2001, www.obesity-treatment.com.

8. M. Theodoro, A. Talebizadeh, and M. Butler, "Body Composition and Fatness Patterns in Prader-Willi Syndrome: Comparison with Simple Obesity," *Obesity* 14, no. 10 (2006): 1685–90.

9. The Mayo Clinic, "Obesity: Causes," www.mayoclinic.com.

10. World Health Organization, "Obesity," 2011, www.who.int/topics /obesity/en/.

11. World Health Organization, "Obesity."

12. U.S. Department of Health and Human Services, "Overweight and Obesity: A Major Public Health Issue," *Prevention Report*, 2001, 16.

13. J. Levine, "Obesity: Mission Possible," *Diabetes* 56, no. 11 (2007): 2653–54.

14. B. Balkau et al., "International Day for the Evaluation of Abdominal Obesity (IDEA): A Study of Waist Circumference, Cardiovascular Disease, and Diabetes Mellitus in 168,000 Primary Care Patients in 63 Countries," *Circulation* 115, no. 17 (2007): 1942–51.

15. World Health Organization, "Obesity."

16. Nestle Corporation, "Nestlé Position on Global Obesity, Diet, Nutrition and Physical Activity," 2003, www.nestle.com.

17. J. Levi et al. "F as in Fat: How Obesity Policies Are Failing in America," *Trust for America's Health* (report), 2009, 3–104.

18. Levi et al., "F as in Fat."

19. BBC News, "US Obesity Problem Intensifies," 2009, www.news.bbc .co.uk.

20. BBC News, "US Obesity Problem Intensifies."

21. Trust for America's Health, "New Report Finds Mississippi Has Most Obese Adults and Highest Obese and Overweight Children in the U.S.," 2009, www.healthyamericans.org.

CHAPTER I

1. World Health Organization, "Global Strategy on Diet, Physical Activity and Health: Obesity and Overweight," 2003, www.who.int.

2. W. Yang, T. Kelly, and J. He, "Genetic Epidemiology of Obesity," *Epidemiologic Reviews* 29 (2007): 49–61.

3. World Health Organization, "Global Strategy on Diet, Physical Activity and Health."

4. R. I. Kosti and D. B. Panagiotakos, "The Epidemic of Obesity in Children and Adolescents in the World," *Central European Journal of Public Health* 14, no. 4 (2006): 151–59.

5. S. Mydans, "Clustering in Cities, Asians Are Becoming Obese," *New York Times*, March 12, 2003.

6. K. R. Hill et al., "Co-residence Patterns in Hunter-Gatherer Societies Show Unique Human Social Structure," *Science* 331, no. 6022 (2011): 1286–89.

7. G. Bray and C. Bouchard, eds., *Handbook of Obesity: Etiology and Pathophysiology* (New York: Informa Health Care, 2004).

8. Bray and Bouchard, *Handbook of Obesity*; European Society of Cardiology, "Egyptian Princess Now Known to Be the First Person in Human History with Diagnosed Coronary Artery Disease: Heart Disease Not Just a Disease of Modern Lifestyle," May 17, 2011, www.escardio.org.

9. K. Keller, *Encyclopedia of Obesity*, 1st ed. (Thousand Oaks, CA: Sage Publications, 2008), 51.

10. Keller, *Encyclopedia of Obesity*, 51.

11. N. Papavramidou and H. Christopoulou-Aletra, "Greco-Roman and Byzantine Views on Obesity," *Obesity Surgery* 17, no. 1 (2007): 112–16.

12. Papavramidou and Christopoulou-Aletra, "Greco-Roman and Byzantine Views on Obesity," 112–16.

13. B. Swanson, "Getting Medieval on Obesity Issue," *Daily Express* (UK), March 6, 2008; Keller, *Encyclopedia of Obesity*, 51.

14. United Nations High Commissioner for Refugees (UNHCR), "Mauritania: Force-Feeding on Decline, but More Dangerous," July 25, 2011, www .unhcr.org.

15. A. Smith, "Girls Being Force-Fed for Marriage as Fattening Farms Revived," *Observer*, March 2009.

16. J. Ross and A. Galen, *Proceedings of the Royal Society of Medicine* 57, no. 8 (1964): 679–81.

17. "Giovanni Alfonso Borelli," *Encyclopedia Britannica*, www.britannica .com (2011); M. H. Pope, "Giovanni Alfonso Borelli—the Father of Biomechanics," *Spine* 30, no. 20 (2005): 2350–55.

18. "Lavoisier, Antoine," *Encyclopedia Britannica*, www.britannica.com (2007); U. Braun, "A. L. Lavoisier and the Anesthetist," *Anesthetist* 37, no. 11 (1988): 664–71.

19. "Obesity: Preventing and Managing the Global Epidemic," 894.

20. P. Klaczynksi, K. Goold, and J. Mudry, "Culture, Obesity Stereotypes, Self-Esteem, and the 'Thin Ideal': A Social Identity Perspective," *Journal of Youth and Adolescence* 33, no. 4 (2004): 307–17.

21. B. Sadock and V. Sadock, "Eating Disorders," in *Synopsis of Psychiatry, Behavioral Sciences/Clinical Psychiatry*, 10th ed., ed. H. Kaplan and B. Sadock (Philadelphia: Lippincott Williams and Wilkins, 2007), 727–35.

22. National Center for Health Statistics (NCHS) Health E Stats, "Prevalence of Overweight, Obesity and Extreme Obesity among Adults: United States, Trends 1960–62 through 2005–2006," December 2008, 1–4.

23. S. Aronson, "A Physician's Lexicon: The Verbiage of Obesity," *Medicine and Health Rhode Island* 86, no. 5 (2003): 154.

24. University of Maryland Medical Center, "Obesity," 2011, www.umm.edu.

25. D. Hensrud, "Dietary Treatment and Long-Term Weight Loss and Maintenance in Type 2 Diabetes," *Obesity Research* 9, no. S4 (2001): S348–S353.

26. Hensrud, "Dietary Treatment and Long-Term Weight Loss," S348–S353.

27. A. Aneja et al., "Hypertension and Obesity," *Recent Progress in Hormone Research* 59 (2004): 169–205; N. Méndez-Sánchez et al., "Obesity-Related Leptin Receptor Polymorphisms and Gallstones Disease," *Annals of Hepatology* 5, no. 2 (2006): 97–102.

28. A. R. Schwartz et al., "Obesity and Obstructive Sleep Apnea: Pathogenic Mechanisms and Therapeutic Approaches," *Proceedings of the American Thoracic Society* 5, no. 2 (2008): 185–92.

29. Méndez-Sánchez et al., "Obesity-Related Leptin Receptor Polymorphisms and Gallstones Disease," 97–102.

30. M. Magliano, "Obesity and Arthritis," *Menopause International* 14, no. 4 (2008): 149–54.

31. H. K. Choi et al., "Obesity, Weight Change, Hypertension, Diuretic Use, and Risk of Gout in Men: The Health Professionals Follow-Up Study," *Archives of Internal Medicine* 165, no. 7 (2005): 742–48.

32. G. A. Bray, "The Underlying Basis of Obesity: Relationship to Cancer," *Journal of Nutrition* 132, no. S11 (2002): S3451–S3455.

33. M. P. St-Onge et al., "Medium-Chain Triglycerides Increase Energy Expenditure and Decrease Adiposity in Overweight Men," *Obesity Research* 11, no. 3 (2003): 395–402.

34. H. Vainio and F. Bianchini, "Occurrence, Trends, and Analysis," in *IARC Handbooks of Cancer Prevention*, vol. 6, *Weight Control and Physical Activity* (Lyon, France: IARC Press, 2002); J. M. Roberts, L. M. Bodnar, and T. E. Patrick, "The Role of Obesity in Preeclampsia," *Pregnancy and Hypertension* 1, no. 1 (2011): 6–16.

35. T. A. Wadden and A. J. Stunkard, "Social and Psychological Consequences of Obesity," *Annals of Internal Medicine* 103, no. 6, pt. 2 (1985): 1062–67.

36. Wadden and Stunkard, "Social and Psychological Consequences of Obesity," 1062–67.

37. K. Fontaine et al., "Years of Life Lost Due to Obesity," *Journal of the American Medical Association* 289, no. 2 (2003): 187–93.

38. North Carolina Department of Health and Human Services, NCHC Policy No. NCHC2010.073, July 1, 2010, www.ncdhhs.gov.

39. A. H. Mokdad et al., "The Continuing Epidemic of Obesity in the United States," *Journal of the American Medical Association* 284, no. 13 (2000): 1650–51.

40. C. Bouchard, "The Magnitude of the Energy Imbalance in Obesity Is Generally Underestimated," *International Journal of Obesity* 32, no. 6 (2008): 879–80; V. Drapeau, N. King, and M. Hetherington, "Appetite Sensations and Satiety Quotient: Predictors of Energy Intake and Weight Loss," *Appetite* 48, no. 2 (2007): 159–66; B. Spiegelman and J. Flier, "Obesity and the Regulation of Energy Balance," *Cell* 104 (2001): 531–43.

41. M. Theodoro, Z. Talebizadeh, and M. Butler, "Body Composition and Fatness Patterns in Prader-Willi Syndrome: Comparison with Simple Obesity," *Obesity* 14, no. 10 (2006): 1685–90; J. B. Croft et al., "Obesity in Heterozygous Carriers of the Gene for the Bardet-Biedl Syndrome," *American Journal of Medical Genetics* 55, no. 1 (1995): 12–15.

42. C. B. Peterson, P. Thuras, and D. M. Ackard, "Personality Dimensions in Bulimia Nervosa, Binge Eating Disorder, and Obesity," *Comprehensive Psychiatry* 51, no. 1 (2010): 31–36.

43. A. Collins, "How the Body Uses Energy," 2009, www.annecollins.net; Drapeau, King, and Hetherington, "Appetite Sensations and Satiety Quotient," 159–66.

44. K. R. Westerterp, "Diet Induced Thermogenesis," *Nutrition and Metabolism* 1 (2004): 5.

45. M. Furnes, C. Zhao, and D. Chen, "Development of Obesity Is Associated with Increased Calories Per Meal Rather Than Per Day: A Study of High-Fat Diet-Induced Obesity in Young Rats," *Obesity Surgery* 19, no. 10 (2009): 1430–38.

46. R. St. Amand and C. Marek, "How Does the Body Make Energy?," in *What Your Doctor May Not Tell You about Fibromyalgia Fatigue: The Powerful Program That Helps You Boost Your Energy and Reclaim Your Life* (New York: Warner Books, 2003); Association of the British Pharmaceutical Industry, "Energy Balance, Fat, Overweight and Body Chemistry," 2009, www.abpi.org.uk.

47. W. W. Wong et al., "Are Basal Metabolic Rate Prediction Equations Appropriate for Female Children and Adolescents?," *Journal of Applied Physiology* 81, no. 6 (1996): 2407–14.

48. J. F. Strauss and R. L. Barbieri, *Yen & Jaffe's Reproductive Endocrinology*, 6th ed. (Philadelphia: W. B. Saunders, 2009), 166.

49. L. Wilson-Fritch et al., "Mitochondrial Remodeling in Adipose Tissue Associated with Obesity and Treatment with Rosiglitazone," *Journal of Clinical Investigation* 114, no. 9 (2004): 1281–89; M. Rogge, "The Role of Impaired Mitochondrial Lipid Oxidation in Obesity," *Biological Research for Nursing* 10, no. 4 (2009): 356–73.

50. J. Maldonado-Valderrama et al., "The Role of Bile Salts in Digestion," *Advances in Colloid and Interface Science* 165, no. 1 (2011): 36–46.

51. M. Badman and J. Flier, "The Gut and Energy Balance: Visceral Allies in the Obesity Wars," *Science* 307 (2005): 1909–14; X. Li et al., "Bile Salt-Stimulated Lipase and Pancreatic Lipase-Related Protein 2 Are the Dominating Lipases in Neonatal Fat Digestion in Mice and Rats," *Pediatric Research* 62, no. 5 (2007): 537–41.

52. Badman and Flier, "The Gut and Energy Balance," 1909–14.

53. St-Onge et al., "Medium-Chain Triglycerides," 395–402.

CHAPTER 2

1. R. C. Rabin, "Risks: Obesity Is Found to Take Toll after Age 40," *New York Times*, May 31, 2010.

2. L. F. Van Gaal, M. A. Wauters, and I. H. De Leeuw, "The Beneficial Effects of Modest Weight Loss on Cardiovascular Risk Factors," *International Journal of Obesity and Related Metabolic Disorders* 21, no. S1 (1997): S5–S9.

3. K. Lee, Y. M. Song, and J. Sung, "Which Obesity Indicators Are Better Predictors of Metabolic Risk? Healthy Twin Study," *Obesity* 16, no. 4 (2008): 834–40.

4. N. H. Durant et al., "Patient Provider Communication about the Health Effects of Obesity," *Patient Education and Counseling* 75, no. 1 (2009): 53–57.

5. L. M. Wen et al., "Family Functioning and Obesity Risk Behaviors: Implications for Early Obesity Intervention," *Obesity* 19, no. 6 (2011): 1252–58.

6. N. V. Christou, "Weight Gain after Short- and Long-Limb Gastric Bypass in Patients Followed for Longer Than 10 Years," *Annals of Surgery* 246, no. 1 (2007): 164.

7. Wen et al., "Family Functioning and Obesity Risk Behaviors," 252–58.

8. Wen et al., "Family Functioning and Obesity Risk Behaviors," 252–58.

9. L. Wang, I. M. Lee, and J. E. Manson, "Alcohol Consumption, Weight Gain, and Risk of Becoming Overweight in Middle-Aged and Older Women," *Archives of Internal Medicine* 170, no. 5 (2010): 453–61; G. E. Swan and D. Carmelli, "Characteristics Associated with Excessive Weight Gain after Smoking Cessation in Men," *American Journal of Public Health* 85, no. 1 (1995): 73–77.

10. D. Biondi, "Cervicogenic Headache: A Review of Diagnostic and Treatment Strategies," *Journal of the American Osteopathic Association* 105, no. S4 (2005): S16–S22.

11. L. K. Jonides, "Polyuria, Polydipsia—Not Always Diabetes," *Journal of Pediatric Health Care* 11, no. 6 (1997): 283, 307–8.

12. C. Thomas et al., "Urinary Calculi Composed of Uric Acid, Cystine, and Mineral Salts: Differentiation with Dual-Energy CT at a Radiation Dose

Comparable to That of Intravenous Pyelography," *Radiology* 257, no. 2 (2010): 402–9.

13. R. Atkinson et al., "Very Low-Calorie Diets," *Journal of the American Medical Association* 270, no. 8 (1993): 967–74.

14. J.-P. Chaputa et al., "Risk Factors for Adult Overweight and Obesity: The Importance of Looking beyond the 'Big Two,'" *Obesity Facts* 3, no. 5 (2010): 320–27.

15. B. Gross et al., "Medical Management of Cushing Disease," *Neurosurgical Focus* 23, no. 3 (2007): E10.

16. K. Hoyt and M. Schmidt, "Polycystic Ovary (Stein-Leventhal) Syndrome: Etiology, Complications, and Treatment," *Clinical Laboratory Science* 17, no. 3 (2004): 155–63.

17. Chaputa et al., "Risk Factors for Adult Overweight and Obesity," 320–27.

18. Y. B. Lee, J. D. Lee, and S. H. Cho, "Unusual Presentation of Obesity-Associated Dermatoses: Acanthosis Nigricans Involving Both Auricles," *Annals of Dermatology* 22, no. 4 (2010): 463–64.

19. G. Bray, *The Metabolic Syndrome and Obesity* (Totowa, NJ: Human Press, 2007).

20. J. Carter and M. Yuhasz, "Skinfolds and Body Composition of Olympic Athletes," in *Physical Structure of Olympic Athletes: Part II, Kinanthropometry of Olympic Athletes* (Basel, Switzerland: Karger, 1984), 107–16.

21. A. S. Jackson et al., "The Effect of Sex, Age and Race on Estimating Percentage Body Fat from Body Mass Index: The Heritage Family Study," *International Journal of Obesity and Related Metabolic Disorders* 26, no. 6 (2002): 789–96.

22. D. D. Hensrud and S. Klein, "Extreme Obesity: A New Medical Crisis in the United States," *Mayo Clinic Proceedings* 81, no. S10 (2006): S5–S10.

23. D. Gallagher, S. B. Heymsfield, and M. Heo, "Healthy Percentage Body Fat Ranges: An Approach for Developing Guidelines Based on Body Mass Index," *American Journal of Clinical Nutrition* 72, no. 3 (2000): 694–701, table 4.

24. G. Marchesini et al., "Obesity-Associated Liver Disease," *Journal of Clinical Endocrinology & Metabolism* 93, no. S1 (2008): S74–S80.

25. R. Atkinson et al., "Very Low-Calorie Diets," *Journal of the American Medical Association* 270, no. 8 (1993): 967–74.

26. A. Wetsman and F. Marlowe, "How Universal Are Preferences for Female Waist-to-Hip Ratios? Evidence from the Hadza of Tanzania," *Evolution and Human Behavior* 20, no. 4 (1999): 219–28; J. E. Brown et al., "Maternal Waist-to-Hip Ratio as a Predictor of Newborn Size: Results of the Diana Project," *Epidemiology* 7, no. 1 (1996): 62–66.

27. National Heart, Lung, and Blood Institute, "What Are the Health Risks of Overweight and Obesity?," n.d., www.nhlbi.nih.gov.

28. World Health Organization, "Obesity: Preventing and Managing the Global Epidemic," *World Health Organization Technical Report Series* 894 (2000): 9, table 2.1.

29. E. Kamel, G. McNeill, and M. Van Wijk, "Usefulness of Anthropometry and DXA in Predicting Intra-abdominal Fat in Obese Men and Women," *Obesity Research* 8 (2000): 36–42; M. Visser, M. Pahor, and F. Tylavsky, "One- and Two-Year Change in Body Composition as Measured by DXA in a Population-Based Cohort of Older Men and Women," *Journal of Applied Physiology* 94, no. 6 (2003): 2368–74.

30. W. Demark-Wahnefried, B. K. Rimer, and E. P. Winer, "Weight Gain in Women Diagnosed with Breast Cancer," *Journal of the American Dietetic Association* 97, no. 5 (1997): 519–29.

31. World Health Organization, "Obesity: Preventing and Managing the Global Epidemic," 9, table 2.1.

32. Visser, Pahor, and Tylavsky, "One- and Two-Year Change in Body Composition," 2368–74; Kamel, McNeill, and Van Wijk, "Usefulness of Anthropometry and DXA," 36–42.

33. J. Ma, L. Xiao, and R. Stafford, "Underdiagnosis of Obesity in Adults in US Outpatient Settings," *Archives of Internal Medicine* 169, no. 3 (2009): 313–14.

34. R. W. Taylor et al., "Gender Differences in Body Fat Content Are Present Well before Puberty," *International Journal of Obesity and Related Metabolic Disorders* 21, no. 11 (1997): 1082–84.

35. B. A. Gross et al., "Medical Management of Cushing Disease," *Neurosurgical Focus* 23, no. 3 (2007): E10.

36. B. A. Swinburn et al., "Body Composition Difference between Polynesians and Caucasians Assessed by Bioelectrical Impedance," *International Journal of Obesity and Related Metabolic Disorders* 20 (1996): 889–94.

37. Visser, Pahor, and Tylavsky, "One- and Two-Year Change in Body Composition," 2368–74.

38. N. S. Sadick, "Predisposing Factors of Varicose and Telangiectatic Leg Veins," *Journal of Dermatologic Surgery & Oncology* 18, no. 10 (1992): 883–86.

39. A. Marcon et al., "Body Mass Index, Weight Gain, and Other Determinants of Lung Function Decline in Adult Asthma," *Journal of Allergy and Clinical Immunology* 123, no. 5 (2009): 1069–74.

40. E. M. Zorn, R. G. Wieland, and M. C. Hallberg, "17beta-ol Androgens and Free Index in Hirsute and Hirsute Obese Women," *Fertility and Sterility* 27, no. 8 (1976): 916–20.

41. Sadick, "Predisposing Factors of Varicose and Telangiectatic Leg Veins," 883–86.

42. M. Lazzaro, K. Krishnan, and S. Prabhakaran, "Detection of Atrial Fibrillation with Concurrent Holter Monitoring and Continuous Cardiac Telemetry Following Ischemic Stroke and Transient Ischemic Attack," *Journal of Stroke and Cerebrovascular Diseases*, 2010, published online ahead of print in *Holter Monitor*, Harvard Medical School, 2010, www.health.harvard.edu/diagnostic-tests/holter-monitor.htm.

43. S. Daniel and M. Marshall, "Evaluation of the Liver: Laboratory Tests," in *Schiff's Diseases of the Liver*, 8th ed. (Philadelphia: J. B. Lippincott, 1999), 205–39; G. Marchesini et al., "Obesity-Associated Liver Disease," *Journal of Clinical Endocrinology & Metabolism* 93, no. S1 (2008): S74–S80; World Health Organization, "Obesity: Preventing and Managing the Global Epidemic," 9, table 2.1.

44. N. Knudsen et al., "Small Differences in Thyroid Function May Be Important for Body Mass Index and the Occurrence of Obesity in the Population," *Journal of Clinical Endocrinology & Metabolism* 90, no. 7 (2005): 4019–24; M. Krotkiewski, "Thyroid Hormones in the Pathogenesis and Treatment of Obesity," *European Journal of Pharmacology* 440, no. 2–3 (2002): 85–98; M. Michalaki, A. Veagenakis, and A. Leonardou, "Thyroid Function in Humans with Morbid Obesity," *Thyroid* 16, no. 1 (2006): 73–78.

45. Gross et al., "Medical Management of Cushing Disease," E10.

46. L. Douyon and D. Schteingart, "Effect of Obesity and Starvation on Thyroid Hormone, Growth Hormone, and Cortisol Secretion," *Endocrinology Metabolism Clinics of North America* 31, no. 1 (2002): 173–89.

47. G. Bray, *The Metabolic Syndrome and Obesity* (Totowa, NJ: Human Press, 2007).

48. K. He et al., "Magnesium Intake and Incidence of Metabolic Syndrome among Young Adults," *Circulation* 113 (2006): 1675–82.

49. L. Charles et al., "Obesity, White Blood Cell Counts, and Platelet Counts among Police Officers," *Obesity* 15 (2007): 2846–54.

CHAPTER 3

1. C. Bouchard, "Current Understanding of the Etiology of Obesity: Genetic and Nongenetic Factors," *American Journal of Clinical Nutrition* 53, no. S6 (1991): S1561–S1565.

2. S. Jebb and M. Moore, "Contribution of a Sedentary Lifestyle and Inactivity to the Etiology of Overweight and Obesity: Current Evidence and Research Issues," *Medicine & Science in Sports & Exercise* 31, no. S11 (1999): S534.

3. R. P. Schwartz, "Super-Size Kids' Meals Lead to Super-Size Kids," *North Carolina Medical Journal* 63, no. 6 (2002): 305–7.

4. D. Molnár and B. Livingstone, "Physical Activity in Relation to Overweight and Obesity in Children and Adolescents," *European Journal of Pediatrics* 159, no. S1 (2000): S45–S55.

5. R. Bertera, "The Effects of Workplace Health Promotion on Absenteeism and Employment Costs in a Large Industrial Population," *American Journal of Public Health* 80, no. 9 (1990): 1101–5; E. Brunner, T. Chandola, and M. Marmot, "Prospective Effect of Job Strain on General and Central Obesity in the Whitehall II Study," *American Journal of Epidemiology* 165, no. 7 (2006): 828–37; E. Brunner, T. Chandola, and M. Marmot, "Chronic Stress at Work and the Metabolic Syndrome: Prospective Study," *British Medical Journal* 332, no. 7540 (2006): 521.

6. Bertera, "The Effects of Workplace Health Promotion," 1101–5.

7. L. Leviton, "Children's Healthy Weight and the School Environment," *Annals of the American Academy of Political and Social Science* 615, no. 1 (2008): 38–55.

8. K. Brownell and F. Kaye, "A School-Based Behavior Modification, Nutrition Education, and Physical Activity Program for Obese Children," *American Journal of Clinical Nutrition* 35, no. 2 (1982): 277–83; B. Caballero et al., "Pathways: A School-Based, Randomized Controlled Trial for the Prevention of Obesity in American Indian Schoolchildren," *American Journal of Clinical Nutrition* 78, no. 5 (2003): 1030–38.

9. Schwartz, "Super-Size Kids' Meals Lead to Super-Size Kids," 305–7.

10. J. J. Wurtman, "The Involvement of Brain Serotonin in Excessive Carbohydrate Snacking by Obese Carbohydrate Cravers," *Journal of the American Dietetic Association*, 84, no. 9 (1984): 1004–7.

11. H. Oh and W. Seo, "The Compound Relationship of Smoking and Alcohol Consumption with Obesity," *Yonsei Medical Journal* 42, no. 5 (2001): 480–87; A. J. Flint et al., "Excess Weight and the Risk of Incident Coronary Heart Disease among Men and Women," *Obesity* 18, no. 2 (2010): 377–83.

12. Flint et al., "Excess Weight and the Risk of Incident Coronary Heart Disease," 377–83.

13. P. M. Suter, E. Jéquier, and Y. Schutz, "Effect of Ethanol on Energy Expenditure," *American Journal of Physiology* 266, no. 4, pt. 2 (1994): R1204–12.

14. J. Kinge and S. Morris, "Socioeconomic Variation in the Impact of Obesity on Health-Related Quality of Life," *Social Science & Medicine* 71, no. 10 (2010): 1864–71.

15. C. Fjeldstad et al., "The Influence of Obesity on Falls and Quality of Life," *Dynamic Medicine* 7 (2008): 4.

16. J. De Mola, "Obesity and Its Relationship to Infertility in Men and Women," *Obstetrics and Gynecology Clinics of North America* 36, no. 2 (2009): 333–46.

17. H. Masuzaki et al., "Human Obese Gene Expression: Adipocyte-Specific Expression and Regional Differences in the Adipose Tissue," *Diabetes* 44, no. 7 (1995): 855–58.

18. C. Grunfeld et al., "Endotoxin and Cytokines Induce Expression of Leptin, the Ob Gene Product, in Hamsters," *Journal of Clinical Investigation* 97, no. 9 (1996): 2152–57.

19. G. Hasler et al., "Depressive Symptoms during Childhood and Adult Obesity: The Zurich Cohort Study," *Molecular Psychiatry* 10, no. 9 (2005): 842–50.

20. W. P. James and P. Trayhurn, "An Integrated View of the Metabolic and Genetic Basis for Obesity," *Lancet* 2, no. 7989 (1976): 770–73.

21. F. Lönnqvist et al., "Overexpression of the Obese (Ob) Gene in Adipose Tissue of Human Obese Subjects," *Nature Medicine* 1 (1995): 950–53.

22. W. C. Knowler et al., "Obesity in the Pima Indians: Its Magnitude and Relationship with Diabetes," *American Journal of Clinical Nutrition* 53, no. S6 (1991): S1543–S1551.

23. D. B. Thompson et al., "Structure and Sequence Variation at the Human Leptin Receptor Gene in Lean and Obese Pima Indians," *Human Molecular Genetics* 6, no. 5 (1997): 675–79.

24. P. Ferre, "Genes and Obesity: The Ob Gene Product and the Beta 3-Adrenergic Receptor," *Diabetes and Metabolism* 22, no. 1 (1996): 77–79; N. Bégin-Heick, "Of Mice and Women: The Beta 3-Adrenergic Receptor Leptin and Obesity," *Biochemistry and Cell Biology* 74, no. 5 (1996): 615–22.

25. S. Farooqi, E. Bullmore, and J. Keogh, "Leptin Regulates Striatal Regions and Human Eating Behavior," *Science* 317, no. 5843 (2007): 1355.

26. M. G. Myers Jr. et al., "The Geometry of Leptin Action in the Brain: More Complicated Than a Simple ARC," *Cell Metabolism* 9, no. 2 (2009): 117–23.

27. C. Bjørbæk, "Central Leptin Receptor Action and Resistance in Obesity," *Journal of Investigative Medicine* 57, no. 7 (2009): 789–94; Grunfeld et al., "Endotoxin and Cytokines Induce Expression of Leptin," 2152–57.

28. T. Kelesidis et al., "Narrative Review: The Role of Leptin in Human Physiology: Emerging Clinical Applications," *Annals of Internal Medicine* 152, no. 2 (2010): 93–100.

29. M. R. Hayes et al., "Comparative Effects of the Long-Acting GLP-1 Receptor Ligands, Liraglutide and Exendin-4, on Food Intake and Body Weight Suppression in Rats," *Obesity* 19, no. 7 (2011): 1342–49.

30. Hayes et al., "Comparative Effects of the Long-Acting GLP-1 Receptor Ligands, Liraglutide and Exendin-4," 1342–49.

31. B. Biondi, "Thyroid and Obesity: An Intriguing Relationship," *Journal of Clinical Endocrinology Metabolism* 95, no. 8 (2010): 3965–72.

32. N. Meunier et al., "Basal Metabolic Rate and Thyroid Hormones of Late-Middle-Aged and Older Human Subjects: The ZENITH Study," *European Journal of Clinical Nutrition* 59, no. S2 (2005): S53–S57.

33. Biondi, "Thyroid and Obesity," 3965–72.

34. H. L. Fehm and K. H. Voigt, "Pathophysiology of Cushing's Disease," *Pathobiology Annual* 9 (1979): 225–55.

35. P. Anderson, "Bidirectional Link between Depression and Obesity Confirmed," *Archives of General Psychiatry* 67 (2010): 220–29; K. N. Boutelle et al., "Obesity as a Prospective Predictor of Depression in Adolescent Females," *Health Psychology* 29, no. 3 (2010): 293–98.

36. N. Vogelzangs et al., "Depressive Symptoms and Change in Abdominal Obesity in Older Persons," *Archives of General Psychiatry* 65, no. 12 (2008): 1386–93.

37. Boutelle et al., "Obesity as a Prospective Predictor of Depression in Adolescent Females," 293–98; J. M. Murphy et al., "Obesity and Weight Gain in Relation to Depression: Findings from the Stirling County Study: Overeating while Depressed," *International Journal of Obesity* 33 (2009): 335–41.

38. F. S. Luppino et al., "Overweight, Obesity, and Depression: A Systematic Review and Meta-Analysis of Longitudinal Studies," *Archives of General Psychiatry* 67, no. 3 (2010): 220–29.

39. A. Lusis, A. Attie, and K. Reue, "Metabolic Syndrome: From Epidemiology to Systems Biology," *Nature Reviews Genetics* 9 (2008): 819–30.

40. K. Rahmouni et al., "Leptin Resistance Contributes to Obesity and Hypertension in Mouse Models of Bardet-Biedl Syndrome," *Journal of Clinical Investigation* 118, no. 4 (2008): 1458–67.

41. G. M. Chertow and T. I. Chang, "Kidney Disease, Hospitalized Hypertension, and Cardiovascular Events: Cause or Consequence?," *Circulation* 121, no. 20 (2010): 2160–61.

42. M. Fava, "Weight Gain and Antidepressants," *Journal of Clinical Psychiatry* 61, no. S11 (2000): S37–S41; A. Serretti and L. Mandelli, "Antidepressants and Body Weight: A Comprehensive Review and Meta-Analysis," *Journal of Clinical Psychiatry* 71, no. 10 (2010): 1259–72.

43. V. L. Holt et al., "Body Mass Index, Weight, and Oral Contraceptive Failure Risk," *Obstetrics & Gynecology* 105, no. 1 (2005): 46–52.

44. N. Vogelzangs et al., "Depressive Symptoms and Change in Abdominal Obesity in Older Persons," *Archives of General Psychiatry* 65, no. 12 (2008): 1386–93.

45. G. Hasler et al., "Depressive Symptoms during Childhood and Adult Obesity: The Zurich Cohort Study," *Molecular Psychiatry* 10, no. 9 (2005): 842–50.

46. A. R. Schwartz et al., "Obesity and Obstructive Sleep Apnea: Pathogenic Mechanisms and Therapeutic Approaches," *Proceedings of the American Thoracic Society* 5, no. 2 (2008): 185–92.

47. T. Mahmood, "Influences of Excess Adiposity on Reproductive Function," *British Journal of Diabetes and Vascular Disease* 9, no. 5 (2009): 197–99.

48. J. Kinge and S. Morris, "Socioeconomic Variation in the Impact of Obesity on Health-Related Quality of Life," *Social Science & Medicine* 71, no. 10 (2010): 1864–71.

49. C. Fjeldstad et al., "The influence of Obesity on Falls and Quality of Life," *Dynamic Medicine* 7 (2008): 4.

50. A. Offer, R. Pechey, and S. Ulijaszek, "Obesity under Affluence Varies by Welfare Regimes: The Effect of Fast Food, Insecurity, and Inequality," *Economics & Human Biology* 8, no. 3 (2010): 297.

51. M. Pompili, P. Girardi, and G. Tatarelli, "Suicide and Attempted Suicide in Eating Disorders, Obesity and Weight-Image Concern," *Eating Behaviors* 7, no. 4 (2006): 384–94.

52. Pompili, Girardi, and Tatarelli, "Suicide and Attempted Suicide in Eating Disorders, Obesity and Weight-Image Concern," 297.

CHAPTER 4

1. L. Nemerson, L. Danowski, and J. Trilling, "The Spectrum of Treatment Options for Obesity," *Family Practice* 21, no. 3 (2004): 324–28.

2. M. Nestle, "Increasing Portion Sizes in American Diets: More Calories, More Obesity," *Journal of the American Dietetic Association* 103, no. 1 (2003): 41–47.

3. P. Chandon and B. Wansink, "Is Obesity Caused by Calorie Underestimation? A Psychophysical Model of Meal Size Estimation," *Journal of Marketing Research* 44, no. 1 (2007): 84–89.

4. K. Melanson et al., "Consumption of Whole-Grain Cereals during Weight Loss: Effects on Dietary Quality, Dietary Fiber, Magnesium, Vitamin B-6, and Obesity," *Journal of the American Dietetic Association* 106, no. 9 (2006): 1380–88; K. He et al., "Changes in Intake of Fruits and Vegetables in Relation to Risk of Obesity and Weight Gain among Middle-Aged Women," *International Journal of Obesity* 28 (2004): 1569–74.

5. B. Draznin and R. Rizza, eds., *Clinical Research in Diabetes and Obesity: Diabetes and Obesity*, 1st ed. (New York: Humana Press, 1997), 213.

6. D. R. Lauren et al., "Chemical Composition and In Vitro Anti-inflammatory Activity of Apple Phenolic Extracts and of Their Sub-fractions," *International Journal of Food Science and Nutrition* 60, no. S7 (2009): S188–S205.

7. R. Köhnke et al., "Thylakoids Suppress Appetite by Increasing Cholecystokinin Resulting in Lower Food Intake and Body Weight in High-Fat Fed Mice," *Phytotherapy Research* 23, no. 12 (2009): 1778–83.

8. B. Singh and U. Singh, "Peanut as a Source of Protein for Human Foods," *Plant Foods for Human Nutrition* 41, no. 2 (1991): 165–77.

9. J. K. Mason, J. Chen, and L. U. Thompson, "Flaxseed Oil-Trastuzumab Interaction in Breast Cancer," *Food and Chemical Toxicology* 48, no. 8–9 (2010): 2223–26; P. Lee and K. Prasad, "Effects of Flaxseed Oil on Serum Lipids and Atherosclerosis in Hypercholesterolemic Rabbits," *Journal of Cardiovascular Pharmacology and Therapeutics* 8, no. 3 (2003): 227–35.

10. A. Pan and F. B. Hu, "Effects of Carbohydrates on Satiety: Differences between Liquid and Solid Food," *Current Opinion in Clinical Nutrition & Metabolic Care* 14, no. 4 (2011): 385–90.

11. C. Berti et al., "Effect on Appetite Control of Minor Cereal and Pseudocereal Products," *British Journal of Nutrition* 94, no. 5 (2005): 850–58.

12. Berti et al., "Effect on Appetite Control of Minor Cereal and Pseudocereal Products," 850–58.

13. J. Levine et al., "The Role of Free-Living Daily Walking in Human Weight Gain and Obesity," *Diabetes* 57, no. 3 (2008): 548–54.

14. R. Browning and R. Kram, "Effects of Obesity on the Biomechanics of Walking at Different Speeds," *Medicine & Science in Sports & Exercise* 39, no. 9 (2007): 1632–41.

15. N. L. Chase, X. Sui, and S. N. Blair, "Swimming and All-Cause Mortality Risk Compared with Running, Walking, and Sedentary Habits in Men," *International Journal of Aquatic Research and Education* 2, no. 3 (2008): 213–23.

16. H. L. Chang, H. L. Wang, and C. H. Kuo, "Effect of Acute Swimming on Heart Rate Variability and HOMA–IR: 2389: Board #268," *Medicine & Science in Sports & Exercise* 42, no. 5 (2010): 609.

17. J. E. Donnelly et al., "Appropriate Physical Activity Intervention Strategies for Weight Loss and Prevention of Weight Regain for Adults," *Medicine & Science in Sports & Exercise* 41, no. 2 (2009): 459–71.

18. Reuters Health Online, "Thirty Minutes a Day of Exercise? Better Think 50," February 10, 2009, www.reuters.com.

19. F. Van Heerden et al., "An Appetite Suppressant from *Hoodia* Species," *Phytochemistry* 68, no. 20 (2007): 2545–53.

20. B. Avula et al., "Determination of the Appetite Suppressant P57 in *Hoodia gordonii* Plant Extracts and Dietary Supplements by Liquid Chromatography/Electrospray Ionization Mass Spectrometry (LC–MSD–TOF) and LC–UV Methods," *Journal of the Association of Analytical Communities (AOAC) International* 89, no. 3 (2006): 606–11.

21. L. Stahl, "New Plant May Fight Obesity" [video], *60 Minutes* Online, June 12, 2008, www.cbsnews.com.

22. I. Vermaak, "Indigenous South African Medicinal Plants Part 9: *Hoodia gordonii*," *South African Pharmaceutical Journal* 75, no. 4 (2008): 37.

23. M. Inchiosa, "Experience (Mostly Negative) with the Use of Sympathomimetic Agents for Weight Loss," *Journal of Obesity*, 2011 (published online ahead of print).

24. M. Guoyi et al., "Pharmacological Effects of Ephedrine Alkaloids on Human Alpha 1- and Alpha 2-Adrenergic Receptor Subtypes," *Journal of Pharmacology and Experimental Therapeutics* 322, no. 1 (2007): 214–21.

25. J. Dwyer, D. Allison, and P. Coates, "Dietary Supplements in Weight Reduction," *Journal of the American Dietetic Association* 105, no. S1 (2005): S80–S86.

26. P. Thaithumyanon, S. Limpongsanurak, and P. Praisuwanna, "Perinatal Effects of Amphetamine and Heroin Use during Pregnancy on the Mother and Infant," *Journal of the Medical Association of Thailand* 88, no. 11 (2005): 1506–13.

27. J. Halford et al., "Serotonergic Drugs: Effects on Appetite Expression and Use for the Treatment of Obesity," *Drugs* 67, no. 1 (2007): 27–55.

28. R. Padwal and S. Majumdar, "Drug Treatments for Obesity: Orlistat, Sibutramine, and Rimonabant," *Lancet* 369, no. 9555 (2007): 71–77.

29. L. Mej, "How Does Sibutramine Work?," *International Journal of Obesity* 25, no. S4 (2001): S8–S11.

30. J. Appolinario et al., "A Randomized, Double-Blind, Placebo-Controlled Study of Sibutramine in the Treatment of Binge-Eating Disorder," *Archives of General Psychiatry* 60, no. 11 (2003): 1109–16.

31. Padwal and Majumdar, "Drug Treatments for Obesity," 71–77.

32. Padwal and Majumdar, "Drug Treatments for Obesity," 71–77.

33. H. G. Preuss et al., "An Overview of the Safety and Efficacy of a Novel, Natural(-)Hydroxycitric Acid Extract (HCA-SX) for Weight Management," *Journal of Medicine* 35, no. 1–6 (2004): 33–48.

34. P. Kopelman, I. Caterson, and W. Dietz, eds., *Clinical Obesity in Adults and Children*, 3rd ed. (Hoboken, NJ: Wiley-Blackwell, 2010), 273.

35. R. B. Rothman et al., "Amphetamine-Type Central Nervous System Stimulants Release Norepinephrine More Potently Than Dopamine and Serotonin," *Synapse* 39, no. 1 (2001): 32–41.

36. R. Magill et al., "Effects of Tyrosine, Phentermine, Caffeine D-Amphetamine, and Placebo on Cognitive and Motor Performance Deficits during Sleep Deprivation," *Nutritional Neuroscience* 6, no. 4 (2003): 237–46.

37. N. Puzziferri et al., "Variations of Weight Loss following Gastric Bypass and Gastric Band," *Annals of Surgery* 248, no. 2 (2008): 233–42.

38. T. Farrell et al., "Clinical Application of Laparoscopic Bariatric Surgery: An Evidence-Based Review," *Surgical Endoscopy* 23, no. 5 (2009): 930–49.

39. V. Moizé et al., "Pica Secondary to Iron Deficiency 1 Year after Gastric Bypass," *Surgery for Obesity and Related Diseases* 6, no. 3 (2010): 316–18.

40. Kopelman, Caterson, and Dietz, *Clinical Obesity in Adults and Children*, 273.

41. M. Stepanoni et al., "The Biliopancreatic Diversion: A Comparison of Laparoscopic and Laparotomic Techniques," *Minerva Chirurgica* 61, no. 3 (2006): 205–13.

42. A. Wittgrove and G. Clark, "Laparoscopic Gastric Bypass, Roux en-Y–500 Patients: Technique and Results, with 3–60 Month Follow-Up," *Obesity Surgery* 10, no. 3 (2000): 233–39.

43. M. Schowalter, A. Benecke, and C. Lager, "Changes in Depression following Gastric Banding: A 5- to 7-Year Prospective Study," *Obesity Surgery* 18, no. 3 (2008): 314–20.

44. R. Pasquali et al., "Clinical and Hormonal Characteristics of Obese Amenorrheic Hyperandrogenic Women Before and After Weight Loss," *Journal of Clinical Endocrinology and Metabolism* 68 (1989): 173–79.

45. M. Lean et al., "Obesity, Weight Loss and Prognosis in Type 2 Diabetes," *Diabetic Medicine* 7 (1990): 416–20.

46. S. Kahn, R. Hull, and K. Utzschneider, "Mechanisms Linking Obesity to Insulin Resistance and Type 2 Diabetes," *Nature* 444, no. 7121 (2006): 840–46; B. Draznin and R. Rizza, eds., *Clinical Research in Diabetes and Obesity: Diabetes and Obesity*, 1st ed. (New York: Humana Press, 1997), 213; Pasquali et al., "Clinical and Hormonal Characteristics of Obese Amenorrheic Hyperandrogenic Women," 173–79.

CHAPTER 5

1. M. Lemonick, "How We Grew So Big: Diet and Lack of Exercise Are Immediate Causes but Our Problem Began in the Paleolithic Era," *Time* 103, no. 23 (2004): 57–71.

2. World Health Organization, "Obesity: Preventing and Managing the Global Epidemic," *World Health Organization Technical Report Series* 894, no. 1–12 (2000): 43, 85–88, 166.

3. Centers for Disease Control and Prevention, "U.S. Obesity Trends," July 21, 2011, www.cdc.gov.

4. D. Lakdawalla and T. Philipson, "The Growth of Obesity and Technological Change," *Economics and Human Biology* 7, no. 3 (2009): 283–93.

5. A. Park, "Study: Too Much Sugar Increases Heart Risks," *Time*, 2010, www.time.com.

6. B. J. Sargent and N. A. Moore, "New Central Targets for the Treatment of Obesity," *British Journal of Clinical Pharmacology* 68, no. 6 (2009): 852–60.

7. E. Finkelstein, I. Fiebelkorn, and G. Wang, "National Medical Spending Attributable to Overweight and Obesity How Much and Who Is Paying," *Health Affairs*, supplement web exclusive (2003): W3–219–26.

8. G. A. Colditz, "Economic Costs of Obesity: The US Perspective," *Pharmacoeconomics* 5, no. S1 (1994): S34–S37.

9. R. Collins and J. Anderson, "Medication Cost Savings Associated with Weight Loss for Obese NIDD Men and Women," *Preventive Medicine* 24 (1995): 369–74.

10. Collins and Anderson, "Medication Cost Savings Associated with Weight Loss," 369–74.

11. Centers for Disease Control and Prevention, "Overweight and Obesity: Data and Statistics," 2009, www.cdc.gov.

12. K. M. Flegal et al., "Prevalence and Trends in Obesity among US Adults, 1999–2000," *Journal of the American Medical Association* 288 (2002): 1723–27.

13. N. Helminch, "Obesity Predicted for 40% of America," *USA Today*, 2003, www.usatoday.com.

14. E. M. Sadler, "The Benefits of Running," Vanderbuilt University Department of Psychology, n.d, www.vanderbilt.edu.

15. D. L. Katz, "Unfattening Our Children: Forks over Feet," *International Journal of Obesity* 35 (2011): 33–37.

16. M. T. Bassett et al., "Purchasing Behavior and Calorie Information at Fast-Food Chains in New York City, 2007," *American Journal of Public Health* 98, no. 8 (2008): 1457–59.

17. C. L. Ogden et al., "Prevalence of High Body Mass Index in US Children and Adolescents 2007–2008," *Journal of the American Medical Association* 303 (2010): 242–49; R. J. Deckelbaum and C. L. Williams, "Childhood Obesity: The Health Issue," *Obesity Research* 9, no. S4 (2001): S239–S243; National Center for Health Statistics (NCHS) Health E Stats, "Prevalence of Overweight, Obesity and Extreme Obesity among Adults: United States, Trends 1960–62 through 2005–2006," December 2008, 1–4.

18. M. K. Serdula et al., "Do Obese Children Become Obese Adults? A Review of the Literature," *Preventative Medicine* 22 (1993): 167–77.

19. D. S. Freedman et al., "Relationship of Childhood Overweight to Coronary Heart Disease Risk Factors in Adulthood: The Bogalusa Heart Study," *Pediatrics* 108 (2001): 712–18.

20. Centers for Disease Control and Prevention, "Overweight and Obesity: Childhood Overweight and Obesity."

21. S. Richardson et al., "Cultural Uniformity in Reaction to Physical Disabilities," *American Social Revolution* 26 (1961): 241–47.

22. L. Irving, "Promoting Size Acceptance in Elementary School Children: The EDAP Puppet Program," *International Journal of Eating Disorders* 8 (2000): 221–32.

23. R. Henig, "Fat Factors," *New York Times Magazine*, August 13, 2006, www.nytimes.com.

24. E. Reisin et al., "The Effect of Weight Loss without Salt Restriction on the Reduction in Blood Pressure of Overweight Hypertensives," *New England Journal of Medicine* 298 (1978): 1–6.

25. Henig, "Fat Factors."

26. P. Brice, "Combating Genetic Predisposition to Obesity," PHG Foundation, April 20, 2010, www.phgfoundation.org.

27. BBC, "Clear Obesity Gene Link Found," *BBC News*, 2007, www.news.bbc.co.uk.

28. A. Drewnowski and S. E. Specter, "Poverty and Obesity: The Role of Energy Density and Energy Costs," *American Journal of Clinical Nutrition* 79, no. 1 (2004): 6–16.

29. J. Seidell and I. Deerenberg, "Obesity in Europe—Prevalence and Consequences for the Use of Medical Care," *Pharmacoeconomics* 5 (1994): 38–44.

30. U. Hakkinen, "The Production of Health and the Demand for Health Care in Finland," *Social Science and Medicine* 33, no. 3 (1991): 225–37.

31. Z. Wang, E. Klipfell, and B. J. Bennett, "Gut Flora Metabolism of Phosphatidylcholine Promotes Cardiovascular Disease," *Nature* 472, no. 7341 (2011): 57–63.

32. World Bank, *World Development Report 1993: Investing in Health: World Development Indicators* (New York: Oxford University Press, 1993).

33. D. V. Schapira et al., "Visceral Obesity and Breast Cancer Risk," *Cancer* 74 (1994): 632–39.

34. D. V. Schapira et al., "Weight as a Risk Factor for Clinical Diabetes in Women," *American Journal of Epidemiology* 132 (1990): 501–13.

35. World Health Organization, "Obesity: Preventing and Managing the Global Epidemic."

36. World Health Organization, "Obesity: Preventing and Managing the Global Epidemic."

37. G. R. Yang, S. Y. Yuan, and H. J. Fu, "Neck Circumference Positively Related with Central Obesity, Overweight, and Metabolic Syndrome in Chinese Subjects with Type 2 Diabetes: Beijing Community Diabetes Study 4," *Diabetes Care* 33, no. 11 (2010): 2465–67.

38. T. P. Gill, "Key Issues in the Prevention of Obesity," *British Medical Bulletin* 53 (1997): 359–88; M. Higgins et al., "Benefits and Adverse Effects of Weight Loss: Observations from the Framingham Study," *Annals of Internal Medicine* 119 (1993): 758–63.

40. World Health Organization, "Obesity: Preventing and Managing the Global Epidemic."

41. World Health Organization, "Obesity: Preventing and Managing the Global Epidemic."

42. World Health Organization, "Obesity: Preventing and Managing the Global Epidemic."

CHAPTER 6

1. M. Ismail, "Prevalence of Obesity and Chronic Energy Deficiency (CED) in Adult Malaysians," *Malaysian Journal of Nutrition* 1 (1995): 1–9.

2. W. C. Willet, W. H. Dietz, and G. A. Colditz, "Guidelines for Healthy Weight," *New England Journal of Medicine* 341, no. 6 (1999): 427–34.

3. Centers for Disease Control and Prevention, "Child and Teen: About BMI, Assessing Your Weight, Healthy Weight," January 27, 2009, www.cdc .gov.

4. D. Lakdawalla and T. Philipson, "The Growth of Obesity and Technological Change," *Economics and Human Biology* 7, no. 3 (2009): 283–93.

5. C. Koebnick et al., "Prevalence of Extreme Obesity in a Multiethnic Cohort of Children and Adolescents," *Journal of Pediatrics* 157, no. 1 (2010): 26–31.

6. World Health Organization, "Prevalence of Overweight and Obesity in Children and Aadolescents," *World Health Organization Europe Fact Sheet* 2.3, 2009, 5–7.

7. World Health Organization, "Obesity: Preventing and Managing the Global Epidemic," *World Health Organization Technical Report Series 894*, no. 1 (2000): 20.

8. A. Musaiger and S. Miladi, eds., "Diet Related Non-communicable Diseases in the Arab Countries of the Gulf," *Cairo: Food and Agriculture Organization of the United Nations*, 1996, 99–117.

9. Willet, Dietz, and Colditz, "Guidelines for Healthy Weight," 427–34.

10. National Health and Medical Research Council (NHMRC), *Acting on Australia's Weight: A Strategic Plan for the Prevention of Overweight and Obesity* (Canberra, Australia: National Health and Medical Research Council, 1997).

11. Ismail, "Prevalence of Obesity and Chronic Energy Deficiency (CED) in Adult Malaysians," 1–9.

12. R. Hughes, "Diet, Food, Supply and Obesity in the Pacific," World Health Organization Regional Office for the Western Pacific, 2003.

13. M. L. Booth et al., "The Epidemiology of Overweight and Obesity among Australian Children and Adolescents, 1995–97," *Australian and New Zealand Journal of Public Health* 25, no. 2 (2001): 162–68.

14. World Health Organization, "Obesity: Preventing and Managing the Global Epidemic," 16.

15. P. Davey and S. Leeder, "The Cost of Cost-of-Illness Studies," *Medical Journal of Australia* 158 (1993): 583–84.

16. S. M. Schwarz, "Obesity," April 13, 2010, www.emedicine.medscape.com.

17. A. Guilherme et al., "Adipocyte Dysfunctions Linking Obesity to Insulin Resistance and Type 2 Diabetes," *Nature Reviews Molecular Cell Biology* 9, no. 5 (2008): 367–77.

18. American Heart Association, "Risk Factors and Coronary Heart Disease," 2008, www.americanheart.org.

19. J. Stamler, J. Neaton, and D. Wentworth, "Blood Pressure (Systolic and Diastolic) and Risk of Fatal Coronary Heart Disease," *Hypertension* 13, no. S5 (1989): S2–S12.

20. Reuters Health, "Obesity Tied to Early Heart Attack," 2008, www.reuters.com/article/2008/10/09/us–obesity-heart–idUSTRE49884O20081009.

21. M. C. Madala et al., "Obesity and Age of First Non-ST-segment Elevation Myocardial Infarction," *Journal of the American College of Cardiology* 52, no. 12 (2008): 979–85.

22. J. Dixon, M. Dixon, and P. O'Brien, "Depression in Association with Severe Obesity: Changes with Weight Loss," *Archives of Internal Medicine* 163, no. 17 (2003): 2058–65.

23. K. E. Friedman et al., "Body Image Partially Mediates the Relationship between Obesity and Psychological Distress," *Obesity Research* 10, no. 1 (2002): 33–41.

24. M. De Zwaan, "Binge Eating Disorder and Obesity," *International Journal Obesity and Related Metabolic Disorders* 25, no. S1 (2001): S51–S55.

25. De Zwaan, "Binge Eating Disorder and Obesity," S51–S55.

26. G. S. Waters et al., "Long-Term Studies of Mental Health after the Greenville Gastric Bypass Operation for Morbid Obesity," *American Journal of Surgery* 161, no. 1 (1991): 154–58.

27. E. Finkelstein, I. Fiebelkorn, and G. Wang, "National Medical Spending Attributable to Overweight and Obesity: How Much, and Who's Paying?," *Health Affairs* W3 (2003): 219–26.

28. S. Solovay, *Tipping the Scales of Injustice: Fighting Weight Based Discrimination* (Amherst, NY: Prometheus Books, 2000).

29. R. Pingitore et al., "Bias against Overweight Job Applicants in a Simulated Employment Interview," *Journal of Applied Psychology* 79 (1994): 909–17.

30. R. Paul and J. Townsend, "Shape Up or Ship Out? Employment Discrimination against the Overweight," *Employee Responsibilities and Rights Journal* 8, no. 2 (1995): 133–45.

31. E. Rothblum et al., "The Relationship between Obesity, Employment Discrimination, and Employment Related Victimization," *Journal of Vocational Behavior* 37, no. 3 (1990): 251–66.

32. J. H. Price et al., "Family Practice Physician's Beliefs, Attitudes and Practices Regarding Obesity," *American Journal of Preventative Medicine* 3, no. 6 (1987): 339–45.

33. C. Bagley et al., "Attitudes of Nurses toward Obesity and Obese Patients," *Perceptual & Motor Skills* 68, no. 3, pt. 1 (1989): 954.

34. L. Irving, "Promoting Size Acceptance in Elementary School Children: The EDAP Puppet Program," *International Journal of Eating Disorders* 8 (2000): 221–32.

35. World Health Organization, "Global Strategy on Diet, Physical Activity and Health," 2004, www.who.int.

36. International Association for the Study of Obesity, "Obesity: Understanding and Challenging the Global Epidemic," 2009, www.iaso.org.

CHAPTER 7

1. The Associated Press, "Fast-Food Fans Clueless about Calories," MSNBC.com, 2006, www.msnbc.msn.com/id/14679909/ns/health-diet_and_nutrition/t/fast-food-fans-clueless-about-calories/.

2. J. Simmonds, "Obesity in Children and Teenagers," *PBS Newshour Extra*, 2001, www.pbs.org.

3. Centers for Disease Control and Prevention, "Childhood Obesity: Healthy Youth," 2010, www.cdc.gov.

4. UCSF Benioff Children's Hospital, "Obesity Causes," 2010, www.ucsfbenioffchildrens.org.

5. Associated Press, "Many Parents of Fat Kids in Denial, Study Finds," *USA Today*, 2007, www.usatoday.com.

6. G. Waters et al., "Long-Term Studies of Mental Health after the Green-ville Gastric Bypass Operation for Morbid Obesity," *American Journal of Surgery* 161, no. 1 (1991): 154–58.

7. Center for Science in the Public Interest, "Food Companies Undermine Parents, Overfeed Kids, Says Report," November 10, 2003, www.cspinet.org.

8. Mayo Foundation for Medical Education and Research, "Gallstones: Complications," Mayo Clinic, 2009, www.mayoclinic.com; R. Mangold et al., "The Effects of Sleep and Lack of Sleep on the Cerebral Circulation and Metabolism of Normal Young Men," *Journal of Clinical Investigation* 34, no. 7, pt. 1 (1955): 1092–1100.

9. P. Heslop et al., "Sleep Duration and Mortality: The Effect of Short or Long Sleep Duration on Cardiovascular and All-Cause Mortality in Working Men and Women," *Sleep Medicine* 3, no. 4 (2002): 305–14.

10. Kaiser Permanente, "Obese People with Asthma Have Nearly Five Times Greater Risk of Hospitalization for Asthma," *ScienceDaily*, September 8, 2008, www.sciencedaily.com.

11. Mayo Foundation for Medical Education and Research, "Gallstones: Complications."

12. C. S. Berkey et al., "Longitudinal Study of Skipping Breakfast and Weight Change in Adolescents," *International Journal of Obesity and Related Metabolic Disorders* 27, no. 10 (2003): 1258–66.

13. About.com, "Obesity, Diabetes on the Increase in US: 44 Million Americans Now Considered Obese—17 million Suffer Diabetes," 2010, www.usgovinfo.about.com.

14. R. J. Ferry, "Diabetes Overview," *E-Medicine*, 2010, www.emedicinehealth.com/diabetes.

15. H. Simon and D. Zieve, "High Blood Cholesterol and Triglycerides," *New York Times*, May 5, 2009, www.health.nytimes.com.

16. P. Belluck, "Children's Life Expectancy Being Cut Short by Obesity," *New York Times*, March 17, 2005, www.nytimes.com.

17. R. Nisenbaum et al., "Variability and Predictors of Negative Mood Intensity in Patients with Borderline Personality Disorder and Recurrent Suicidal Behavior: Multilevel Analyses Applied to Experience Sampling Methodology," *Journal of Abnormal Psychology* 119, no. 2 (2010): 433–39.

18. N. Hellmich, "An Overweight America Comes with a Hefty Price Tag," *USA Today*, 2003, www.usatoday.com; National Center for Health Statistics, "Overweight Prevalence," Centers for Disease Control and Prevention, June 18, 2010, www.cdc.gov

19. P. Orenstein, "The Way We Live Now: The Fat Trap," *New York Times Magazine*, 2010, www.nytimes.com.

20. Simon and Zieve, "High Blood Cholesterol and Triglycerides."

21. Berkey et al., "Longitudinal Study of Skipping Breakfast and Weight Change in Adolescents," 1258–66.

22. Center for Science in the Public Interest, "Food Companies Undermine Parents, Overfeed Kids, Says Report."

CHAPTER 8

1. M. G. Sawyer et al., "Is There a Relationship between Overweight and Obesity and Mental Health Problems in 4- to 5-Year-Old Australian Children?," *Ambulatory Pediatrics* 6, no. 6 (2006): 306–11.

2. A. Fabricatore, "Behavior Therapy and Cognitive-Behavioral Therapy of Obesity: Is There a Difference?," *Journal of the American Dietetic Association* 107, no. 1 (2007): 92–99.

3. F. Koch, A. Sepa, and J. Ludvigsson, "Psychological Stress and Obesity," *Journal of Pediatrics* 153, no. 6 (2008): 839–44; L. E. Kuo et al., "Chronic Stress, Combined with a High-Fat/High-Sugar Diet, Shifts Sympathetic Signaling toward Neuropeptide Y and Leads to Obesity and the Metabolic Syndrome," *Annals of New York Academy of Science* 1148 (2008): 232–37.

4. D. Stein, "Obsessive-Compulsive Disorder," *Lancet* 360, no. 9330 (2002): 397–405.

5. M. Jenike, "Clinical Practice: Obsessive-Compulsive Disorder," *New England Journal of Medicine* 350, no. 3 (2004): 259–65.

6. G. Maina et al., "Weight Gain during Long-Term Treatment of Obsessive-Compulsive Disorder: A Prospective Comparison between Serotonin Reuptake Inhibitors," *Journal of Clinical Psychiatry* 65, no. 10 (2004): 1365–71.

7. C. Jacobi, G. Schmitz, and W. Agras, "Is Picky Eating an Eating Disorder?," *International Journal of Eating Disorders* 41, no. 7 (2008): 626–34.

8. S. Kirchner et al., "Prenatal Exposure to the Environmental Obesogen Tributyltin Predisposes Multipotent Stem Cells to Become Adipocytes," *Molecular Endocrinology* 24, no. 3 (2010): 526–39.

9. M. Bongiovi-Garcia et al., "Comparison of Clinical and Research Assessments of Diagnosis, Suicide Attempt History and Suicidal Ideation in Major Depression," *Journal of Affective Disorders* 115, no. 1–2 (2009): 183–88.

10. B. M. Appelhans et al., "Time to Abandon the Notion of Personal Choice in Dietary Counseling for Obesity?," *Journal of the American Dietetic Association* 111, no. 8 (2011): 1130–36.

11. L. F. Faulconbridge et al., "Changes in Symptoms of Depression with Weight Loss: Results of a Randomized Trial," *Obesity* 17, no. 5 (2009): 1009–16.

12. A. Biswas et al., "Obesity in People with Learning Disabilities: Possible Causes and Reduction Interventions," *Nursing Times* 106, no. 31 (2010): 16–18.

13. S. Cortese et al., "Attention-Deficit/Hyperactivity Disorder (ADHD) and Obesity: A Systematic Review of the Literature," *Critical Reviews in Food Science and Nutrition* 48, no. 6 (2008): 524–37; R. Yang, "ADHD and Obesity," *Canadian Medical Association Journal* 182, no. 5 (2010): 482.

14. S. Cortese and C. Morcillo Peñalver, "Comorbidity between ADHD and Obesity: Exploring Shared Mechanisms and Clinical Implications," *Postgraduate Medicine* 122, no. 5 (2010): 88–96.

15. C. Curtin et al., "Prevalence of Overweight in Children and Adolescents with Attention Deficit Hyperactivity Disorder and Autism Spectrum Disorders: A Chart Review," *BMC (BioMed Central) Pediatrics* 5 (2005): 48.

16. Biswas et al., "Obesity in People with Learning Disabilities," 16–18.

17. L. E. Kuo et al., "Chronic Stress, Combined with a High-Fat/High-Sugar Diet, Shifts Sympathetic Signaling toward Neuropeptide Y and Leads to Obesity and the Metabolic Syndrome," *Annals of New York Academy of Science* 1148 (2008): 232–37.

18. R. Dishman and P. O'Connor, "Lessons in Exercise Neurobiology: The Case of Endorphins," *Mental Health and Physical Activity* 2, no. 1 (2009): 4–9.

19. R. Pandit, J. W. de Jong, and L. J. Vanderschuren, "Neurobiology of Overeating and Obesity: The Role of Melanocortins and Beyond," *European Journal of Pharmacology* 660, no. 1 (2011): 28–42.

20. C. Fairburn and P. Harrison, "Eating Disorders," *Lancet* 361, no. 9355 (2003): 407–16.

21. S. S. Wang, "No Age Limit on Picky Eating," *Wall Street Journal*, July 5, 2010, online.wsj.com.

22. A. Stunkard, K. Allison, and J. O'Reardon, "The Night Eating Syndrome: A Progress Report," *Appetite* 45, no. 2 (2005): 182–86.

23. W. Zhong et al., "Depression and Anxiety: Obesity and Depression Symptoms in the Beaver Dam Offspring Study Population," *Obesity Symptoms & Warning* 27, no. 9 (2010): 846–51.

24. C. Evers, F. Marijn Stok, and D. de Ridder, "Feeding Your Feelings: Emotion Regulation Strategies and Emotional Eating," *Personality and Social Psychology Bulletin* 36, no. 6 (2010): 792–804.

25. R. Leverence et al., "Obesity Counseling and Guidelines in Primary Care: A Qualitative Study," *American Journal of Preventative Medicine* 32, no. 4 (2007): 334–39.

26. K. Phillips, "Body Dysmorphic Disorder: Recognizing and Treating Imagined Ugliness," *World Psychiatry* 3, no. 1 (2004): 12–17.

27. J. Kornbeck, "Why Social Work Can't Ignore Obesity," *Professional Social Work*, Feb. 2009, 20–21.

28. Jacobi, Schmitz, and Agras, "Is Picky Eating an Eating Disorder?," 626–34.

29. S. Becker, N. Rapps, and S. Zipfel, "Psychotherapy in Obesity—a Systematic Review," *Psychotherapie, Psychosomatik, medizinische Psychologie* 57, no. 11 (2007): 420–27.

30. W. Miller and T. Miller, "Attitudes of Overweight and Normal Weight Adults Regarding Exercise at a Health Club," *Journal of Nutrition Education and Behavior* 42, no. 1 (2010): 2–9.

31. T. Lang and G. Rayner, "Corporate Responsibility in Public Health," *BMJ* 341 (2010): c3758.

32. L. H. Epstein, J. N. Roemmich, and H. A. Raynor, "Behavioral Therapy in the Treatment of Pediatric Obesity," *Pediatric Clinics of North America* 48, no. 4 (2001): 981–93; C. A. Johnston, C. Tyler, and J. P. Foreyt, "Behavioral Management of Obesity," *Current Atherosclerosis Reports* 9, no. 6 (2007): 448–53; G. D. Foster, A. P. Makris, and B. A. Bailer, "Behavioral Treatment of Obesity," *American Journal of Clinical Nutrition* 82, no. S1 (2005): S230–S235.

33. M. Bongiovi-Garcia et al., "Comparison of Clinical and Research Assessments of Diagnosis, Suicide Attempt History and Suicidal Ideation in Major Depression," *Journal of Affective Disorders* 115, no. 1–2 (2009): 183–88.

34. P. W. Pace, M. P. Bolton, and R. S. Reeves, "Ethics of Obesity Treatment: Implications for Dietitians," *Journal of the American Dietetic Association* 91, no. 10 (1991): 1258–60.

35. T. McAlindon and D. T. Felson, "Nutrition: Risk Factors for Osteoarthritis," *Annals of the Rheumatic Diseases* 56, no. 7 (1997): 397–400.

36. V. Raisová, "The Work of the Dietitian in the Outpatient Obesity Unit," *Sb Lek* (English abstract) 99, no. 3 (1998): 329–31.

37. N. P. Quinlan et al., "Psychosocial Outcomes in a Weight Loss Camp for Overweight Youth," *International Journal of Pediatric Obesity* 4, no. 3 (2009): 134–42.

38. S. Bitton and J. Roth, "Addressing Food Insecurity: Freedom from Want, Freedom from Fear," *Journal of the American Medical Association* 304, no. 21 (2010): 2405–6.

39. M. Navarro-Díaz et al., "Effect of Drastic Weight Loss after Bariatric Surgery on Renal Parameters in Extremely Obese Patients: Long-Term Follow-Up," *Journal of the American Society of Nephrology* 17, no. S3 (2006): S213–S217.

40. B. M. Appelhans et al., "Time to Abandon the Notion of Personal Choice in Dietary Counseling for Obesity?," *Journal of the American Dietetic Association* 111, no. 8 (2011): 1130–36.

41. G. E. Faulkner, P. F. Gorczynski, and T. A. Cohn, "Psychiatric Illness and Obesity: Recognizing the 'Obesogenic' Nature of an Inpatient Psychiatric Setting," *Psychiatric Services* 60, no. 4 (2009): 538–41.

42. W. Zhong et al., "Depression and Anxiety: Obesity and Depression Symptoms in the Beaver Dam Offspring Study Population," *Obesity Symptoms & Warning* 27, no. 9 (2010): 846–51.

CHAPTER 9

1. L. J. Aronne, "Classification of Obesity and Assessment of Obesity-Related Health Risks," *Obesity Research* 10, no. S2 (2002): S105–S115.

2. R. Leung, "The Subway Diet," *CBS News*, December 5, 2007, www.cbsnews.com.

3. G. Jackson, "How Many Calories Are in an Empty Subway Foot Long Sandwich?," November 8, 2010, www.livestrong.com.

4. "Chemicals in Food Can Make You Fat," *CBS News*, 2010, www.cbsnews.com.

5. S. Branch, "Food Makers Get Defensive about Gains in U.S.," *Wall Street Journal*, 2002.

6. USDA Center for Nutrition Policy and Promotion, "Is Total Fat Consumption Really Decreasing?," *Nutrition Insights* 5 (1998): 1–2.

7. K. M. Flegal et al., "Overweight and Obesity in the United States: Prevalence and Trends, 1960–1994," *Internal Journal of Obesity and Related Metabolic Disorders* 22 (1998): 39–47.

8. USDA Center for Nutrition Policy and Promotion, "Is Total Fat Consumption Really Decreasing?"

9. C. L. Ogden et al., "Obesity among Adults in the United States—No Statistically Significant Chance Since 2003–2004," *National Center for Health Statistics (NCHS) Data Brief* 1 (2007): 1–8.

10. National Institutes of Health, "Fat," *Medline Plus*, August 2, 2009.

11. M. Enig, *Know Your Fats: The Complete Primer for Understanding the Nutrition of Fats, Oils and Cholesterol*, 1st ed. (Silver Spring, MD: Bethesda Press, 2001).

12. Enig, *Know Your Fats*.

13. S. M. Teegala et al., "Consumption and Health Effects of Trans Fatty Acids: A Review," *Journal of AOAC International* 92 (2009): 1250.

14. Enig, *Know Your Fats*.

15. Walgreens, "Gatorade G2 Low Calorie Electrolyte Beverage Orange," 2011, www.walgreens.com.

16. Associated Press, "PepsiCo Spent $1.2 Million Lobbying Gov't in 2Q," *ABC News*, July 26, 2010, www.abcnews.go.com.

17. Ecosystems, Ltd., "Industry Lobbying Sees EU Reject 'Traffic Light' Food Labeling," *The Ecologist*, June 17, 2010, www.theecologist.org/News.

18. US Food and Drug Administration, "How to Understand and Use the Nutrition Facts Label," March 11, 2011, www.fda.gov.

19. W. M. Pride and O. C. Ferrell, "Marketing: Concepts and Strategies" (Boston: Houghton Mifflin Co., 2006), 93.

20. Encyclopedia.com, "Human Nutrition: Sugars, Preserves, and Syrups," n.d, www.britannica.com.

21. K. C. Hayes and A. Pronczuk, "Replacing Trans Fat: The Argument for Palm Oil with a Cautionary Note on Interesterification," *Journal of the American College of Nutrition* 29, no. S3 (2010): S253–S284.

22. L. Layton, "FDA Warns 17 Food Companies of Misleading Claims on Label," *Washington Post*, 2010, www.washingtonpost.com.

23. B. McKevith, "Is Salmon Salmon Pink? The Use of Canthaxanthin in Animal Feeds," *Nutrition Bulletin* 28, no. 3 (2003): 243–45.

24. Hong Kong Center for Food Safety, "Canthaxanthin in Food," January 2009, www.cfs.gov.hk/english; S. Gradelet et al., "Effects of Canthaxanthin, Astaxanthin, Lycopene and Lutein on Liver Xenobiotic-Metabolizing Enzymes in the Rat," *Xenobiotica* 26, no. 1 (1996): 49–63.

25. USDA Center for Nutrition Policy and Promotion, "Is Total Fat Consumption Really Decreasing?," 1–2.

26. "Chemicals in Food Can Make You Fat," *CBS News*; F. Grün, "Obesogens: Current Opinion in Endocrinology," *Diabetes Obesity* 17, no. 5 (2010): 453–59.

27. P. H. Weis, "Obesity: The Real Cause," *True Health*, www.truehealth.org/obesity.html.

28. Center for Science in the Public Interest, "Food Companies Undermine Parents, Overfeed Kids, Says Report," November 10, 2003, www.cspinet.org.

29. J. Hill and L. Radimer, "A Content Analysis of Food Advertisements in Television for Australian Children," *Australian Journal of Nutrition and Diet* 54 (1997): 174–81.

30. D. Green, "How Much Weight Can You Lose Not Drinking Sodas or Eating Junk Food?," January 17, 2011, www.livestrong.com.

31. C. Hellerman, "Nutritionists: Soda Making Americans Drink Themselves Fat," *CNN*, 2007, www.edition.cnn.com.

32. S. Malik, F. McGlone, and D. Bedrossian, "Ghrelin Modulates Brain Activity in Areas That Control Appetitive Behavior," *Cell Metabolism* 7, no. 5 (2008): 400–409.

33. G. Bray, S. Nielsen, and B. Popkin, "Consumption of High-Fructose Corn Syrup in Beverages May Play a Role in the Epidemic of Obesity," *American Journal of Clinical Nutrition* 79, no. 4 (2004): 537–43.

34. D. Benton, "The Plausibility of Sugar Addiction and Its Role in Obesity and Eating Disorders," *Clinical Nutrition* 29, no. 3 (2010): 288–303.

35. M. Takahashi et al., "Behavioral and Pharmacological Studies on Gluten Exorphin A5, a Newly Isolated Bioactive Food Protein Fragment, in Mice," *JJP: The Japanese Journal of Pharmacology* 84, no. 3 (2000): 259–65; S. Fukudome and M. Yoshikawa, "Gluten Exorphin C: A Novel Opioid Peptide Derived from Wheat Gluten," *Federation of the Societies of Biochemistry and Molecular Biology (FEBS) Letters* 316, no. 1 (1993): 17–19.

36. A. Morabia and M. C. Costanza, "Sodas, High Fructose Corn Syrup, and Obesity: Let's Focus on the Right Target," *Preventative Medicine* 51, no. 1 (2010): 1–2.

37. C. Alford, H. Cox, and R. Wescott, "The Effects of Red Bull Energy Drink on Human Performance and Mood," *Amino Acids* 21, no. 2 (2001): 139–50; E. Rush et al., "Are Energy Drinks Contributing to the Obesity Epidemic?," *Asia Pacific Journal of Clinical Nutrition* 15, no. 2 (2006): 242–44.

38. H. Karppanen and E. Mervaala "Sodium Intake and Hypertension," *Progress in Cardiovascular Diseases* 49, no. 2 (2006): 59–75.

39. Karppanen and Mervaala "Sodium Intake and Hypertension," 59–75.

40. K. Ortolon, "Gatorade or Water?," *Texas Medical Association Journal* 99, no. 6 (2003): 31–33.

41. K. He et al., "Association of Monosodium Glutamate Intake with Overweight in Chinese Adults: The INTERMAP Study," *Obesity* 16, no. 8 (2008): 1875–80.

CHAPTER 10

1. A. Wolf and G. Colditz, "Current Estimates of the Economic Cost of Obesity in the United States," *Obesity Research* 6 (1998): 97–106.

2. J. Bhattacharya and N. Sood, "Health Insurance and the Obesity Externality," *Advances in Health Economics and Health Services Research* 17 (2007): 279–318.

3. S. A. Seelig, "Rising Interest Rates and Cost Push Inflation," *Journal of Finance* 29, no. 4 (1974): 1049–61.

4. D. Bessesen, "Update on Obesity," *Journal of Clinical Endocrinology and Metabolism* 93, no. 6 (2008): 2027–34.

5. J. H. Merriam, "Coincident and Lagging Indicators," *Nebraska Journal of Economics and Business* 10, no. 3 (1971): 37–50.

6. Merriam, "Coincident and Lagging Indicators," 37–50.

7. N. E. Adler and J. M. Ostrove, "Socioeconomic Status and Health: What We Know and What We Don't," *Annals of New York Academy of Science* 896 (1999): 3–15; T. Dam, J. Jensen, and N. Kaergard, "Obesity, Social Inequality and Economic Rationality: An Overview," *Food Economics—Acta Agriculturae Scandinavica, Section C* 5, no. 3 (2008): 124–37.

8. Virginia Commonwealth University Medical Center, "Facts about Obesity," n.d., www.vcu.edu.

9. US Census Bureau, "US & World Population Clocks," n.d., www.census.gov.

10. D. Bessesen, "Update on Obesity," *Journal of Clinical Endocrinology and Metabolism* 93, no. 6 (2008): 2027–34.

11. T. F. Gary and F. Brancati, "Strategies to Curb the Epidemic of Diabetes and Obesity in Primary Care Settings," *Journal of General Internal Medicine* 19, no. 12 (2004): 1242–43.

12. A. Adams, "Obesity Epidemic Threatens to Bankrupt US Economy and Threatens Financial Stability of the World," *Natural News*, 2004, www.naturalnews.com.

13. P. Elmer et al., "Effects of Weight Gain on Medical Care Costs," *International Journal of Obesity* 28 (2004): 1365–73.

14. Gary and Brancati, "Strategies to Curb the Epidemic of Diabetes and Obesity in Primary Care Settings," 1242–43.

15. E. Ross-Thomas, "Obesity Could Hit Economies as Hard as Malnutrition," *Reuters Health*, November 15, 2006, www.reutershealth.com.

16. California Health and Human Services Agency, "The Obesity Epidemic in California," *2010 Summit on Health, Nutrition, and Obesity: Actions for Healthy Living*, n.d.

17. Ross-Thomas, "Obesity Could Hit Economies as Hard as Malnutrition."

18. Wolf and Colditz, "Current Estimates of the Economic Cost of Obesity in the United States," 97–106.

19. Wolf and Colditz, "Current Estimates of the Economic Cost of Obesity in the United States," 97–106.

20. Wolf and Colditz, "Current Estimates of the Economic Cost of Obesity in the United States," 97–106.

21. West Virginia Health and Human Services, "Obesity: Facts, Figures, and Guidelines," 2002, www.wvdhhr.org.

22. C. Quesenberry, B. Caan, and A. Jacobson, "Obesity, Health Services Use, and Health Care Costs among Members of a Health Maintenance Organization," *Archives of Internal Medicine* 158 (1998): 466–72.

23. D. Thompson et al., "Body Mass Index and Future Healthcare Costs: A Retrospective Study," *Obesity Research* 9 (2001): 210–18.

24. B. Snowdon and H. R. Vane, *An Encyclopedia of Macroeconomics* (Northhamptom, MA: Edward Elgar Publishing, 2002).

25. "Economic Factors: Monetary Policy," *Investopedia*, 2009, www .investopedia.com.

26. A. B. Hoskins, "Occupational Injuries, Illnesses, and Fatalities among Nursing, Psychiatric, and Home Health Aides, 1995–2004," Bureau of Labor Statistics, June 30, 2006, www.bls.gov.

27. J. Ma, L. Xiao, and R. Stafford, "Underdiagnosis of Obesity in Adults in US Outpatient Settings," *Archives of Internal Medicine* 169, no. 3 (2009): 313–14.

28. D. Olick, "Fats Take a Toll on US Economy," *MSNBC*, 2003, www.msnbc .msn.com.

29. S. Devi, "Progress on Childhood Obesity Patchy in the USA," *Lancet* 371, no. 9607 (2008): 105–6.

30. A. M. Minino et al., "Deaths: Final Data for 2004," *National Vital Statistics Reports* 55, no. 19 (2007): 8, table C.

31. R. Sturm, "The Effects of Obesity, Smoking, and Drinking on Medical Problems and Costs," *Health Affairs* 21, no. 2 (2002): 245–53.

32. Sturm, "The Effects of Obesity, Smoking, and Drinking," 245–53.

33. Sturm, "The Effects of Obesity, Smoking, and Drinking," 245–253; R. Sturm and K. Wells, "Does Obesity Contribute as Much to Morbidity as Poverty or Smoking?," *Public Health* 115, no. 3 (2001): 229–35.

34. M. Daviglus et al., "Relation of Body Mass Index in Young Adulthood and Middle Age to Medicare Expenditures in Older Age," *Journal of the American Medical Association* 292, no. 22 (2004): 2243–749.

35. D. E. Wiener, "Causes and Consequences of Chronic Kidney Disease: Implications for Managed Healthcare," *Journal of Managed Care Pharmacy* 13, no. S3 (2007): S1–S9.

36. Wiener, "Causes and Consequences of Chronic Kidney Disease," S1–S9.

37. J. Bhattacharya and N. Sood, "Health Insurance and the Obesity Externality," *Advances in Health Economics and Health Services Research* 17 (2007): 279–318.

38. J. Bhattacharya et al., "Does Health Insurance Make You Fat?," in *Economic Aspects of Obesity*, ed. M. Grossman and N. Mocan (Chicago: University of Chicago Press, 2011), 35–64; E. Finkelstein, C. Ruhm, and K. Kosa, "Economic Causes and Consequences of Obesity," *Annual Review of Public Health* 26 (2005): 239–57.

39. Finkelstein, Ruhm, and Kosa, "Economic Causes and Consequences of Obesity," 239–57.

40. Daviglus et al., "Relation of Body Mass Index in Young Adulthood and Middle Age to Medicare Expenditures in Older Age," 2243–749.

41. D. Thompson et al., "Body Mass Index and Future Healthcare Costs: A Retrospective Study," *Obesity Research* 9 (2001): 210–18.

42. K. Fontaine et al., "Years of Life Lost Due to Obesity," *Journal of the American Medical Association* 289, no. 2 (2003): 187–93.

43. J. Stevens et al., "The Effect of Age on the Association between Body-Mass Index and Mortality," *New England Journal of Medicine* 338, no. 1 (1998): 1–7.

44. Daviglus et al., "Relation of Body Mass Index in Young Adulthood and Middle Age to Medicare Expenditures in Older Age," 2243–749.

45. L. McLaren and J. Godley, "Social Class and BMI among Canadian Adults: A Focus on Occupational Prestige," *Obesity* 17, no. 2 (2009): 290–99.

46. Sturm, "The Effects of Obesity, Smoking, and Drinking," 245–53.

47. L. Barrington and B. Rosen, "Weights and Measures: What Employers Should Know about Obesity—Key Findings," *The Conference Board*, 2008.

48. Barrington and Rosen, "Weights and Measures."

49. E. B. York and K. Skiba, "Healthier Food Finds New Ally in Wal-Mart Initiative," *Chicago Tribune*, January 20, 2011, www.articles.chicagotribune.com.

50. New York City Department of Health and Mental Hygiene, "Health Department's New TV Spot Shows How a Day's Worth of Sugary Drinks Adds Up to a Whopping 93 Sugar Packets: Latest Installment of City's 'Pouring on the Pounds' Campaign Debuts New Don't Drink Yourself Sick Televised Ad, Subway Posters," January 31, 2011, www.nyc.gov.

CHAPTER 11

1. K. Borer, E. Wuorinen, and C. Burant, "Loss of Exercise-Associated Suppression of Hunger and Plasma Leptin in Obese but Not Lean Women" (paper presented at the 90th Annual Meeting of the Endocrine Society, San Francisco, California, 2008).

2. S. Guven, A. El-Bershawi, and G. E. Sonnenberg, "Plasma Leptin and Insulin Levels in Weight-Reduced Obese Women with Normal Body Mass Index: Relationships with Body Composition and Insulin," *Diabetes* 48, no. 2 (1999): 347–52.

3. Borer, Wuorinen, and Burant, "Loss of Exercise-Associated Suppression of Hunger and Plasma Leptin."

4. B. Balkau et al., "Physical Activity and Insulin Sensitivity: The RISC Study," *Diabetes* 57, no. 10 (2008): 2613–18; N. Hamburg et al., "Physical Inactivity Rapidly Induces Insulin Resistance and Microvascular Dysfunction in Healthy Volunteers," *Arteriosclerosis, Thrombosis, and Vascular Biology* 27, no. 12 (2007): 2650–56; M. Williams et al., "Resistance Exercise in Individuals with and without Cardiovascular Disease: 2007 Update: A Scientific Statement from the American Heart Association Council on Clinical Cardiology and Council on Nutrition, Physical Activity, and Metabolism," *Circulation* 116, no. 5 (2007): 572–84.

5. C. L. Davis, J. Tkacz, and M. Gregoski, "Aerobic Exercise and Snoring in Overweight Children: A Randomized Controlled Trial," *Obesity* 14, no. 11 (2006): 1985–91.

6. Balkau et al., "Physical Activity and Insulin Sensitivity," 2613–18.

7. A. Nikolai et al., "Cardiovascular and Metabolic Responses to Water Aerobics Exercise in Middle-Age and Older Adults," *Journal of Physical Activity and Health* 6, no. 3 (2009): 333–38.

8. J. Eckerson and T. Anderson, "Physiological Response to Water Aerobics," *Journal of Sports Medicine and Physical Fitness* 32, no. 2 (1992): 255–61.

9. *New York Times* Company, "Calories Burned with Running: 8.6 mph (7 Min/mile)," www.caloriecount.about.com.

10. L. Burke et al., "Guidelines for Daily Carbohydrate Intake: Do Athletes Achieve Them?," *Sports Medicine* 31 (2001): 267–99.

11. Harvard Medical School, "Obesity Keeps Climbing for U.S. Adults," *Harvard Health Publications*, www.harvardhealthcontent.com.

12. L. J. Whyte, J. M. Gill, and A. J. Cathcart, "Effect of 2 Weeks of Sprint Interval Training on Health-Related Outcomes in Sedentary Overweight/Obese Men," *Metabolism* 59, no. 10 (2010): 1421–28.

13. H. Pasternak, *The 5 Factor Diet* (New York: Ballantine, 2009).

14. Harvard Medical School, "Obesity Keeps Climbing for U.S. Adults."

15. M. Kennedy and M. Newton, "Effect of Exercise Intensity on Mood in Step Aerobics," *Journal of Sports Medicine and Physical Fitness* 37, no. 3 (1997): 200–204.

16. J. Raglin and M. Wilson, "State Anxiety following 20-Minutes of Bicycle Ergometer Exercise at Selected Intensities," *International Journal of Sports Medicine* 17 (1996): 467–71.

17. R. Thayer, *Calm Energy: How People Regulate Mood with Food and Exercise* (New York: Oxford University Press, 2003).

18. M. Meissner et al., "Exercise Enhances Whole-Body Cholesterol Turnover in Mice," *Medicine & Science in Sports & Exercise* 42, no. 8 (2010): 1460–68.

19. J. M. Zmuda et al., "Exercise Training Has Little Effect on HDL Levels and Metabolism in Men with Initially Low HDL Cholesterol," *Atherosclerosis* 137, no. 1 (1998): 215–21.

20. H. Steinberg et al., "Exercise Enhances Creativity Independently of Mood," *British Journal of Sports Medicine* 31, no. 3 (1997): 240–45.

21. J. Drake et al., "Do Exercise Balls Provide a Training Advantage for Trunk Extensor Exercises? A Biomechanical Evaluation," *Journal of Manipulative and Physiological Therapeutics* 29, no. 5 (2006): 354–62.

22. S. McGill, N. Kavcic, and E. Harvey, "Sitting On a Chair or an Exercise Ball: Various Perspectives to Guide Decision Making," *Clinical Biomechanics* 21, no. 4 (2006): 353–60.

23. R. Rydeard, A. Leger, and D. Smith, "Pilates-Based Therapeutic Exercise: Effect on Subjects with Nonspecific Chronic Low Back Pain and Functional Disability: A Randomized Controlled Trial," *Journal of Orthopaedic & Sports Physical Therapy* 36, no. 7 (2006): 472–84.

24. I. Moinuddin and D. Leehey, "A Comparison of Aerobic Exercise and Resistance Training in Patients with and without Chronic Kidney Disease," *Advanced Chronic Kidney Disease* 15, no. 1 (2008): 83–96.

25. W. Campbell et al., "Resistance Training Preserves Fat-Free Mass without Impacting Changes in Protein Metabolism after Weight Loss in Older Women," *Obesity* 17, no. 7 (2009): 1332–39; E. Kirk et al., "Minimal Resistance Training Improves Daily Energy Expenditure and Fat Oxidation," *Medicine & Science in Sports & Exercise* 41, no. 5 (2009): 1122–29.

26. M. Anderson et al., "The Relationships among Isometric, Isotonic, and Isokinetic Concentric and Eccentric Quadriceps and Hamstring Force and Three Components of Athletic Performance," *Journal of Orthopedic & Sports Physical Therapy* 14, no. 3 (1991): 114–20.

27. T. Hallage et al., "The Effects of 12 Weeks of Step Aerobics Training on Functional Fitness of Elderly Women," *Journal of Strength & Conditioning Research* 24, no. 8 (2010): 2261–66.

28. I. Stewart and K. Stewart, "Energy Balance during Two Days of Continuous Stationary Cycling," *Journal of the International Society of Sports Nutrition* 4 (2007): 15.

29. M. Dehghan et al., "Childhood Obesity, Prevalence and Prevention," *Nutrition Journal* 4 (2005): 24.

30. K. Slavin, "Why Am I Watching This?," *Human Architecture: Journal of the Sociology of Self-Knowledge* 4, no. 1–2 (2005): 63–68.

31. A. Page, A. Cooper, and E. Stamatakis, "Physical Activity Patterns in Nonobese and Obese Children Assessed Using Minute-by-Minute Accelerometry," *International Journal of Obesity* 29, no. 9 (2005): 1070–76.

32. T. Baechle and R. Earle, *Essentials of Strength Training and Conditioning*, 2nd ed. (Champaign, IL: Human Kinetics, 2000).

33. S. Telles et al., "Short Term Health Impact of a Yoga and Diet Change Program on Obesity," *Medical Science Monitor* 16, no. 1 (2010): CR35–40.

34. K. Fox and L. Edmunds, "Understanding the World of the 'Fat Kid': Can Schools Help Provide a Better Experience?," *Reclaim Child Youth* 9 (2000): 177–81.

35. B. Mittendorfer, D. Fields, and S. Klein, "Excess Body Fat in Men Decreases Plasma Fatty Acid Availability and Oxidation during Endurance Exercise," *American Journal of Physiology—Endocrinology and Metabolism* 286, no. 3 (2004): E354–E362.

36. J. O'Hora et al., "Efficacy of Static Stretching and Proprioceptive Neuromuscular Facilitation Stretch on Hamstrings Length after a Single Session," *Journal of Strength & Conditioning Research* 25, no. 6 (2011): 1586–91.

37. T. You et al., "Addition of Aerobic Exercise to Dietary Weight Loss Preferentially Reduces Abdominal Adipocyte Size," *International Journal of Obesity* 30, no. 8 (2006): 1211–16.

38. You et al., "Addition of Aerobic Exercise to Dietary Weight Loss," 1211–16.

39. P. Neighmond, "Sitting All Day: Worse for You Than You Might Think," *NPR News*, April 25, 2011, www.npr.org.

40. S. Ziebland et al., "Lack of Willpower or Lack of Wherewithal? 'Internal' and 'External' Barriers to Changing Diet and Exercise in a Three Year Follow-Up of Participants in a Health Check," *Social Science & Medicine* 46, no. 4–5 (1998): 461–65.

41. C. Barlow et al., "Physical Fitness, Mortality, and Obesity," *International Journal of Obesity and Related Metabolic Disorders* 19, no. S4 (1995): S41–S44.

CHAPTER 12

1. O. Ousova et al., "Corticosteroid Binding Globulin: A New Target for Cortisol-Driven Obesity," *Molecular Endocrinology* 18, no. 7 (2004): 1687–96.

2. G. D. Foster, T. A. Wadden, and A. P. Makris, "Primary Care Physicians' Attitudes about Obesity and Its Treatment," *Obesity Research* 11, no. 10 (2003): 1168–77.

3. T. Gurley-Calvez and A. Higginbotham, "Childhood Obesity, Academic Achievement, and School Expenditures," *Public Finance Review* 38, no. 5 (2010): 619–46.

4. Ousova et al., "Corticosteroid Binding Globulin," 1687–96.

5. P. Kopelman, I. Caterson, and W. Dietz, eds., *Clinical Obesity in Adults and Children*, 3rd ed. (Hoboken, NJ: Wiley-Blackwell, 2010), 28.

6. R. Puhl, "Understanding the Stigma of Obesity and Its Consequences," Obesity Action Coalition, n.d., www.obesityaction.org.

7. C. Adams et al., "The Relationship of Obesity to the Frequency of Pelvic Examinations: Do Physician and Patient Attitudes Make a Difference?," *Women Health* 20, no. 2 (1993): 45–57.

8. R. Puhl and K. Brownell, "Bias, Discrimination, and Obesity," *Obesity Research* 9 (2001): 788–805.

9. Kopelman, Caterson, and Dietz, *Clinical Obesity in Adults and Children*, 28.

10. J. L. Kristeller and R. A. Hoerr, "Physician Attitudes toward Managing Obesity: Differences among Six Specialty Groups," *Preventative Medicine* 26, no. 4 (1997): 542–49.

11. G. D. Foster, T. A. Wadden, and A. P. Makris, "Primary Care Physicians' Attitudes about Obesity and Its Treatment," *Obesity Research* 11, no. 10 (2003): 1168–77.

12. Adams et al., "The Relationship of Obesity to the Frequency of Pelvic Examinations," 45–57.

13. C. Olson, H. Schumaker, and B. Yawn, "Overweight Women Delay Medical Care," *Archives of Family Medicine* 3, no. 10 (1994): 888–92.

14. S. Kirkey, "Bias against Obese People Increasing, Study Says," Canada .com, 2009, www.canada.com.

15. C. Rand and A. Macgregor, "Morbidly Obese Patients' Perceptions of Social Discrimination Before and After Surgery for Obesity," *Southern Medical Journal* 83, no. 12 (1990): 1390–95.

16. M. Makara-Studzinska and A. Zaborska, "The Influence of Obesity on Self-Esteem and Body Image," *Zdrow Publiczne* 117, no. 1 (2007): 59–62.

17. L. Heisler et al., "Serotonin Reciprocally Regulates Melanocortin Neurons to Modulate Food Intake," *Neuron* 51, no. 2 (2006): 239–49.

18. E. King et al., "The Stigma of Obesity in Customer Service: A Mechanism for Remediation and Bottom-Line Consequences of Interpersonal Discrimination," *Journal of Applied Psychology* 91, no. 3 (2006): 579–93.

19. K. M. Carpenter et al., "Relationships between Obesity and DSM-IV Major Depressive Disorder, Suicide Ideation, and Suicide Attempts: Results from a General Population Study," *American Journal of Public Health* 90, no. 2 (2000): 251–57.

20. R. Puhl and K. Brownell, "Ways of Coping with Obesity Stigma: Review and Conceptual Analysis," *Eating Behaviors* 4, no. 1 (2003): 53–78.

21. Carpenter et al., "Relationships between Obesity and DSM-IV Major Depressive Disorder, Suicide Ideation, and Suicide Attempts."

22. A. Meyer et al., "Initial Development and Reliability of a Motivation for Weight Loss Scale," *Obesity Facts* 3, no. 3 (2010): 205–11.

23. L. Kravitz and V. H. Heyward, "Getting a Grip on Body Composition," University of New Mexico Department of Exercise Science, n.d., www.unm.edu.

24. J. Huh, N. Riggs, and D. Spruijt-Metz, "Identifying Patterns of Eating and Physical Activity in Children: A Latent Class Analysis of Obesity Risk," *Obesity* 19, no. 3 (2010): 652–58.

25. K. Presnell, S. K. Bearman, and E. Stice, "Risk Factors for Body Dissatisfaction in Adolescent Boys and Girls: A Prospective Study," *International Journal of Eating Disorders* 36, no. 4 (2004): 389–401.

26. K. Webber et al., "The Effect of a Motivational Intervention on Weight Loss Is Moderated by Level of Baseline Controlled Motivation," *International Journal of Behavioral Nutrition and Physical Activity* 7 (2010): 4.

27. Webber et al., "The Effect of a Motivational Intervention on Weight Loss," 4.

28. Webber et al., "The Effect of a Motivational Intervention on Weight Loss," 4.

29. D. West et al., "A Motivation-Focused Weight Loss Maintenance Program Is an Effective Alternative to a Skill-Based Approach," *International Journal of Obesity*, 2010 (published online ahead of print).

30. C. Davis et al., "From Motivation to Behavior: A Model of Reward Sensitivity, Overeating, and Food Preferences in the Risk Profile for Obesity," *Appetite* 48, no. 1 (2007): 12–19.

31. Example: Lane Bryant, www.lanebryant.com.

32. A. M. Prentice, "Overeating: The Health Risks," *Obesity Research* 9, no. S11 (2001): S234–S238.

33. C. Davis and J. C. Carter, "Compulsive Overeating as an Addiction Disorder: A Review of Theory and Evidence," *Appetite* 53, no. 1 (2009): 1–8.

34. Y. Liu et al., "Food Addiction and Obesity: Evidence from Bench to Bedside," *Journal of Psychoactive Drugs* 42, no. 2 (2010): 133–45.

35. L. Heisler et al., "Serotonin Reciprocally Regulates Melanocortin Neurons to Modulate Food Intake," *Neuron* 51, no. 2 (2006): 239–49.

36. S. Simpson and L. Bennett, "Big and Beautiful," *Indianapolis Monthly*, January 2002, 91–93.

37. Simpson and Bennett, "Big and Beautiful," 91–93.

GLOSSARY

acanthosis nigricans. A very specific condition of the skin where, at the folds of the body, the skin becomes dark.

adenosine triphosphate. Molecule that stores energy in the body for future use.

adiponectin. Protein hormone that controls glucose-lipid metabolic activity and influences the body's response to insulin.

agoraphobia. Excessive fear of a situation, an activity, or something that leads one to avoid it.

anorexia. Lack of appetite that results in inability to eat.

antidepressants. Medicines used to treat depressions, which enhance your mood, appetite, sleep, and concentration.

antipsychotics. Medicines that reduce the psychotic impacts of the condition of schizophrenia.

android obesity. Excessive accumulation of fat in the abdominal section of the body, giving your body the shape of an apple.

atherosclerosis. When fat pockets in the walls of the arteries lead to plaque buildup.

Bardet-Biedl syndrome. A genetic disorder affecting various parts of the body, such as vision loss, obesity, possessing extra fingers and toes, learning disability, impaired speech, sexual inadequacies, and delayed motor development.

Basal Metabolic Rate (BMR). The minimum amount of calories that a body burns just to remain alive.

body dysmorphic disorder. An illness caused by preoccupied thoughts of physical disabilities in the body.

body mass index (BMI). A measurement of a person's body weight against height, which helps identify whether he or she is healthy or overweight.

bulimia. An eating disorder involving psychological distress, binging and purging of food, depression, or issues related with self-esteem.

cardiovascular diseases. Diseases of the heart, arteries, or veins. Can be treated and cured even with long family history. Examples include aneurysm, angina, stroke, and heart attack.

catastrophic disease. An acute, severe disease requiring immediate care toward the patient suffering, incurring heavy and often distressful medical expenses.

cerebral edema. Excessive amount of water accumulating in the intracellular spaces of the brain.

cervical spondylitis. Arthritis of the neck.

childhood obesity. Severe overweightness in children with excessive amount of body fat, often resulting in diabetes, cholesterol problems, hypertension, and numerous psychological disorders.

chronic clinical depression. A severe state of psychological imbalance which affects a person's way of thinking, actions, and behaviors negatively for a prolonged period.

Cohen syndrome. A rare genetic disorder which causes the skeletal muscles to become weak, apart from resulting in childhood obesity, and other malfunctions.

coronary heart disease (CHD). A heart condition sprung by the collection of fatty materials within arterial walls, affecting the normal blood flow in the body.

Cushing's disease. Disease caused by too much activity of the pituitary gland, located near the base of the head.

cyanosis. A condition where the skin of different parts of the body might turn blue due to insufficient supply of oxygen in the hemoglobin within the body.

diabetes mellitus. A collective term used to represent a group of diseases characterized by high sugar, too much urination, excessive thirst, and extreme hunger in an individual.

diaphragm. A partition made up of muscular membrane that separates the abdominal cavity from the thoracic cavity. Very important for breathing functions.

Down's syndrome. Mental and physical symptoms that occurs in an individual due to the presence of an extra chromosome 21.

dual-energy X-ray absorptiometry (DEXA or DXA). A medical screening test used to check the density of the bones and identify any premature decline in bone density.

duodenum. The part of the small intestine that lies between the middle part of the small intestine and the stomach.

dyslipidemia. Presence of excessive amounts of fats and cholesterols in the blood.

dyspnea. A disease of the lungs, heart, or the airways that causes difficulty in breathing.

edema. Swelling caused in different parts of the body due to excessive accumulation of fluid collection.

energy imbalance. Refers to disparity in the amount of energy consumed than used.

estrogen. Important hormone involved in reproduction.

gallstones. Small particles formed either due to too much accumulation of bilirubin present in the bile or too much cholesterol that, when deposited, cause immense pain.

genetics. The branch of study that tells us about the hereditary patterns of inheritance of organisms with similarity.

gout. Disease caused by accumulation of excessive uric acid in the body, causing consistent joint inflammation, kidney stones, and declining function of the kidney.

gynecomastia. Male disorder where one or both the breasts are found to be in an enlarged state.

gynoid fat distribution. Excessive amount of fat distributed in the hips, buttocks, and thighs.

heart attack (myocardial infarction). A condition of the heart when the muscles start dying due to shortage of oxygen obtained from blood flow. Can be a result of cholesterol buildup in the blood vessels.

heart failure. A gradual disorder of the heart due to damage caused, which weakens the cardiovascular system and reduces the amount of blood flow to the tissues.

hirsutism. A phenomenon in women characterized by excessive hair growth in places where hair is normally absent or appearing at a minimum level.

hypercortisolism. A condition caused by the excessive production of adrenocorticotropic hormone, produced by the pituitary glands. Leads to a number of symptoms such as weight gain, weakness, backaches, and headache.

hyperinsulinism. A condition that arises from excessive insulin production in the body, going beyond normal range, and lowers the level of sugar. Leads to symptoms such as emotional instability, headache, weakness, and dizziness.

hypertension. The state of the body, when the heart pumps more blood than usual, increasing its pressure on the walls of the artery.

hypogastric region. The area of the abdomen, found in the region below the navel area.

hypothalamic obesity. Weight gain that results from the damage of the hypothalamus region of the brain. Sometimes due to brain tumors.

hypothalamus. Area of the brain that produces hormones that affect the temperature of the body, moods, hunger, sexual drive, thirst, and sleep hormones released from the pituitary gland.

hypothyroidism. A physical condition reflecting a lack of production of thyroid hormone, a hormone responsible for physical development, growth, and other functions.

intertrigo. An inflammation or a rash in the body that develops as a result of fungal, bacterial, or viral infection that occurs in moist folds of the body.

left ventricular hypertrophy (LVH). A condition of the heart where the muscles of the left ventricle, the main chamber of the heart, becomes thicker and loses elasticity. Leads to the gradual inability to pump the necessary amount of blood.

leptin. A hormone that alerts the brain of the presence of fat in the body and helps in reducing it.

lymphatic system. One of the body's transport systems that is responsible for carrying lymph using lymphatic vessels and lymphoid tissues.

metabolic syndrome. Term used to define a series of metabolic risk factors that may be found in an individual simultaneously, such as high blood pressure, insulin resistance, abnormalities in cholesterol, a high risk of clotting, and so forth.

monosodium glutamate (MSG). A food additive commonly used in fast food restaurants as a flavor enhancer.

myocardial infarction. Term used interchangeably with *heart attack*. Happens when blood supply ceases to go to a certain part of the heart.

neuropeptide. Protein-like, small molecule that neurons (nerve cells) use to communicate with each other.

neurotransmitters. Chemicals that spread signals or information to a particular cell from a neuron across a synapse.

obesogen. Fattening, obesity-causing chemicals suspected of being added to commercialized food.

obsessive compulsive disorder. An anxiety disorder involving uncontrollable repetitive thoughts and actions.

Orlistat. A drug that treats obesity by preventing fat absorption from regular diets, resulting in a reduction of calorie intake.

osteoarthritis. A series of disorders leading to structural or functional failure of the joints, affecting the surrounding muscles, ligaments, and joint coverings.

polycystic ovarian syndrome (POS). A disease in women due to multiple small cysts growing within the ovaries, leading to a variety of metabolic as well as other disorders such as irregularity in menstrual cycles, resistance to insulin, abnormal hair growth, inability to conceive, and weight gain.

preeclampsia. A severe medical condition typically found in pregnant women, usually during the twentieth week of pregnancy. Revealed by increased blood pressure and abnormal levels of protein and/or fat in urine. The mother's brain, liver, kidney, and placenta are affected.

Prader-Willi syndrome. An uncommon, incurable genetic disorder that causes poor muscle building, a constant feeling of hunger, and a very little amount of sex hormone. Babies with Prader-Willi Syndrome overeat and are obese since their hunger control systems are imbalanced.

pulmonary diseases. Severe disease of the lung, which brings about a difficulty in breathing, shortness of breath, chronic cough as well as other sleeping disorders such as sleep apnea.

resting metabolism. The rate at which the body burns its calories to serve essential functions such as breathing, brain functioning, and pumping blood.

rhinoscopy. The process of diagnosing the nasal passage of an individual with a rhinoscope.

Sibutramine. A drug used previously for treating obesity. Side effects include severe heart complications such as stroke.

sleep apnea. A sleeping disorder that hinders regular breathing patterns. Reduces mental alertness, energy level, reflexes, and productivity of an individual.

Stein-Leventhal disease. A disorder in women marked by creation of an excessive level of male hormones in the body. Irregular or absent ovulation is also involved.

subcutaneous fat. The layer of fat found just under the skin.

thermogenesis. The process by which heat is generated in warm blooded animals.

thylakoids. Sac-like structures that house other important structures involved in a plant's energy production process.

tophi. Excessive deposition of uric acid stones in patients suffering from gout, leading to fibrous growths, frequently around the joint areas.

triglyceride. A molecule with three fatty acids attached. It is found in both animals and plants.

Type 2 diabetes. A state of diabetes when the affected person becomes resistant to insulin.

urinary calculi. Presence of hard particles in the urinary tracts that causes immense pains, vomiting, fever or chills, and nausea.

varicose veins. Enlarged and painful veins. The veins are unable to perform their primary function of keeping blood from flowing backwards. Results in thickening of the veins.

xanthelasmas. A common type of cholesterol deposition near the eyelids.

Yuhasz skinfold test. A test for measuring extra fat; measurement is achieved by pinching the subcutaneous layer of fat in the body using specialized calipers.

RESOURCES

A Healthier You: Based on the Dietary Guidelines for Americans
US Department of Health and Human Services
Washington, DC: Government Printing Office, 2005

Active at Any Size
www.win.niddk.nih.gov/publications/active.htm

Aim for a Healthy Weight
DHHS, NIH, National Heart, Lung and Blood Institute (NHLBI)
NHLBI Publication No. 05-5213
www.nhlbi.nih.gov/health/public/heart/obesity/aim_hwt.htm

Finding Your Way to a Healthier You: Based on the *Dietary Guidelines for Americans*
Department of Health and Human Services, US Department of Agriculture
www.health.gov/dietaryguidelines/dga2005/document/html/brochure.htm

Fit and Fabulous as You Mature
www.win.niddk.nih.gov/publications/mature.htm

Just Enough for You: About Food Portions
www.win.niddk.nih.gov/publications/just_enough.htm

Mayo Clinic Healthy Weight for Everybody
Donald Hensrud, MD (editor), and the Mayo Clinic
Rochester, MN: Mayo Clinic Health Information, 2005
ISBN: 1-8930-0534-8

Mindless Eating: Why We Eat More Than We Think
Brian Wansink, PhD
New York: Bantam Dell, 2006
ISBN: 978-0-553-38448-2

No-Fad Diet: A Personal Plan for Healthy Weight Loss
New York: Clarkson Potter, 2005
ISBN: 1-4000-5159-2

The Complete Food Counter, Third Edition
Annette B. Natow, PhD, and Jo-Ann Heslin
New York: Pocket Books, 2009
ISBN: 1-4165-6666-X

The Calorie Counter, Fourth Edition
Annette B. Natow, PhD, and Jo-Ann Heslin
New York: Pocket Books, 2007
ISBN: 1-4165-0982-8

The Step Diet Book: Count Steps, Not Calories, to Lose Weight and Keep It off Forever
James O. Hill, PhD, John C. Peters, PhD, and Bonnie T. Jortberg
New York: Workman Publishing Company, 2004
ISBN: 0761133240

The Volumetrics Eating Plan: Techniques and Recipes for Feeling Full on Fewer Calories
Barbara Rolls, PhD
New York: HarperCollins, 2005
ISBN: 0-0607-3730-1

The Way to Eat
David L. Katz, MD, and Maura Gonzalez
Naperville, IL: Sourcebooks, Inc., 2002
ISBN: 1-4022-0264-4

Watch Your Weight! (Available in English and Spanish)
DHHS, NIH, National Heart, Lung and Blood Institute (NHLBI) NHLBI
    Publication No. 96-4047
www.nhlbi.nih.gov/health/public/heart/other/sp_wt.htm

What Are Overweight and Obesity?
DHHS, NIH, National Heart, Lung and Blood Institute
www.nhlbi.nih.gov/health/dci/Diseases/obe/obe_whatare.html

What Are the Health Risks of Overweight and Obesity?
DHHS, NIH, National Heart, Lung and Blood Institute
www.nhlbi.nih.gov/health/dci/Diseases/obe/obe_risks.html

Weight and Waist Measurement: Tools for Adults
www.win.niddk.nih.gov/publications/tools.htm

Overweight, Obesity & Weight Management
International Food Information Council Foundation, 2007–2009 IFIC Foun-
    dation Media Guide on Food Safety and Nutrition, chapter 5
www.ific.org/nutrition/obesity/upload/obesitybackgrounder.pdf

**Real Fitness for Real Women: A Unique Workout Program for the Plus-
    Size Woman**
Rochelle Rice
Warner Books, 2001
www.rochellerice.com

Tips to Help You Get Active
NIH Publication No. 06–5578, 2009
www.win.niddk.nih.gov/publications/tips.htm

Walking . . . a Step in the Right Direction
NIH Publication No. 07–4155, 2007
www.win.niddk.nih.gov/publications/walking.htm

SELECTED BIBLIOGRAPHY

American Psychiatric Association. "Obsessive-Compulsive Personality Disorder." In *Diagnostic and Statistical Manual of Mental Disorders*, 4th ed., 725–29. Washington, DC: American Psychiatric Association, 2000.

Anandacoomarasamy, A., M. Fransen, and L. March. "Obesity and the Musculoskeletal System." *Current Opinion in Rheumatology* 21, no. 1 (2009): 71–77.

Andrews, J., R. Netemeyer, and S. Burton. "The Nutrition Elite: Do Only the Highest Levels of Caloric Knowledge, Obesity Knowledge, and Motivation Matter in Processing Nutrition Claims and Disclosures?" *Journal of Public Policy & Marketing* 28, no. 1 (2009): 41–55.

Angulo, P. "Obesity and Nonalcoholic Fatty Liver Disease." *Nutrition Reviews* 65, no. S6 (2007): S57– S63.

Anzman, S., and L. Birch. "Low Inhibitory Control and Restrictive Feeding Practices Predict Weight Outcomes." *Journal of Pediatrics* 155 (2009): 651–56.

Anzman, S., B. Rollins, and L. Birch. "Parents' Influence on Children's Early Eating Environments and Obesity Risk: Implications for Prevention." *International Journal of Obesity* 32 (2010): 1116–24.

Archivos de Cirgía general y Digestiva. "Physiology and Consequences of Obesity." 2009. www.cirugest.com.

Base-Smith, V., and J. Campinha-Bacote. "The Culture of Obesity." *Journal of the National Black Nurses Association* 14, no. 1 (2003): 52–56.

Bauer, J. "10 Ways to Prevent Raising a Fat Kid." *MSNBC*. 2007. www.today.msnbc.msn.com.

Birch, L., and S. Anzman. "Learning to Eat in an Obesogenic Environment: A Developmental Systems Perspective on Childhood Obesity." *Child Development Perspectives* 4, no. 2 (2010): 138–43.

Blokstra, A., C. Burns, and J. Seidell. "Perception of Weight Status and Dieting Behavior in Dutch Men and Women." *International Journal of Obesity Related Metabolic Disorders* 23, no. 1 (1999): 7–17.

Bouchard, C. "Spouse Resemblance in Body Mass Index: Effects on Adult Obesity Prevalence in the Offspring Generation." *American Journal of Epidemiology* 165 (2007): 101–8.

Brownell, K., and R. Puhl. "Stigma and Discrimination in Weight Management and Obesity." *Permanente Journal* 7 (2003): 21–23.

Business First of Louisville. "Obesity Bad for Economy, Business." 2006. www .louisville.bizjournals.com.

Caballero, B. "The Global Epidemic of Obesity: An Overview." *Epidemiologic Reviews* 29 (2007): 1–5.

Carels, R. A., L. Darby, H. M. Cacciapaglia, K. Konrad, C. Coit, J. Harper, M. E. Kaplar, K. Young, C. A. Baylen, and A. Versland. "Using Motivational Interviewing as a Supplement to Obesity Treatment: A Stepped-Care Approach." *Health Psychology* 26, no. 3 (2007): 369–74.

Caro, J. F. "Definitions and Classification of Obesity." Endotext, 2002. www .endotext.org.

Carr, D., and M. Friedman. "Is Obesity Stigmatizing? Body Weight, Perceived Discrimination, and Psychological Well-Being in the United States." *Journal of Health and Social Behavior* 46, no. 3 (2005): 244–25.

Centers for Disease Control and Prevention. "About BMI for Children and Teens." 2009. www.cdc.gov.

———. "Obesity and Overweight Center for Disease Control." 2009. www .cdc.gov.

The Cochrane Collaboration. "Psychological Interventions for Overweight and Obesity." 2005. www.cochrane.org.

Coltidz, G. "Economic Costs of Obesity and Inactivity." *Medicine & Science in Sports & Exercise* 31, no. S11 (1999): S663–S667.

Counts, C. R., C. Jones, C. L. Frame, G. J. Jarvie, and C. C. Strauss. "The Perception of Obesity by Normal-Weight versus Obese School-Age Children." *Child Psychiatry and Human Development* 17, no. 2 (1986): 113–20.

Crouch, L. "New Tax Break May Motivate Obese Americans to Shed a Few Pounds." *13 News*, 2002. www.wvec.com.

Cutler, D., E. Glaeser, and J. Shapiro. "Why Have Americans Become More Obese?" *Journal of Economic Perspectives* 17, no. 3 (2003): 93–118.

Devlin, M., S. Yanovski, and G. Wilson. "Obesity: What Mental Health Professionals Need to Know." *American Journal of Psychiatry* 157 (2000): 854–66.

"Diagnosing Obesity." Health Reserve. 2003. www.healthreserve.com/obesity/diagnosing_obesity.htm.

Dierk, J. M., M. Conradt, E. Rauh, P. Schlumberger, J. Hebebrand, and W. Rief. "What Determines Well-Being in Obesity? Associations with BMI, Social Skills, and Social Support." *Journal of Psychosomatic Research* 60, no. 3 (2006): 219–27.

Domínguez-Vásquez, P., S. Olivares, and J. Santos. "Eating Behavior and Childhood Obesity: Family Influences." *Archivos Latino Americanos de Nutrición (Latin American Archives of Nutrition)* 58, no. 3 (2008): 249–55.

Eagle, L., and R. Brennan. "Beyond Advertising: In-Home Promotion of 'Fast Food.'" *Young Consumers: Insight and Ideas for Responsible Marketers* 8, no. 4 (2007): 278–88.

Enriori, P. J., A. E. Evans, P. Sinnayah, E. E. Jobst, L. Tonelli-Lemos, S. K. Billes, M. M. Glavas, et al. "Diet-Induced Obesity Causes Severe but Reversible Leptin Resistance in Arcuate Melanocortin Neurons." *Cell Metabolism* 5, no. 3 (2007): 181–94.

Feld, S. "War on Obesity: Obesity and the Economy." Wellsphere, 2008. www.stanford.wellsphere.com.

Flodmark C. "Childhood Obesity." *Clinical Child Psychology and Psychiatry* 2, no. 2 (1997): 283–95.

Finkelstein, E., I. Fiebelkorn, and G. Wang. "National Medical Spending Attributable to Overweight and Obesity: How Much, and Who's Paying?" *Health Affairs* W3 (2003): 219–26.

Finucane, M. M., G. A. Stevens, M. J. Cowan, G. Danaei, J. K. Lin, C. J. Paciorek, G. Singh, et al. "National, Regional, and Global Trends in Body-Mass Index Since 1980: Systematic Analysis of Health Examination Surveys and Epidemiological Studies with 960 Country-Years and 91 Million Participants." *Lancet* 377, no. 9765 (2011): 557–67.

Gennuso, J., L. H. Epstein, R. A. Paluch, and F. Cerny. "The Relationship between Asthma and Obesity in Urban Minority Children and Adolescents." *Archives of Pediatrics and Adolescent Medicine* 152, no. 12 (1998): 1197–200.

Georgiadis, M., S. Biddle, and N. Stavrou. "Motivation for Weight-Loss Diets: A Clustering, Longitudinal Field Study Using Self-Esteem and Self-Determination Theory Perspectives." *Health Education Journal* 65, no. 1 (2006): 53–72.

Greenhouse, S. "Obese People Are Taking Their Bias Claims to Court." *New York Times*, 2003. www.nytimes.com.

Haller, C., and J. Schwartz. "Pharmacologic Agents for Weight Reduction." *Journal of Gender-Specific Medicine* 5, no. 5 (2002): 16–21.

Hart, W., and D. Albarracín. "The Effects of Chronic Achievement Motivation and Achievement Primes on the Activation of Achievement and Fun Goals." *Journal of Personality and Social Psychology* 97, no. 6 (2009): 1129–41.

Health Reserve. "Treatment of Obesity." 2003. www.healthreserve.com.

Hill, J., and H. Wyatt. "Role of Physical Activity in Preventing and Treating Obesity." *Journal of Applied Physiology* 99, no. 2 (2005): 765–70.

Iwase, M., M. Yamamoto, K. Iino, K. Ichikawa, N. Shinohara, M. Yoshinari, and M. Fujishima. "Obesity Induced by Neonatal Monosodium Glutamate Treatment in Spontaneously Hypertensive Rats: An Animal Model of Multiple Risk Factors." *Hypertension Research: Official Journal of the Japanese Society of Hypertension* 21, no. 1 (1998): 1–6.

Jia, W. P., C. Wang, S. Jiang, and J. M. Pan. "Characteristics of Obesity and Its Related Disorders in China." *Biomedical and Environmental Sciences* 23, no. 1 (2010): 4–11.

Kaplan, L. "Pharmacologic Therapies for Obesity." *Gastroenterology Clinics of North America* 39, no. 1 (2010): 69–79.

Kemper, K. "Stratifying Patients for Weight Loss Counseling." *Nurse Practitioner* 35, no. 8 (2010): 33–38.

Koch, F., A. Sepa, and J. Ludvigsson. "Psychological Stress and Obesity." *Journal of Pediatrics* 153, no. 6 (2008): 839–44.

Kopelman, P., I. Caterson, and W. Dietz. *Clinical Obesity in Adults and Children*. Malden, MA: Wiley-Blackwell, 2009.

Kristeller, J., and R. Hoerr. "Physician Attitudes toward Managing Obesity: Differences among Six Specialty Groups." *Preventative Medicine* 26, no. 4 (1997): 542–49.

Kuczmarski, R., and K. Flegal. "Criteria for Definition of Overweight in Transition: Background and Recommendations for the United States." *American Journal of Clinical Nutrition* 72, no. 5 (2000): 1067–68.

Lam, D., A. Garfield, and O. Marston. "Brain Serotonin System in the Coordination of Food Intake and Body Weight." *Pharmacology Biochemistry and Behavior* 91, no. 1 (2010): 84–91.

Lobstein, T., L. Baur, and R. Uauy. "Obesity in Children and Young People: A Crisis in Public Health." *Obesity Reviews* 5, no. S1 (2004): S4–S104.

Lopez, R. "Neighborhood Risk Factors for Obesity." *Obesity* 15 (2007): 2111–19.

Mallick, M. "Health Hazards of Obesity and Weight Control in Children: A Review of the Literature." *American Journal of Public Health* 73, no. 1 (1983): 78–82.

Martin, K., and A. Ferris. "Food Insecurity and Gender Are Risk Factors for Obesity." *Journal of Nutrition Education and Behavior* 39, no. 1 (2007): 31–36.

Mayo Clinic. "Obesity: Causes." 2009. www.mayoclinic.com.

Mayo Clinic. "Obesity: Treatments and Drugs." 2009. www.mayoclinic.com.

Mazzocchi, M., and W. Traill. "Calories, Obesity, and Health in OECD Countries." Paper presented at the 81st Annual Conference of the Agricultural Economics Society, 2007.

Melnyk, B. M., L. Small, D. Morrison-Beedy, A. Strasser, L. Spath, R. Kreipe, H. Crean, D. Jacobson, and S. Van Blankenstein. "Mental Health Correlates of Healthy Lifestyle Attitudes, Beliefs, Choices, and Behaviors in Overweight Adolescents." *Journal of Pediatric Health Care* 20, no. 6 (2006): 401–6.

Monografías. "History of Obesity in the World." 2009. www.monografias.com.

Montague, M. "The Physiology of Obesity." *ABNF Journal* 14, no. 3 (2003): 56–60.

Morabia, A., and M. Costanza. "Does Walking 15 Minutes Per Day Keep the Obesity Epidemic Away? Simulation of the Efficacy of a Population Wide Campaign." *American Journal of Public Health* 94, no. 3 (2004): 437–40.

Moreno, L., and G. Rodríguez. "Dietary Risk Factors for Development of Childhood Obesity." *Current Opinion in Clinical Nutrition & Metabolic Care* 10, no. 3 (2007): 336–41.

"Mechanisms of Leptin Action and Leptin Resistance." *Annual Review of Physiology* 70 (2008): 537–56.

Musich, S., C. Lu, T. McDonald, L. Champagne, and D. Edington. "Association of Additional Health Risks on Medical Charges and Prevalence of Diabetes within Body Mass Index Categories." *American Journal of Health Promotion* 18, no. 3 (2004): 264–68.

My Overweight Child. "Simple Steps for Increasing Physical Activity." 2009. www.myoverweightchild.com.

NHS Careers. "Dietitian's Role." 2010. www.nhscareers.nhs.uk.

Nowicka, P., and C. Foldmark. "Family in Pediatric Obesity Management: A Literature Review." *International Journal of Pediatric Obesity* 3, no. S1 (2008): S44–S50.

Oracle Thinkquest. "Self-Esteem." 2009. www.library.thinkquest.org/06aug /00014/id21.htm.

Pagan, J., and A. Davila. "Obesity, Occupational Attainment, and Earnings." *Social Science Quarterly* 78, no. 3 (1997): 756–70.

Powers, S., and E. Howley. *Exercise Physiology: Theory and Application to Fitness and Performance.* 7th ed. New York: McGraw Hill, 2009.

Prescription Medications for the Treatment of Obesity. "Weight-Control Information Network." www.win.niddk.nih.gov.

Raebel, M. A., D. C. Malone, D. A. Conner, S. Xu, J. A. Porter, and F. A. Lanty. "Health Services Use and Health Care Costs of Obese and Nonobese Individuals." *Archives of Internal Medicine* 164 (2002): 2135–40.

Sacks, F. M., G. A. Bray, V. J. Carey, S. R. Smith, D. H. Ryan, S. D. Anton, K. McManus, et al. "Comparison of Weight-Loss Diets with Different Compositions of Fat, Protein, and Carbohydrates." *New England Journal of Medicine* 360, no. 9 (2009): 859–73.

Science Daily. "MSG Use Linked to Obesity." 2008. www.sciencedaily.com.

———. "Salt Intake Is Strongly Associated with Obesity." 2006. www.sciencedaily.com.

Selko, A. "Obesity Costs US Companies as Much as $45 Billion a Year." *Industry Week*, 2008. www.industryweek.com

Sharma, A., V. Madaan, and F. Petty. "Exercise for Mental Health." *Primary Care Companion to the Journal of Clinical Psychiatry* 8, no. 2 (2006): 106.

Shoelson, S., L. Herrero, and A. Naaz. "Obesity, Inflammation, and Insulin Resistance." *Gastroenterology* 132, no. 6 (2007): 2169–80.

Signal, L., T. Lanumata, J. A. Robinson, A. Tavila, J. Wilton, and C. Ni Mhurchu. "Perceptions of New Zealand Nutrition Labels by Māori, Pacific and Low-Income Shoppers." *Public Health Nutrition* 11, no. 7 (2008): 706–13.

Silva, M. N., D. Markland, E. V. Carraça, P. N. Vieira, S. R. Coutinho, C. S. Minderico, M. G. Matos, L. B. Sardinha, and P. J. Teixeira. "Exercise Autonomous Motivation Predicts Three-Year Weight Loss in Women." *Medicine & Science in Sports & Exercise*, 2010.

Sim, L. A., D. E. McAlpine, K. B. Grothe, S. M. Himes, R. G. Cockerill, and M. M. Clark. "Identification and Treatment of Eating Disorders in the Primary Care Setting." *Mayo Clinic Proceedings* 85, no. 8 (2010): 746–51.

Srinivasan, K., and P. Ramarao. "Animal Models in Type 2 Diabetes Research: An Overview." *Indian Journal of Medical Research* 125, no. 3 (2007): 451–72.

Taras, H., and W. Potts-Datema. "Obesity and Student Performance at School." *Journal of School Health* 75, no. 8 (2005): 291–95.

Taras, H. L., J. F. Sallis, T. L. Patterson, P. R. Nader, and J. A. Nelson. "Television's Influence on Children's Diet and Physical Activity." *Journal of Developmental & Behavioral Pediatrics* 10 (1989): 176–80.

Tsai, A., and T. Wadden. "Treatment of Obesity in Primary Care Practice in the United States: A Systematic Review." *Journal of General Internal Medicine* 24, no. 9 (2009): 1073–79.

UCSF Benioff Children's Hospital. "Obesity Causes, Conditions & Treatments." 2010. www.ucsfhealth.org.

Uwaifo, G., and E. Arioglu. "Obesity." Emedicine, 2010. www.emedicine.medscape.com.

Vainio, H., and F. Bianchini. "Occurrence, Trends, and Analysis." In *IARC Handbooks of Cancer Prevention: Weight Control and Physical Activity*, vol. 6. Lyon, France: IARC Press, 2002.

Wang, Y., and M. Beydoun. "The Obesity Epidemic in the United States—Gender, Age, Socioeconomic, Racial/Ethnic, and Geographic Characteristics: A Systematic Review and Metaregression Analysis." *Epidemiologic Reviews* 29 (2007): 6–28.

Webb, B. "Seven Rules of Motivation." 2001. www.motivation-tools.com.

Weiner, D. E. "Public Health Consequences of Chronic Kidney Disease." *Clinical Pharmacology & Therapeutics* 86 (2009): 566–69.

Wharton, C., and J. Hampl. "Beverage Consumption and Risk of Obesity among Native Americans in Arizona." *Nutrition Reviews* 62, no. 4 (2004): 153–59.

Wolf, A., and G. Colditz. "The Cost of Obesity: The US Perspective." *Pharmacoeconomics* 5, no. S1 (1994): 34–37.

World Health Organization. "Controlling the Global Obesity Epidemic." 2011. www.who.int.

———. "Obesity: Preventing and Managing the Global Epidemic." *World Health Organization Technical Report Series* 894 (2000): 85–88.

Wren, A., and S. Bloom. "Gut Hormones and Appetite Control." *Gastroenterology* 132, no. 6 (2007): 2116–30.

INDEX

blood sampling procedures. *See* complete blood count
BMI. *See* body mass index
BMR. *See* basal metabolic rate
body dysmorphic disorder, 157
body mass index (BMI), xiii, 8–10, 12, 30–36, 62, 86, 88, 97, 101, 103, 106, 114, 119, 122, 146, 165, 197, 199, 201–3, 238, 248, 255, 265
Borelli, Giovanni Alfonso, 7
breakfast, 48, 146–47
bulimia, 9, 12, 14, 48, 123, 155, 261; nervosa, 123

caffeine, 15, 77, 184–85
cancer, 11, 59, 72, 92, 103, 196
cardio exercise, 212, 225
cardiovascular disease (CVD), 10, 36, 39, 95, 103, 121, 173, 228
CAT scan. *See* computerized axial tomography
catabolism, 16
causes and symptoms of obesity: lifestyle, 26–27; work system, 47–48; diet, 48–50
CBC. *See* complete blood count
CDC. *See* Centers for Disease Control and Prevention
cell functions, 19–20
Centers for Disease Control and Prevention (CDC), 95–97
cerebral edema, 59
cervical spondylitis, 27
CHD. *See* coronary heart disease
chemical effects, 178
childhood obesity, xvi, 4, 109, 115–16, 126, 133–34, 136–37, 139, 141–46, 148–50, 193, 227–28; health problems, 140–142; overcoming, 137–38

China, 118
cholesterol dilemma, 141
chronic renal disease (CRD), 200
classification of obesity, 32
clinical depression, chronic, 13,
Cohen syndrome, 59
coincident indicators, 192
Colorado, 96
comfort foods, 49–50
complete blood count, 42
comprehensive health assessment, 110
computerized axial tomography (CAT scan), 35–36, 38
compulsive overeating, 155–56, 249
conditions leading to obesity, 27–28
Consumer Price Index (CPI), 190–91
coronary heart disease (CHD), 10, 110, 196
corticosteroids, 60, 236
cortisol, 28, 38, 41, 55, 60–61, 139
cost-push inflation, 190
costs of obesity-related disease to the economy, *196*, 201, 203–5, 207
counseling, 61, 67, 153, 156, 159, 166
CPI. *See* Consumer Price Index
CRD. *See* chronic renal disease
Cushing's disease, xiv, 13, 28, 36, 41, 54–55
Cushing's syndrome. *See* Cushing's disease
CVD. *See* cardiovascular disease
cyanosis, 28, 64

deflation, 190–191
demand-pull inflation, 190
depression, xiv, 12–13, 41, 54–56, 62, 65–67, 84, 89, 91, 98, 123, 126, 143, 153, 156–157, 168, 169, 194, 240, 250. *See also* clinical depression, chronic

DEXA or DXA. *See* dual-energy X-ray absorptiometry
diabetes, xi, xiii–xv, 5, 10, 12, 24, 27, 31–33, 36–37, 41–42, 50, 64–65, 86, 88, 90, 95, 103–5, 107, 110, 114, 117, 120–21, 124, 130, 140–42, 164–65, 178, 193–94, 196–98, 200–203, 208, 213–14, 217, 228, 231, 244–45, 253, 258–59. *See also* Type 2 diabetes
diagnosis of obesity, 8, 23, 25–27, 30, 32–34, 36–38, 56, 62, 114, 126, 196–97; tests, 28
diet control, 249–250
diet club, 160–61
dieticians, 163–164
Down's syndrome, 59
drugs, 165
dual-energy X-ray absorptiometry (DEXA or DXA), 34
duodenum, 19–20, 34–35, 88
dyslipidemia,24, 32, 105
dyspnea, 27

eating disorders, 12, 98, 155–56, 167, 183, 235, 261, 263
economics of obesity, 179, 189, 194, 197, 200, 223; costs of obesity-related diseases, *196*
economic indicators for obesity, 191–92
economic status, 192
economist conclusion, 205
edema, 37–38, 59
electrolytes, 42
emotions, 6, 153, 156–57, 252
empty calories, 148
endurance training, 230
energy, 14–18, 220–21, 230, 245, 252; imbalance of, 3, 13, 17–18

ephedra, 77
ephedrine alkaloids, 77–78
epidemics in the US, 103
erythro-sedimentation rate (ESR), 42
ESR. *See* erythro-sedimentation rate
estrogen, 31, 50, 61
estrone, 51
Europe, 116, 118
exercise, xiii–xiv, 3, 6, 11, 13, 15, 18, 26, 47, 61, 69, 72–75, 77, 83–84, 90, 93–94, 96, 98, 100–102, 104, 108–11, 114, 119–20, 122–23, 127–28, 137–38, 140, 142, 144–45, 149, 154, 162, 164–65, 168, 172, 195, 206, 211–33, 242, 247, 253; aerobic, 18, 72, 74, 216–17; and children, 226–29
exorphins, 184

face-to-face counseling, 166–67
factors of obesity, 13, 24
false nutrition, 174–76
fast food, 3, 13–14, 47–49, 70, 93, 97, 133–34, 146, 181–82, 206–7
fats, 12, 15, 52, 55, 79, 96, 106, 113, 115, 119, 128, 152, 172–174, 176–177, 181–182, 187, 216, 244, 245; types of, 173; gynoid distribution and, 115; subcutaneous, 20, 29–30,
fat-mass and obesity-associated gene (FTO), 101
fatteners, 178
Federal Reserve Board, 191
fiber, 16, 19, 72, 78, 148
fitness trainers, 229
flexibility training, 230
food corporations, 161, 171, 176–77, 179–80, 187–88, 195, 207
food hormones, 178

ABOUT THE AUTHOR

Naheed Ali, M.D., is the author of the highly revered book *Diabetes and You: A Comprehensive, Holistic Approach*. Dr. Ali began writing professionally while still an undergrad in college, when he was published as the sole author of a high-impact academic journal article. Since then, he has appeared as a special guest on numerous talk shows and has been quoted in many national print magazines and TV websites across the United States. Additional information is available online at NaheedAli.com.